Diseases of the Salivary Glands—Part II

Diseases of the Salivary Glands—Part II

Editor

Margherita Sisto

MDPI • Basel • Beijing • Wuhan • Barcelona • Belgrade • Manchester • Tokyo • Cluj • Tianjin

Editor
Margherita Sisto
University of Bari "Aldo Moro"
Italy

Editorial Office
MDPI
St. Alban-Anlage 66
4052 Basel, Switzerland

This is a reprint of articles from the Special Issue published online in the open access journal *Journal of Clinical Medicine* (ISSN 2077-0383) (available at: https://www.mdpi.com/journal/jcm/special_issues/Salivary_Glands_Part_II).

For citation purposes, cite each article independently as indicated on the article page online and as indicated below:

LastName, A.A.; LastName, B.B.; LastName, C.C. Article Title. *Journal Name* **Year**, *Volume Number*, Page Range.

ISBN 978-3-0365-5567-6 (Hbk)
ISBN 978-3-0365-5568-3 (PDF)

Cover image courtesy of Margherita Sisto

Contents

About the Editor . . . . **vii**

Margherita Sisto
Special Issue "Diseases of the Salivary Glands-Part II"
Reprinted from: *J. Clin. Med.* **2022**, *11*, 5567, doi:10.3390/jcm11195567 . . . . **1**

José Mário Matos-Sousa, Leonardo Oliveira Bittencourt, Maria Karolina Martins Ferreira, Vinicius Ruan Neves dos Santos, Karolyny Martins Balbinot, Sérgio Alves-Júnior, João de Jesus Viana Pinheiro, Senda Charone, Juliano Pelim Pessan and Rafael Rodrigues Lima
Fluoride Exposure and Salivary Glands: How Is Glandular Morphology Susceptible to Long-Term Exposure? A Preclinical Study
Reprinted from: *J. Clin. Med.* **2022**, *11*, 5373, doi:10.3390/jcm11185373 . . . . **3**

Margherita Sisto, Domenico Ribatti, Giuseppe Ingravallo and Sabrina Lisi
The Expression of Follistatin-like 1 Protein Is Associated with the Activation of the EMT Program in Sjögren's Syndrome
Reprinted from: *J. Clin. Med.* **2022**, *11*, 5368, doi:10.3390/jcm11185368 . . . . **13**

Giuseppe Campagna, Luz Kelly Anzola, Michela Varani, Chiara Lauri, Guido Gentiloni Silveri, Lorenzo Chiurchioni, Francesca Romana Spinelli, Roberta Priori, Fabrizio Conti and Alberto Signore
Imaging Activated-T-Lymphocytes in the Salivary Glands of Patients with Sjögren's Syndrome by ^{99m}Tc-Interleukin-2: Diagnostic and Therapeutic Implications
Reprinted from: *J. Clin. Med.* **2022**, *11*, 4368, doi:10.3390/jcm11154368 . . . . **25**

Cheng-Yu Hsieh, Chuan-Jen Hsu, Hung-Pin Wu and Chuan-Hung Sun
Comparison Benefit between Hydrogen Peroxide and Adrenaline in Tonsillectomy: A Randomized Controlled Study
Reprinted from: *J. Clin. Med.* **2022**, *11*, 2723, doi:10.3390/jcm11102723 . . . . **37**

Shivai Gupta, Danmeng Li, David A. Ostrov and Cuong Q. Nguyen
Epitope Mapping of Pathogenic Autoantigens on Sjögren's Syndrome-Susceptible Human Leukocyte Antigens Using In Silico Techniques
Reprinted from: *J. Clin. Med.* **2022**, *11*, 1690, doi:10.3390/jcm11061690 . . . . **45**

Micaela F. Beckman, Elizabeth J. Brennan, Chika K. Igba, Michael T. Brennan, Farah B. Mougeot and Jean-Luc C. Mougeot
A Computational Text Mining-Guided Meta-Analysis Approach to Identify Potential Xerostomia Drug Targets
Reprinted from: *J. Clin. Med.* **2022**, *11*, 1442, doi:10.3390/jcm11051442 . . . . **75**

Anzola Luz Kelly, Rivera Jose Nelson, Ramírez Sara and Signore Alberto
Sjögren Syndrome: New Insights in the Pathogenesis and Role of Nuclear Medicine
Reprinted from: *J. Clin. Med.* **2022**, *11*, 5227, doi:10.3390/jcm11175227 . . . . **91**

Yuka Matsumiya-Matsumoto, Yoshihiro Morita and Narikazu Uzawa
Pleomorphic Adenoma of the Salivary Glands and Epithelial–Mesenchymal Transition
Reprinted from: *J. Clin. Med.* **2022**, *11*, 4210, doi:10.3390/jcm11144210 . . . . **107**

Margherita Sisto, Domenico Ribatti and Sabrina Lisi
Sjögren's Syndrome-Related Organs Fibrosis: Hypotheses and Realities
Reprinted from: *J. Clin. Med.* **2022**, *11*, 3551, doi:10.3390/jcm11123551 . . . . **121**

Margherita Sisto, Domenico Ribatti and Sabrina Lisi
E-Cadherin Signaling in Salivary Gland Development and Autoimmunity
Reprinted from: *J. Clin. Med.* **2022**, *11*, 2241, doi:10.3390/jcm11082241 . . . . **131**

About the Editor

Margherita Sisto

Margherita Sisto is a Professor of Human Anatomy at the Faculty of Medicine, University of Bari, Italy, with a Biological Degree cum laude, and a PhD in "Human and Experimental Morphology (macroscopic, microscopic and ultrastructural)", University of Bari, Italy. Professor Sisto's research interests are primarily in the area of pathophysiology and molecular immunology applied to immunological research lines, with an emphasis on the elucidation of molecular processes underlying the interaction between receptors of the immune response, inflammation and characterization of new anti-inflammatory molecules. Her particle research has involved the in-vitro analysis of dysregulated immunological responses during the pathogenesis of chronic inflammatory diseases such as the autoimmune Sjögren's syndrome. Professor Sisto's innovative research has been featured in high-prestige peer-reviewed journals.

Journal of
Clinical Medicine

MDPI

Editorial

Special Issue "Diseases of the Salivary Glands-Part II"

Margherita Sisto

Department of Basic Medical Sciences, Neurosciences and Sense Organs, Section of Human Anatomy and Histology, University of Bari Medical School, 70124 Bari, Italy; margherita.sisto@uniba.it

Citation: Sisto, M. Special Issue "Diseases of the Salivary Glands-Part II". *J. Clin. Med.* **2022**, *11*, 5567. https://doi.org/10.3390/jcm11195567

Received: 19 September 2022
Accepted: 20 September 2022
Published: 22 September 2022

This Special Issue, "Diseases of Salivary Gland-Part II", was born as a continuation of the volume "Diseases of the Salivary Gland", published, with great success, in 2021 in the prestigious *Journal of Clinical Medicine* (JCM) (https://www.mdpi.com/journal/jcm/special_issues/Salivary_Glands, accessed on 3 April 2021). The management of salivary gland (SGs) disorders encompasses a broad array of diseases, both benign and malignant, and the great international interest in this topic has led to the publication of the second part of the Special Issue, thusly entitled "Diseases of the Salivary Glands-Part II", which reflects the diverse nature of SG dysfunction and is focused on various topics ranging from diagnosis and therapeutic implications to the study of the molecular mechanisms underlying autoimmune and neoplastic diseases of the salivary glands.

The first part of this Special Issue concerns research articles focused on new discoveries in the diagnostic field of SG diseases [1–6] and on the identification of molecular mechanisms that could correlate the state of chronic inflammation that characterizes autoimmune SG diseases with the dysfunction of the glands themselves [1–6]. SGs are of the utmost importance for maintaining the health of the oral cavity and carrying out physiological functions such as mastication, the protection of teeth, the perception of taste, and speech. José Mário Matos-Sousa and colleagues from the Federal University of Pará, Brazil, examined whether fluoride—known to be effective in preventing and controlling caries—damages SGs by inducing biochemical and proteomic changes; interestingly, the research group demonstrated that fluoride does not cause any morphological or biochemical changes in the SGs and so reinforced the effectiveness of a low-dose fluoride treatment for the maintenance of cavity homeostasis [1]. Moreover, a comparative study from Taiwanese researchers comparing the effectiveness of hydrogen peroxide and adrenaline during tonsillectomy was included, which aimed at safeguarding the integrity of the SGs of the entire oral mucosa [4]. Among the research papers, a portion of this Special Issue is dedicated to the study of the molecular mechanisms underlying Sjögren's syndrome (SS), a chronic inflammatory disease, with a varied and still partly unknown etiology, which leads to the dysfunction of the SGs and xerostomia. The Special Issue collects the most recent discoveries made by the Sisto and Lisi group that correlate the inflammatory degree of SGs with the Epithelial to Mesenchymal Transition (EMT) program activation in SS, underlining the possibility of a fibrotic evolution of the glandular tissue [2]. Furthermore, a recent study of Campagna et al., resulting from an international collaboration between Italy and Colombia, investigated and clarified the role of T lymphocytes in SS, universally accepted as actors in the pathogenesis of SS [3]; in addition, an interesting study by Gupta and colleagues from the University of Florida enriched this Special Issue by contributing an article describing the possibility of mapping the epitopes of pathogenic autoantigens on SS leukocytes [5]. Other authors, such as the group of Micaela F. Beckman and Farah and Jean-Luc Mougeot (conducted at Carolinas Medical Center, Charlotte, NC, USA), analyzed data relating to the expression of specific antigens associated with SS in order to identify new therapeutic targets for xerostomia [6]. The etiology of SS remains poorly understood; however, as evidenced by the section of this Special Issue dedicated to reviews [7–10], the findings are becoming increasingly interesting and lately they correlate SS with the activation of an EMT program that could explain the altered function of the SGs in SS with a reduction in saliva secretion. It is interesting to underline that, up to now, the EMT is a process related to neoplastic transformation, as also reported for SG tumors by Yuka Matsumiya-Matsumoto from Osaka University [8]; however, in recent years, vast amounts of evidence have been collected that highlights the activation of the EMT even in situations of chronic inflammation, similar to that which occurs in autoimmune diseases [7,9,10].

Given the scientific importance of the articles collected, I am thrilled to reiterate that this Special Issue aims to provide insights into SGs diseases and summarizes the current knowledge of underlying pathophysiological mechanisms, yielding surprising results.

Funding: This research received no external funding.

Acknowledgments: As the Guest Editor, I would like to give special thanks to the reviewers who have spent some of their time to provide extremely helpful suggestions to improve the quality of the articles collected, and to the Journal Editorial Team for their robust support. Finally, a dutiful thanks goes to all the authors who with dedication, professionalism, originality, and enthusiasm have accepted my invitation and contributed to the publication of this Special Issue.

Conflicts of Interest: The authors declare no conflict of interest.

References

1. Matos-Sousa, J.; Bittencourt, L.; Ferreira, M.; dos Santos, V.; Balbinot, K.; Alves-Júnior, S.; Pinheiro, J.; Charone, S.; Pessan, J.; Lima, R. Fluoride Exposure and Salivary Glands: How Is Glandular Morphology Susceptible to Long-Term Exposure? A Preclinical Study. *J. Clin. Med.* **2022**, *11*, 5373. [CrossRef]
2. Sisto, M.; Ribatti, D.; Ingravallo, G.; Lisi, S. The Expression of Follistatin-Like 1 Protein Is Associated with the Activation of the EMT Program in Sjögren's Syndrome. *J. Clin. Med.* **2022**, *11*, 5368. [CrossRef]
3. Campagna, G.; Anzola, L.; Varani, M.; Lauri, C.; Gentiloni Silveri, G.; Chiurchioni, L.; Spinelli, F.; Priori, R.; Conti, F.; Signore, A. Imaging Activated-T-Lymphocytes in the Salivary Glands of Patients with Sjögren's Syndrome by 99mTc-Interleukin-2: Diagnostic and Therapeutic Implications. *J. Clin. Med.* **2022**, *11*, 4368. [CrossRef] [PubMed]
4. Hsieh, C.; Hsu, C.; Wu, H.; Sun, C. Comparison Benefit between Hydrogen Peroxide and Adrenaline in Tonsillectomy: A Randomized Controlled Study. *J. Clin. Med.* **2022**, *11*, 2723. [CrossRef] [PubMed]
5. Gupta, S.; Li, D.; Ostrov, D.; Nguyen, C. Epitope Mapping of Pathogenic Autoantigens on Sjögren's Syndrome-Susceptible Human Leukocyte Antigens Using In Silico Techniques. *J. Clin. Med.* **2022**, *11*, 1690. [CrossRef] [PubMed]
6. Beckman, M.; Brennan, E.; Igba, C.; Brennan, M.; Mougeot, F.; Mougeot, J. A Computational Text Mining-Guided Meta-Analysis Approach to Identify Potential Xerostomia Drug Targets. *J. Clin. Med.* **2022**, *11*, 1442. [CrossRef]
7. Kelly, A.; Nelson, R.; Sara, R.; Alberto, S. Sjögren Syndrome: New Insights in the Pathogenesis and Role of Nuclear Medicine. *J. Clin. Med.* **2022**, *11*, 5227. [CrossRef]
8. Matsumiya-Matsumoto, Y.; Morita, Y.; Uzawa, N. Pleomorphic Adenoma of the Salivary Glands and Epithelial–Mesenchymal Transition. *J. Clin. Med.* **2022**, *11*, 4210. [CrossRef] [PubMed]
9. Sisto, M.; Ribatti, D.; Lisi, S. Sjögren's Syndrome-Related Organs Fibrosis: Hypotheses and Realities. *J. Clin. Med.* **2022**, *11*, 3551. [CrossRef] [PubMed]
10. Sisto, M.; Ribatti, D.; Lisi, S. E-Cadherin Signaling in Salivary Gland Development and Autoimmunity. *J. Clin. Med.* **2022**, *11*, 2241. [CrossRef] [PubMed]

Journal of
Clinical Medicine

MDPI

Article

Fluoride Exposure and Salivary Glands: How Is Glandular Morphology Susceptible to Long-Term Exposure? A Preclinical Study

José Mário Matos-Sousa [1], Leonardo Oliveira Bittencourt [1], Maria Karolina Martins Ferreira [1], Vinicius Ruan Neves dos Santos [1], Karolyny Martins Balbinot [2], Sérgio Alves-Júnior [2], João de Jesus Viana Pinheiro [2], Senda Charone [1], Juliano Pelim Pessan [3] and Rafael Rodrigues Lima [1,*]

1 Laboratory of Functional and Structural Biology, Institute of Biological Sciences, Federal University of Pará, Belém 66075-110, PA, Brazil
2 School of Dentistry, Federal University of Pará, Belém 66075-110, PA, Brazil
3 Department of Preventive and Restorative Dentistry, School of Dentistry, São Paulo State University, Araçatuba 14801-385, SP, Brazil
* Correspondence: rafalima@ufpa.br

Abstract: Despite a strong body of evidence attesting to the effectiveness of fluoride (F) in preventing and controlling caries, some studies have sought to investigate the influence of F exposure on the salivary glands, organs that are essential for the maintenance of cavity homeostasis through salivary production, finding that exposure to F can cause biochemical and proteomic changes. Thus, this study aimed to investigate the morphological effects of prolonged exposure to F on the salivary glands of mice, at concentrations that would correspond to optimally fluoridated water (suitable for human consumption) and to fluorosis-endemic regions. Twenty-four male mice (*Mus musculus*) were divided into three groups, according to F levels in the drinking water: 0 (control), 10, or 50 mg F/L, with an exposure period of 60 days. The glands were morphometrically analyzed for the total acinar area, parenchyma area, and stromal area, as well as for the immunohistochemical analysis of myoepithelial cells. The results showed that prolonged exposure to F at 10 mg F/L did not promote significant changes in the morphometry of the salivary glands of mice, which reinforces the safety of the chronic use of F in low doses.

Keywords: fluoride; sodium fluoride; salivary glands

Citation: Matos-Sousa, J.M.; Bittencourt, L.O.; Ferreira, M.K.M.; dos Santos, V.R.N.; Balbinot, K.M.; Alves-Júnior, S.; Pinheiro, J.d.J.V.; Charone, S.; Pessan, J.P.; Lima, R.R. Fluoride Exposure and Salivary Glands: How Is Glandular Morphology Susceptible to Long-Term Exposure? A Preclinical Study. *J. Clin. Med.* **2022**, *11*, 5373. https://doi.org/10.3390/jcm11185373

Academic Editor: Margherita Sisto

Received: 22 July 2022
Accepted: 14 August 2022
Published: 13 September 2022

1. Introduction

Fluorine is a non-metallic element with high electronegativity, which can be found naturally in the forms of fluoride (F). The exposure to this ion can occur both naturally (through volcanic activity, coal combustion, dissolution of minerals, and marine aerosols) and anthropogenically (when F is released as waste from industrial activity or from manufactured products) [1,2]. Due to its unquestionable effects on caries prevention and control, F is also incorporated into vehicles available at a population level (water, salt, milk, sugar, and supplements), as well as at an individual level for professional (gels, foams, and varnishes) and home application (dentifrices and mouthwashes), which are known to contribute to the overall systemic exposure to fluoridated compounds [3].

Considering the possibility of bioaccumulation in organic systems, previous studies indicate that F ingested at excessive doses is capable of causing damage to the central nervous system [4], reduced immunity [5], male reproductive system dysfunction [6], liver damage [7], alterations in the antioxidant systems of kidney [8], and skeletal and dental manifestations [9,10]. Furthermore, F may interact with various cellular processes, such as gene expression, cell cycle, proliferation and migration, respiration, metabolism, ion transport, vesicular transport, oxidative stress, and cell death [11].

Moreover, F has been shown to impair the metabolism of key organs that ensure the physiological balance of the oral environment, including the salivary glands. These are secretory organs that contribute to the homeostasis of the oral cavity, and whose products play a substantial role in the regulation of physiological properties and maintenance of soft tissue integrity [12,13]. Total salivary production and composition vary according to different physiological conditions [14]. The major salivary glands, represented by three pairs of glands (parotid, submandibular, and sublingual), produce on average 90% of the saliva secreted in the oral cavity, while the remainder is produced by minor salivary glands dispersed in the mucosa [15]. Thus, total saliva becomes a complex of multiglandular secretions composed of gingival fluid, desquamated epithelial cells, microorganisms, products of bacterial metabolism, food remnants, leukocytes, and mucus from the nasal cavity and the pharynx [16].

In a previous study, the biochemical parameters of the submandibular salivary glands of mice under F exposure were evaluated through proteomic analysis, showing changes in the protein profile of the groups exposed to F at 10 mg F/L or 50 mg F/L, which were especially related to the structural constituents of the cytoskeleton and actin-myosin filaments [17]. Furthermore, a similar study on the parotid salivary glands reached similar results in the proteomic analysis, but also reported alterations in proteins associated with the anatomical structure of the glands [17,18]. Based on the aforementioned studies, the question on the effects of these biochemical alterations on the morphological structure of the salivary glands can be raised. Thus, considering that possible tissue-level repercussions of biochemical, proteomic, and genotoxic changes in salivary glands caused by prolonged exposure to F have not yet been addressed, there is a need to investigate the effects of F on the morphology of the salivary glands, thus seeking a better understanding of the possible risks to human health.

Within the context above, this study aimed to investigate the effects of systemic and chronic exposure to F on the morphometric parameters of the major salivary glands of mice. The study's hypothesis was that the molecular damages caused by F exposure reported in the literature would be associated with histological alterations in the salivary glands of the exposed animals.

2. Materials and Methods

2.1. Experimental Animals

The experimental procedures were performed after approval by the Ethics Committee on Experimental Animals of the Federal University of Pará (UFPA), project No. 7360181219, following the recommendations of the NIH Guide for Care and Use of Laboratory Animals. A total of 24 male Swiss albino mice (21 days old) were randomly divided into three groups of 8 animals each, which were fed ad libitum with chow and water, and housed inside an air conditioned room, with a 12 h light/dark cycle. For 60 days, all animals received deionized water containing 10 mg F/L and 50 mgF/L (as NaF, Sigma-Aldrich—San Luis, AZ, USA), to mimic chronic F ingestion from water by humans at concentrations corresponding to ≅2 mg F/L (roughly equivalent to the concentration of drinking water)) and 10 mg F/L (equivalent to water from areas endemic to fluorosis). This concentration is justified by the metabolism of rodents being 5 times higher than that of humans [19–21]. The control group received only deionized water without NaF for the same period. The weight of the animals and the volume of water ingested per cage were measured weekly. Other studies by our research group used this same exposure protocol [17–19], which found increased fluoride concentrations in the submandibular and parotid glands, and in blood plasma. The results from these initial studies were that F levels in the group receiving the highest exposure dose (50 mg F/L) were significantly higher (0.19 ± 0.01 μg/mL) than the levels in the control group ($0.05 \pm 0.\ 01$ μg/mL) in the submandibular glands [17], as well as in the parotid glands, with similar results as the levels in the group receiving the highest exposure dose (50 mg F/L) were significantly higher (0.14 ± 0.01 μg/mL) than the levels in the control group (0.06 ± 0.01 μg/mL) [18]. Furthermore, an increase in plasma fluoride concentration, finding statistically higher results in the groups exposed to 10 mg/L NaF (0.122 μg F/mL) and 50 mg/L NaF (0.142 μg F/mL) when compared to the control group (0.081 μg F/mL) mL) [19]. This led us to devise the present experimental design.

2.2. Euthanasia and Salivary Glands Collection

All animals were anesthetized with a solution of ketamine hydrochloride (90 mg/kg) and xylazine (9 mg/kg) for the perfusion protocol [22]. Then, the collections of the glands were performed for histological analysis, as described below and represented in Figure 1.

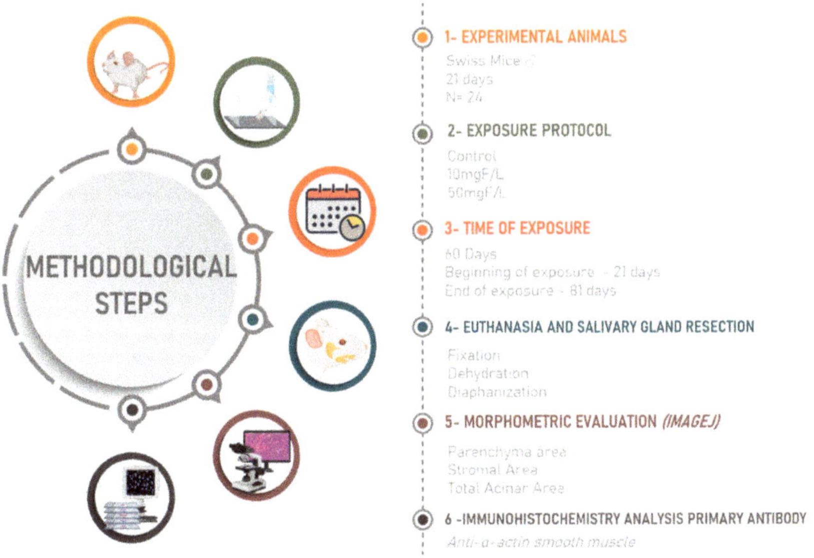

Figure 1. Experimental protocol of the study. In 1, description of experimental animals; in 2, the method of exposure to fluoride (F) at 0, 10 or 50 mg F/L; in 3, time of exposure and age at which experiment started and ended; in 4, euthanasia, salivary glands resection and histological processing steps; in 5, morphometric evaluation; and 6, immunohistochemical analyses.

2.3. Histopathological and Morphological Evaluations

After the surgical process for the collection of the parotid, submandibular and sublingual salivary glands, all samples were immersed in 10% formalin for 48 h for further tissue analysis.

To assess and quantify morphological and tissue changes, morphometric and immunohistochemical analyses were performed. For this, after the period of fixation of the samples in formalin, the glands of each animal were post-fixed in 6% formaldehyde until processing. The glands were dehydrated in increasing solutions of ethanol (70%, 80%, 90%, absolute 1, and absolute 2) cleared in xylene, and included in Paraplast for subsequent 5 μm-thick sections.

Twenty sagittal sections of the glands previously included in Paraplast were made, with a thickness of 5 μm, and then stained with Hematoxylin and Eosin. To perform this analysis, images were taken by a color digital camera (Cyber-Shot DSC W-230, Sony, Tokyo, Japan) coupled to a microscope (Eclipse E200, Nikon, Tokyo, Japan; at a magnification of 40×) of 4 random sagittal sections of the glands being evaluated, on average, 4 fields from each section. The tissue morphometric evaluation variables, expressed in μm^2, were: Total Acinar Area (TAA), Total Duct Area (TDA), Parenchyma Area (PA), and Stromal Area (SA) [23,24].

Variable values were obtained using a digital image analyzer (ImageJ software, v. 1.53, NIMH, NIH, Bethesda, MD, USA, http://rsbweb.nih.gov/ij/ (accessed on 1 June 2022).

Immunohistochemistry Analysis

The immunohistochemical analysis was performed because myoepithelial cells (present around the acini of the salivary glands) are difficult to observe when stained by Hematoxylin and Eosin. Due to the great importance of this group of cells for the functioning of the salivary glands, immunohistochemistry was used to overcome the limitations of conventional staining techniques. For this analysis, the slides were deparaffinized in xylene and hydrated in decreasing concentrations of alcohol. Antigen retrieval was performed in citrate buffer (pH 6.0) in a Pascal pressure chamber (Dako, Carpinteria, CA, USA) for 30 s. Then, they were immersed in 6% H_2O_2 and methanol at a ratio of 1:1 for 30 min to inhibit the activity of endogenous peroxidase. Non-specific binding was blocked with 1% bovine serum albumin (BSA) (Sigma-Aldrich Corp., St. Louis, MI, USA) in phosphate-buffered saline (1× PBS) for 1 h.

After this step, primary anti-α-smooth muscle actin antibodies (DAKO, 1:350) to actin filaments of myoepithelial cells were incubated for 1 h. Then, the slides were incubated for 30 min with the Immunohistoprobe plus detection system (Advance Biosystems, San Francisco, CA, USA). Diaminobenzidine (DAB) (ScyTek, Logan, UT, USA) was used as a chromogen. Slides were counterstained with hematoxylin (Sigma®), dehydrated, divinized, and mounted with Permount (Fisher Scientific, Fair Lawn, NJ, USA).

The immunostaining was carried out by evaluating the area measurement (μm) and a fraction (%) of the marking of the analyses performed. Brightfield images of 3 randomly selected areas from each sample were acquired using the same magnifications (40×).

The areas revealed by diaminobenzidine (DAB) were separated and segmented using the "color deconvolution" tool (Gabriel Landini, http://www.dentistry.bham.ac.uk/landinig/software/software.html (accessed on 1 June 2022) available in the ImageJ software (NIMH, NIH, Bethesda, MD, USA). After image segmentation, the total area and total staining fraction were measured. The immunostaining differences found in the studied groups were analyzed.

2.4. Statistical Analyses

Data were statistically analyzed using the GraphPad Prism v. 8.0 software (San Diego, CA, USA), using one-way ANOVA (for parametric data) or Kruskal–Wallis test (for non-parametric data), and Tukey's post hoc test, assuming a statistical significance value of $p < 0.05$. Parametric results are expressed mean ± standard error (Supplementary Table S1), while non-parametric results were expressed as median, interquartile range (Supplementary Table S2).

3. Results

3.1. Long-Term F Exposure Is Not Able to Alter the Morphology of Mice Salivary Glands

The three major salivary glands showed a pattern of morphological normality, with intact acini and grouped in lobes, close to the ducts, with uniformity of the areas of parenchyma and stroma for the three experimental groups, as shown in Figure 2.

For the quantitative analyses (Figure 3), no statistically significant differences were observed among the three groups regarding the measured areas of parenchyma (Figure 3A), stroma (Figure 3B), and total acinar area (Figure 3C) of the parotid glands.

A similar trend was observed for the submandibular glands, i.e., no statistical differences among the groups, considering the parenchyma area (Figure 3D), stromal area (Figure 3E), and total acinar area (Figure 3F).

For the sublingual glands, on the other hand, despite no statistical differences were observed among the three groups for the parenchyma area (Figure 3G) and the acinar area (Figure 3I), exposure to 50 mg F/L water led to significant increases in the stromal area (Figure 3H) compared with the groups exposed to 0 (control) or 10 mg F/L drinking water.

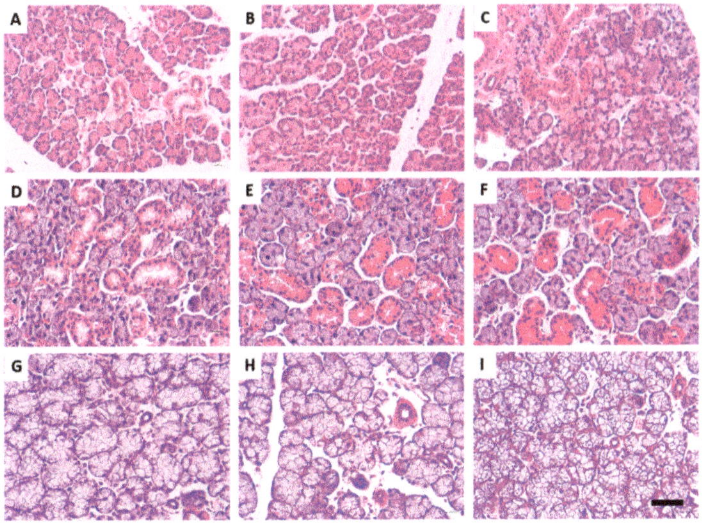

Figure 2. Effects of 60-day exposure to 0, 10, or 50 mg F/L from the drinking water on the histologic characteristics of the salivary glands of mice. Photomicrographs were obtained from the parotid (**A–C**), submandibular (**D–F**), and sublingual (**G–I**) glands, which were stained with hematoxylin and eosin. From left to right, exposure to 0 mg F/L (control), 10 mg F/L, and 50 mg F/L. 50 μm scale bar. (n = 8 animals/group).

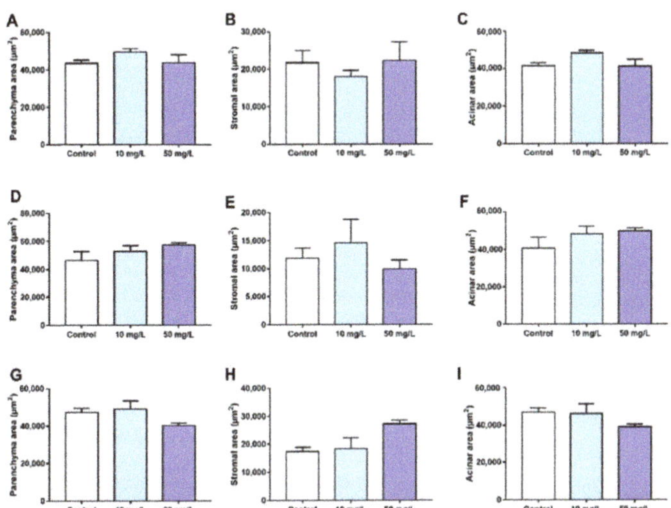

Figure 3. Effects of 60-day exposure to 0, 10, or 50 mg F/L from the drinking water on the morphometric parameters of the mice salivary glands. Graphs represent the morphometric analyses of the parotid glands (parenchyma, stromal, and acini areas represented by (**A–C**), respectively), submandibular glands (parenchyma, stromal, and acini areas represented by (**D–F**), respectively), and sublingual glands (parenchyma, stromal, and acini areas represented by (**G–I**), respectively). The results are expressed as mean ± standard error of mean. Different superscript letters indicate statistical differences among the groups. The absence of letters indicates that there was no statistical difference. One-way ANOVA and Tukey's post hoc test. ($p < 0.05$, n = 8 animals/group).

3.2. *Long-Term F Exposure Did Not Affect the Immunostained Area Fraction of the Smooth Muscle Actin Filaments in Myoepithelial Cells of Mice Salivary Glands*

The immunostaining pattern was fairly uniform among the control, 10 mg F/L and 50 mg F/L groups, showing a morphological normal pattern of myoepithelial cells, as presented in Figure 4. No statistical differences were observed among the groups (0, 10, or 50 50 mg F/L) regarding the parotid (Figure 4D), the submandibular (Figure 4H), and the sublingual (Figure 4L) glands.

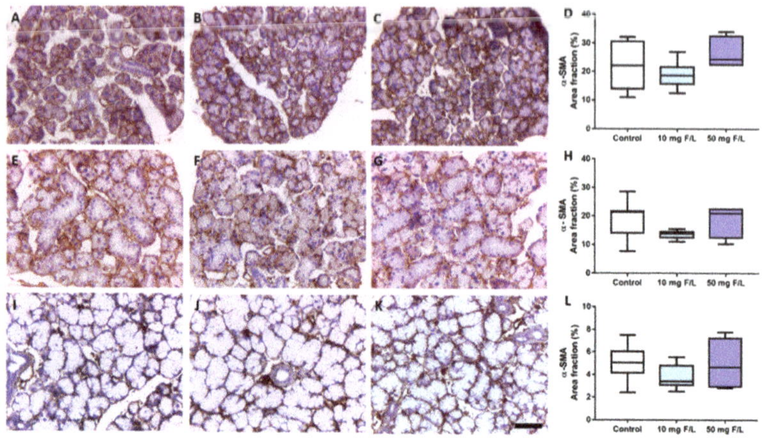

Figure 4. Effects of 60 days exposure to 0, 10, or 50 mg F/L on smooth muscle actin immunostaining area fraction in mice salivary glands, represented by photomicrographs of each group and graphs of the area fraction analysis. Letters (**A–D**) represent the parotid gland; (**E–H**), the submandibular gland; (**I–L**), the sublingual gland. From left to right (columns), control, 10 mg F/L, and 50 mg F/L groups and area fraction graphs. Brown areas indicate positive labeling for the antibody by DAB reaction, while blue areas are counterstained by Harris' hematoxylin. Results are expressed as median and interquartile range. Different superscript letters indicate a statistical difference between the groups. The absence of letters indicates that there was no statistical difference. Kruskal–Wallis test, followed by Tukey's post hoc test, $p < 0.05$. 50 μm scale bar. (n = 8 animals/group).

4. Discussion

This study gathered morphological evidence about long-term exposure to F, and the repercussions on the salivary glands of adult mice. Our findings pointed out that F, under the present experimental conditions, does not pose a significant threat to the major salivary glands' morphological organization in adult organisms, especially considering the data from the glandular functional unit, the acini, and the myoepithelial cells.

The F concentrations adopted were based on previous studies investigating F exposure from the drinking water, which somehow mimicked the F concentrations to which humans may be exposed to [21,25], then, from the known mean human ingestion doses of F, the resulting concentrations for exposure in this study were 10 mg F/L and 50 mg F/L [20].

In previous studies, we showed that systemic and prolonged exposure to F at 10 mg F/L and 50 mg F/L resulted in significant increases in F bioavailability in the blood plasma at both concentrations, however, only higher concentrations increased the levels of F in the parotid and submandibular glands of mice [17–19]. Despite these differences in F distribution among different organs, this evidence ensures the reliability in establishing a dose–response in our experimental protocol. Furthermore, it is worth mentioning that the exposure concentrations used were still above the optimal indication values [26].

In our morphometric results, we found an increase in the stromal area in the sublingual glands of animals exposed to 50 mg F/L, while no statistical differences were observed among the groups for this parameter for the other glands. In this context, it is important to emphasize that although the major salivary glands are fundamentally involved in the same role (i.e., saliva production), they have different morphological development and organization. The parotid gland has its terminal acini-like secretory units consisting of serous cells. The submandibular gland, on the other hand, is characterized as mixed, with serous predominance, but with the presence of mucous terminals. The sublingual glands have their composition substantially formed by tubular mucosal terminals, with the presence of some serous semilunas [27]. These structural differences may help to explain the increase in the stromal area of the sublingual gland of mice exposed to 50 mg F/L compared to the other glands.

Considering the peculiarities of the morphology of the salivary glands, the myoepithelial cells (which are attached to the basal lamina of the serous acinous secretory units) structurally resemble smooth muscle cells, and are composed of filament bodies of actin, myosin, and dense bodies, containing a central body with its nucleus and four to eight processes surrounding the secretory unit, as well as the proximal portion of the duct system. These cells are contractile, and their function is to facilitate and better promote the excretion of the secretory product from the acini glands to the duct system [27,28]. This ability is mediated by alpha-actin filaments, which are used as good cell markers for this cell population. Our findings showed that chronic exposure to F is not associated with the modulation in the immunostaining of smooth muscle actin filaments in the salivary glands, suggesting, therefore, that no impairment in salivary flow might be caused by F at the levels tested.

The functional and structural maintenance of the glands, demonstrated in our morphometric results, is essential to oral cavity homeostasis, considering that saliva contributes to the maintenance of a wide range of physiological needs. In the digestive tract, for example, saliva plays an important role in the digestive process and in the protection of gastric cells. In the oral cavity, saliva participates in mastication, speech, swallowing, and tissue lubrication, in addition to having antibacterial, antifungal, and antiviral activity. It also has buffering capacity and acts as a carrier of essential ions, such as calcium, phosphate, and fluorine itself, which have an essential role in enamel remineralization [29,30].

In this perspective, a recent study from our group showed that F exposure at the same concentrations as in the present work, during the pre- and post-natal periods, elicited morphological changes in the duct area of the parotid and submandibular glands in animals exposed to 50 mg F/L [31]. These findings prompted the present investigation, which assessed the morphological changes of the salivary glands of exposed mice from the end of the lactation period (21st day after birth), until the adult phase (at 81 days of life) [32]. Therefore, the exposure period of 60 days occurred during the stage of differentiation of the glands until the consolidated adult phase [28]. Differently from the prenatal studies [31], in this model of postnatal exposure to F no morphological changes were found. This different response suggests that susceptibility to damage is age-dependent and that the salivary glands show greater resistance to morphological damage that could be triggered by F after their full development.

The trend above, however, should be viewed with caution. Scientific evidence suggests that excess F leads to increases in reactive oxygen species production, accelerated consumption of antioxidant enzymes, and accumulation of lipid peroxidation products [33,34]. Previous studies have also shown that F is able to modulate oxidative biochemistry, such as increased GSH and TBARS, in addition to genotoxic changes in the submandibular gland in the group exposed to the highest concentration (50 mg F/L) and modulation in the proteomic profile [17,18]. Thus, it is possible to interpret the morphological results presented here in two ways: (1) the molecular changes did not result in changes in the tissues, and/or (2) chronic exposure over 60 days did not allow enough time for any molecular changes to have an effect on the tissues.

Other factors must also be considered, such as the fact that F exposure may occur from multiple sources and can be influenced by the length of exposure and by the specific developmental phases. Thus, other forms of exposure to F should be considered, as well as other time windows, for a closer assessment of the risks of F exposure to these organs. Further research seeking longer exposure times, and at doses representative of human exposure may better reinforce the safety of F use. Finally, it must be emphasized that there is no evidence to support that F can bring any harm to human health when used at recommended levels [35].

5. Conclusions

From the results presented, it can be concluded that chronic exposure to F by mice over a 60-day period (from the end of the lactation period to adult life) led to no significant changes in the morphology of adult rat salivary glands. Nonetheless, the present results should be interpreted with caution, considering that chronic F exposure at earlier developmental stages was previously shown to increase the systemic bioavailability of F, as well as to promote proteomic modulations in important cell cycle processes, cytoskeleton regulation, and cellular metabolism. The simultaneous analysis of the present and previous studies cited above clearly point to the need to further address this important research question, whose results might guide future translational research.

Supplementary Materials: The following supporting information can be downloaded at: https://www.mdpi.com/article/10.3390/jcm11185373/s1, Table S1: Parametric results of the morphometric analysis of the parenchyma area, stromal area, and total acinar area, of parotid, submandibular and sublingual glands of mice exposed to 10mg F/L and 50mgF/L for 60 days. Results were expressed as mean ± standard error of mean.; Table S2: Nonparametric results of the analysis of the immunostained area fraction of the smooth muscle actin filaments of the myoepithelial cells of the salivary glands of mice exposed to 10mgF/L and 50mg F/L for 60 days. Results are expressed as median and interquartile ranges.

Author Contributions: Conceptualization, J.M.M.-S., M.K.M.F. and R.R.L.; methodology, J.M.M.-S., M.K.M.F., V.R.N.d.S., L.O.B., K.M.B., J.d.J.V.P. and S.A.-J.; data curation, J.M.M.-S., M.K.M.F., L.O.B., K.M.B., S.A.-J., J.d.J.V.P. and R.R.L.; draft writing preparation, J.M.M.-S., M.K.M.F. and L.O.B.; reviewing and editing R.R.L., J.P.P. and S.C. All authors have read and agreed to the published version of the manuscript.

Funding: This work was supported by the Research Pro-Rectory of Federal University of Pará (PROPESP, UFPA, Brazil) by the APC payment. This study was also financed in part by the CAPES—Finance Code 001. R.R.L is a researcher from Brazilian National Council for Scientific and Technological Development (CNPq) and received a grant under the numbers 435093/2018-5 and 312275/2021-8.

Institutional Review Board Statement: The experimental protocol was approved by the Ethics Committee on the Use of Experimental Animals (CEUA), under opinion number 7360181219, and was executed following the Guidelines for the Care and Use of Laboratory Animals and Animal Research: Reporting of In Vivo Experiments (ARRIVE).

Informed Consent Statement: Not applicable.

Data Availability Statement: The quantitative and qualitative data used to support the findings of this study are included in the article.

Conflicts of Interest: The authors declare no conflict of interest.

References

1. Miranda, G.H.N.; Ferreira, M.K.M.; Bittencourt, L.O.; Lima, L.A.D.O.; Puty, B.; Lima, R.R. The role of oxidative stress in fluoride toxicity. In *Toxicology*; Academic Press: Cambridge, MA, USA, 2021; pp. 157–163. [CrossRef]
2. WHO. *World Health Organization. Fluorides. Environmental Health Criteria227*; World Health Organization: Geneva, Switzerland, 2002.
3. Buzalaf, M.A.R.; Whitford, G.M. Fluoride metabolism. In *Fluoride and the Oral Environment*; Karger: Basel, Switzerland, 2011; Volume 22, pp. 20–36.
4. Dec, K.; Łukomska, A.; Maciejewska, D.; Jakubczyk, K.; Baranowska-Bosiacka, I.; Chlubek, D.; Wąsik, A.; Gutowska, I. The Influence of Fluorine on the Disturbances of Homeostasis in the Central Nervous System. *Biol. Trace Element Res.* **2017**, *177*, 224–234. [CrossRef] [PubMed]
5. Kuang, P.; Deng, H.; Cui, H.; Chen, L.; Guo, H.; Fang, J.; Zuo, Z.; Deng, J.; Wang, X.; Zhao, L. Suppressive effects of sodium fluoride on cultured splenic lymphocyte proliferation in mice. *Oncotarget* **2016**, *7*, 61905–61915. [CrossRef] [PubMed]

. Saumya, S.M.; Basha, P.M. Fluoride exposure aggravates the testicular damage and sperm quality in diabetic mice: Protec-tive role of ginseng and banaba. *Biol. Trace Elem. Res.* **2017**, *177*, 331–344.
. Bouaziz, H.; Ketata, S.; Jammoussi, K.; Boudawara, T.; Ayedi, F.; Ellouze, F.; Zeghal, N. Effects of sodium fluoride on hepatic toxicity in adult mice and their suckling pups. *Pestic. Biochem. Physiol.* **2006**, *86*, 124–130. [CrossRef]
. Iano, F.G.; Ferreira, M.C.; Quaggio, G.B.; Fernandes, M.S.; Oliveira, R.C.; Ximenes, V.F.; Buzalaf, M.A.R. Effects of chronic fluoride intake on the antioxidant systems of the liver and kidney in rats. *J. Fluor. Chem.* **2014**, *168*, 212–217. [CrossRef]
. Revelo-Mejía, I.A.; Hardisson, A.; Rubio, C.; Gutiérrez, J.; Paz, S. Dental Fluorosis: The Risk of Misdiagnosis—A Review. *Biol. Trace Element Res.* **2020**, *199*, 1762–1770. [CrossRef]
0. Srivastava, S.; Flora, S.J.S. Fluoride in Drinking Water and Skeletal Fluorosis: A Review of the Global Impact. *Curr. Environ. Health Rep.* **2020**, *7*, 140–146. [CrossRef]
1. Barbier, O.; Arreola-Mendoza, L.; Del Razo, L.M. Molecular Mechanisms of Fluoride Toxicity. *Chem. -Biol. Interact.* **2010**, *188*, 319–333. [CrossRef]
2. Yamaguchi, P.M.; Simões, A.; Ganzerla, E.; Souza, D.N.; Nogueira, F.N.; Nicolau, J. Effects of a single exposure of sodium fluoride on lipid peroxidation and antioxidant enzymes in salivary glands of rats. *Oxid. Med. Cell. Longev.* **2013**, *2013*, 674593.
3. Nascimento, P.C.; Aragão, W.; Bittencourt, L.O.; Silva, M.; Crespo-Lopez, M.E.; Lima, R.R. Salivary parameters alterations after early exposure to environmental methylmercury: A preclinical study in offspring rats. *J. Trace Elem. Med. Biol.* **2021**, *68*, 126820. [CrossRef]
4. Castagnola, M.; Scarano, E.; Passali, G.; Messana, I.; Cabras, T.; Iavarone, F.; Di Cintio, G.; Fiorita, A.; De Corso, E.; Paludetti, G. Salivary biomarkers and proteomics: Future diagnostic and clinical utilities. *Acta Otorhinolaryngol. Ital.* **2017**, *37*, 94–101. [CrossRef] [PubMed]
5. Humphrey, S.P.; Williamson, R.T. A review of saliva: Normal composition, flow, and function. *J. Prosthet. Dent.* **2001**, *85*, 162–169. [CrossRef] [PubMed]
6. Falcão, D.P.; Da Mota, L.M.H.; Pires, A.L.; Bezerra, A.C.B. Sialometry: Aspects of clinical interest. *Rev. Bras. Reum.* **2013**, *53*, 525–531. [CrossRef]
7. Lima, L.A.D.O.; Miranda, G.H.N.; Aragão, W.A.B.; Bittencourt, L.O.; dos Santos, S.M.; de Souza, M.P.C.; Nogueira, L.S.; de Oliveira, E.H.C.; Monteiro, M.C.; Dionizio, A.; et al. Effects of Fluoride on Submandibular Glands of Mice: Changes in Oxidative Biochemistry, Proteomic Profile, and Genotoxicity. *Front. Pharmacol.* **2021**, *12*, 1–13. [CrossRef] [PubMed]
8. Miranda, G.H.N.; Lima, L.A.D.O.; Bittencourt, L.O.; dos Santos, S.M.; de Souza, M.P.C.; Nogueira, L.S.; de Oliveira, E.H.C.; Monteiro, M.C.; Dionizio, A.; Leite, A.L.; et al. Effects of long-term fluoride exposure are associated with oxidative biochemistry impairment and global proteomic modulation, but not genotoxicity, in parotid glands of mice. *PLoS ONE* **2022**, *17*, e0261252. [CrossRef]
19. Miranda, G.H.N.; Gomes, B.A.Q.; Bittencourt, L.O.; Aragão, W.; Nogueira, L.S.; Dionizio, A.; Buzalaf, M.A.R.; Monteiro, M.C.; Lima, R.R. Chronic Exposure to Sodium Fluoride Triggers Oxidative Biochemistry Misbalance in Mice: Effects on Peripheral Blood Circulation. *Oxidative Med. Cell. Longev.* **2018**, *2018*, 8379123. [CrossRef]
20. Dionizio, A.S.; Melo, C.G.S.; Sabino-Arias, I.T.; Ventura, T.M.S.; Leite, A.L.; Souza, S.R.G.; Santos, E.X.; Heubel, A.D.; Souza, J.G.; Perles, J.V.C.M.; et al. Chronic treatment with fluoride affects the jejunum: Insights from proteomics and enteric innervation analysis. *Sci. Rep.* **2018**, *8*, 3180. [CrossRef]
21. Dunipace, A.; Brizendine, E.; Zhang, W.; Wilson, M.; Miller, L.; Katz, B.; Warrick, J.M.; Stookey, G.K. Effect of aging on animal response to chronic fluoride exposure. *J. Dent. Res.* **1995**, *74*, 358–368. [CrossRef]
22. Lima, L.A.D.O.; Bittencourt, L.O.; Puty, B.; Fernandes, R.M.; Nascimento, P.C.; Silva, M.C.F.; Alves-Junior, S.M.; Pinheiro, J.D.J.V.; Lima, R.R. Methylmercury Intoxication Promotes Metallothionein Response and Cell Damage in Salivary Glands of Rats. *Biol. Trace Element Res.* **2018**, *185*, 135–142. [CrossRef]
23. Bohl, L.; Merlo, C.; Carda, C.; De Ferraris, M.E.G.; Carranza, M. Morphometric analysis of the parotid gland affected by alcoholic sialosis. *J. Oral Pathol. Med.* **2008**, *37*, 499–503. [CrossRef]
24. Merlo, C.; Bohl, L.; Carda, C.; de Ferraris, M.E.G.; Carranza, M. Parotid sialosis: Morphometrical analysis of the glandular parenchyma and stroma among diabetic and alcoholic patients. *J. Oral Pathol. Med.* **2010**, *39*, 10–15. [CrossRef] [PubMed]
25. Angmar-Månsson, B.; Whitford, G.M. Enamel fluorosis related to plasma F levels in the rat. *Caries Res.* **1984**, *18*, 25–32. [CrossRef] [PubMed]
26. WHO. *WHO Guidelines Approved by the Guidelines Review Committee. Guidelines for Drinking-Water Quality: Fourth Edition Incorporating the First Addendum*; World Health Organization: Geneva, Switzerland, 2017.
27. De Paula, F.; Teshima, T.H.N.; Hsieh, R.; Souza, M.M.; Nico, M.M.S.; Lourenco, S.V. Overview of Human Salivary Glands: Highlights of Morphology and Developing Processes. *Anat. Rec.* **2017**, *300*, 1180–1188. [CrossRef] [PubMed]
28. Tucker, A. Salivary gland development. *Semin. Cell Dev. Biol.* **2007**, *18*, 237–244. [CrossRef] [PubMed]
29. Lima, D.P.; Diniz, D.G.; Moimaz, S.A.S.; Sumida, D.H.; Okamoto, A.C. Saliva: Reflection of the body. *Int. J. Infect. Dis.* **2010**, spects of clinical interes *14*, e184–e188. [CrossRef]
30. Farooq, I.; Bugshan, A. The role of salivary contents and modern technologies in the remineralization of dental enamel: A narrative review. *F1000Research* **2020**, *9*, 171. [CrossRef]

31. Dos Santos, V.R.N.; Ferreira, M.K.M.; Bittencourt, L.O.; Mendes, P.F.S.; Souza-Monteiro, D.; Balbinot, K.M.; Pinheiro, J.D.J.V Charone, S.; Pessan, J.P.; Lima, R.R. Maternal Fluoride Exposure Exerts Different Toxicity Patterns in Parotid and Submandibula Glands of Offspring Rats. *Int. J. Mol. Sci.* **2022**, *23*, 7217. [CrossRef]
32. Dutta, S.; Sengupta, P. Men and mice: Relating their ages. *Life Sci.* **2016**, *152*, 244–248. [CrossRef]
33. Guan, Z. Role of oxidative stress in molecular pathogenesis of endemic fluorosis. *Chin. J. Endem.* **2016**, *16*, 79–82.
34. Zhong, N.; Yao, Y.; Ma, Y.; Meng, X.; Sowanou, A.; Pei, J. Effects of Fluoride on Oxidative Stress Markers of Lipid, Gene, and Protein in Rats. *Biol. Trace Element Res.* **2020**, *199*, 2238–2246. [CrossRef]
35. Cury, J.A.; Ricomini-Filho, A.P.; Berti, F.L.P.; Tabchoury, C.P. Systemic Effects (Risks) of Water Fluoridation. *Braz. Dent. J.* **2019** spects of clinical interes *30*, 421–428. [CrossRef] [PubMed]

Journal of
Clinical Medicine

MDPI

Article

The Expression of Follistatin-like 1 Protein Is Associated with the Activation of the EMT Program in Sjögren's Syndrome

Margherita Sisto [1,*], Domenico Ribatti [1], Giuseppe Ingravallo [2] and Sabrina Lisi [1]

1 Department of Basic Medical Sciences, Neurosciences and Sensory Organs (SMBNOS), Section of Human Anatomy and Histology, University of Bari "Aldo Moro", 70121 Bari, Italy
2 Department of Emergency and Organ Transplantation (DETO), Pathology Section, University of Bari "Aldo Moro", 70121 Bari, Italy
* Correspondence: margherita.sisto@uniba.it; Tel.:+39-080-547-8315; Fax: +39-080-547-8327

Abstract: Background: The activation of the epithelial to mesenchymal transition (EMT) program is a pathological response of the Sjögren's syndrome (SS) salivary glands epithelial cells (SGEC) to chronic inflammation. Follistatin-like 1 protein (FSTL1) is a secreted glycoprotein induced by transforming growth factor-β1 (TGF-β1), actively involved in the modulation of EMT. However, the role of FSTL1 in the EMT program activation in SS has not yet been investigated. Methods: TGF-β1-stimulated healthy human SGEC, SS SGEC, and SS salivary glands (SGs) biopsies were used to assess the effect of FSTL1 on the activation of the EMT program. FSTL1 gene activity was inhibited by the siRNA gene knockdown technique. Results: Here we reported that FSTL1 is up-regulated in SS SGs tissue in a correlated manner with the inflammatory grade. Blockage of FSTL1 gene expression by siRNA negatively modulates the TGF-β1-induced EMT program in vitro. We discovered that these actions were mediated through the modulation of the SMAD2/3-dependent EMT signaling pathway. Conclusions: Our data suggest that the TGF-β1-FSTL1-SMAD2/3 regulatory circuit plays a key role in the regulation of EMT in SS and targeting FSTL1 may be a strategy for the treatment of SGs EMT-dependent fibrosis.

Keywords: EMT; Sjögren's syndrome; Follistatin-like 1 protein; TGF-β1; SMAD2/3

Citation: Sisto, M.; Ribatti, D.; Ingravallo, G.; Lisi, S. The Expression of Follistatin-like 1 Protein Is Associated with the Activation of the EMT Program in Sjögren's Syndrome. *J. Clin. Med.* **2022**, *11*, 5368. https://doi.org/10.3390/jcm11185368

Academic Editor: Giuseppe Magliulo

Received: 9 August 2022
Accepted: 8 September 2022
Published: 13 September 2022

1. Introduction

Follistatin-like protein 1 (FSTL1) is a secreted glycoprotein with extensive glycosylation modifications, produced primarily by cells of the mesenchymal phenotype [1–3]. FSTL1 is composed of the presence of a follistatin (FS)-like domain and an extracellular calcium-binding (EC) motif and belongs to the SPARC (secreted protein acidic and rich in cysteine) family of matricellular proteins whose members participate in fine cellular functions [4]. Although the role in the progression of most pathological processes remains unclear, recent studies have described the involvement of FSTL1 in several pathological and physiological processes, such as embryonic development, tissue remodeling/repair, and organ fibrosis [5,6].

Converging lines of evidence have suggested an intrigant key role of FSTL1 in epithelial-mesenchymal transition (EMT) [7], a dynamic and reversible process in which cells gradually lose their epithelial phenotype and transform into a mesenchymal phenotype; moreover, sustained activation of EMT, in the context of the response to injury, promotes inflammation, triggering the fibrotic pathology of multiple organs [8,9]. Interesting studies have underlined as FSTL1 promotes EMT in concert with TGF-β1 [10,11]. Indeed, TGF-β1 regulates epithelial injury, myofibroblasts proliferation and differentiation, collagen production, and deposition. For this reason, it is indicated as a "master switch" in the initiation of the cascade of events that characterizes the EMT-dependent organ fibrosis [12–15].

Interestingly, there is additional evidence describing FSTL1 as a downstream effector of TGF-β1-induced fibrotic responses, and it is demonstrated that FSTL1 is upregulated in several fibrotic tissues, and promotes fibrogenesis through facilitating TGF-β1 signaling [10,16].

In recent years, a number of published reports have identified a new role for FSTL1 in the regulation of immune cell function, demonstrating overexpression of FSTL1 in several autoimmune diseases [16,17]. An interesting study performed by Li and colleagues [16] demonstrated that by targeting FSTL1, the attenuation of bleomycin-induced pulmonary and dermal fibrosis in vivo and TGF-β1-induced dermal fibrosis ex vivo in human skin was detected, a finding also confirmed by experimental models. In addition, elevated serum levels of FSTL1 were detected in patients with rheumatoid arthritis, and Sjögren's syndrome (SS), levels which are much higher than the levels observed in other chronic inflammatory diseases such as ulcerative colitis, systemic lupus erythematosus, systemic sclerosis, and polymyositis/dermatomyositis which, however, show altered levels of FSTL1 [17]. According to these literature data, elevated FSTL1 serum levels were detected in patients affected by primary Sjögren's syndrome (pSS) [16,17]. pSS is a chronic, systemic autoimmune disorder, commonly linked with dry eyes and dry mouth [18] and characterized by the trigger of the TGF-β1/SMAD-dependent EMT process in response to chronic inflammatory factors release [13].

In fact, the role of FSTL1 in the pathogenic pSS EMT has not yet been investigated [10,11,16]. In this report, we analyze the expression of FSTL1 in pSS salivary glands (SGs) biopsies and study the induction of FSTL1 by TGF-β1 treatment in human healthy salivary gland epithelial cells (SGEC); in addition, we evaluate the ability of FSTL1 to activate SMAD2/3-regulated TGF-β1-dependent EMT cascade in pSS.

2. Materials and Methods

2.1. Cell Treatment and Antibodies

Recombinant human TGF-β1 was purchased from R&D Systems (Minneapolis, MN, USA). Mouse anti-human TGF-β1 monoclonal antibody (mAb) (1:50, Santa Cruz Biotechnology, Santa Cruz, CA, USA), goat anti-human SMAD2/3 polyclonal Ab (pAb) (1:100, R&D Systems, Minneapolis, MN, USA), goat anti-humanp-SMAD2/3 (Ser 423/425) pAb (1:100, Santa Cruz Biotechnology), mouse anti-human β-actin mAb clone AC-15 (1:100, Sigma-Aldrich, St. Louis, MO, USA), mouse anti-human E-cadherin mAb (1:100, Dako, Santa Clara, CA, USA), mouse anti-human vimentin mAb (1:100, Thermo Fisher Scientific, Waltham, MA, USA), human Follistatin-like 1/FSTL1 polyclonal Antibody (pAb) (1 μg/mL, R&D Systems) were used in the experimental procedure.

2.2. Bioptic Samples Collection

The Department of Pathology, University of Bari Medical School, selected 30 labial SGs biopsies from pSS patients (aged 66.8 ± 2.3 years) according to the ACR/EULAR classification criteria for pSS [19], (using an absolutely anonymous form). The slides relating to 20 biopsies were already present in the archive. In addition, slides, and small glandular fragments from 10 SS patients who had to undergo a biopsy for diagnostic purposes were collected, maintaining anonymity. Five items were evaluated for the selection: anti-SSA/Ro antibody positivity and focal lymphocytic sialadenitis with a focus score of ≥1 foci/4 mm^2, each scoring 3, and an abnormal ocular staining score of ≥5 (or van Bijsterveld score of ≥4), a Schirmer's test result of ≥5 mm/5 min, and an unstimulated salivary flow rate of ≥0.1 mL/min, each scoring 1. On the basis of these parameters, biopsies were subdivided into three inflammatory groups: I, low; II, intermediate; III, advanced. Healthy volunteers (aged 60.1 ± 1.4 years, n = 10) with no salivary condition were included in the study as controls. Controls are healthy individuals awaiting the removal of salivary mucoceles from the lower lip [20]. The healthy subjects had no complaints of oral dryness, no autoimmune disease, and normal salivary function. LSG samples were collected from the lower lip under local anesthesia through normal mucosa. The cell cultures of SS SGEC were obtained using pieces of biopsy samples from SGs biopsies, a process which the patients underwent for diagnostic purposes, and the patients agreed that we could use a small piece of the gland to prepare the cultures. Similarly, the cells of healthy subjects were obtained from individuals who underwent the removal of the glands for mucoceles and not for purely experimental purposes.

2.3. Histochemistry

Representative serial 3 μm sections of healthy and pSS formalin-fixed, paraffin-embedded minor SG (MSG) tissues were rehydrated and deparaffinized in graded alcohol. (1 h in 70% ethanol supplemented with 0.25% NH_3 and immersion in 50% ethanol for 10 min). The slides were washed in phosphate-buffered saline (PBS) (pH 7.6 3 × 10 min) and immersed in EDTA buffer (0.01 M, pH 8.0) for 20 min to unmask antigens. The immunolabeling was performed by blocking the endogenous peroxidase by treatment with 3% hydrogen peroxide solution in water for 10 min at room temperature (RT) and carrying out a preincubation in non-immune donkey serum (Dako LSAB Kit, Dako, CA, USA). Then, the slides were incubated overnight at 4 °C with primary Abs. The relative secondary Abs (Santa Cruz Biotechnology, Dallas, TX, USA) diluted 1:200 in PBS for 1 h at RT followed by the streptavidin-peroxidase complex (Vector Laboratories, Newark, CA, USA) for 1 h at RT were applied to the sections. Then, 3,3-diaminobenzidine tetrahydrochloride (DAB) was used as chromogen (Vector Laboratories), and hematoxylin (Merck Eurolab, Dietikon, Switzerland) for counterstaining. Negative controls of the immunoreactions were performed by replacing the primary Ab with donkey serum. After the addition of the secondary Ab, no specific immunostaining was observed in the negative controls.

2.4. FSTL1 Immunohistochemical Analysis and Quantification

For immunohistochemistry image quantification, representative areas of the sections were viewed using a ×20 objective and photographed using a Zeiss Axio Cam HRc (Zeiss, Oberkochen, Germany). For each image of stained slides, ten representative visual fields, each 586 μm × 439 μm in area, were randomly acquired by the computerized image-acquisition (ImageJ, version 1.46c; WS Rasband, National Institutes of Health, Bethesda, MD, USA) connected to the microscope. SGEC were identified on the captured images and the number of SGEC positive for FSTL1 and the area occupied by these cells were measured. Positive areas were expressed as a percentage of the total tissue area examined.

2.5. SGEC Culture and Treatment

Healthy and pSS glandular fragments belonging to each classification group were dissociated by enzymatic and mechanical means into a suspension of single cells and plated onto a culture flask. Cells were used to obtain the experimental material (RNA and proteins) used to carry out our evaluations. After dissociation pSS dispersal cells were resuspended in McCoy's 5a modified medium supplemented with 10% heat-inactivated (56 °C for 30 min) FCS, 1% antibiotic solution, 2 mM L-glutamine, 50 ng mL^{-1} epidermal growth factor (EGF, Promega, Madison, WI, USA), and 0.5 μg mL^{-1} insulin (Novo, Bagsværd, Denmark) and incubated at 37 °C, 5% CO_2 in the air. The contaminating fibroblasts were selectively removed using 0.02% EDTA treatment. Immunocytochemical confirmation of the epithelial origin of cultured cells was routinely performed, as previously described [21]. Healthy human SGEC were grown in the same modified McCoy's 5A medium (Invitrogen, Waltham, MA, USA) supplemented with 1% heat-inactivated FCS (to avoid excessive growth during treatment with TGF-β1). Healthy SGEC were stimulated with 10 ng/mL of TGF-β1 in the growth medium for 24–48 h and then harvested for FSTL1 analysis. To inhibit FSTL1, siRNA gene knockdown technique was used. All experiments were performed in triplicate and repeated three times.

2.6. *Reverse Transcriptase Polymerase Chain Reaction (RT-PCR) and Quantitative Real-Time PCI (q-RT-PCR)*

Total RNA from all experimental samples was isolated using the TRIzol reagen (Invitrogen Corp., Waltham, MA, USA). First-strand cDNA was synthesized by M-MLV reverse transcriptase (Promega, Madison, WI, USA) with 1 μg each of DNA-free tota RNA sample and oligo-(dT)15 (Life Technologies, Grand Island, NY, USA). Equal amount of cDNA were subsequently amplified by PCR in a 20 μL reaction mixture containin 2 μM of each sense and antisense primer, PCR buffer, 2.4 mM MgCl2, 0.2 mM each dNTP, 10 μL of transcribed cDNA, and 0.04 U/μL Taq DNA polymerase. The primers used to amplify cDNA fragments were as follows: 5′-GGGAACTGCTGGCTCC-3′ anc 5′-TTTACAGGGGATGCAG-3′ were used for FSTL1 gene amplification, SMAD2, forwar 5′-ACTAACTTCCCAGCAGGAAT-3′ and reverse 5′-GTTGGTCACTTGTTTCTCCA-3′ SMAD3, forward 5′-ACCAAGTGCATTACCATCC-3′ and reverse 5′-CAGTAGATAACGTC AGGGAGCCC-3′; E-cadherin, forward 5′-TTCCCTGCGTATACCCTGGT-3′ and reverse 5′ GCGAAGATACCGGGGGACACTCATGAG-3′; vimentin, forward 5′-AGGAAATGGCTCC TCACCTTCGTGAATA-3′ and reverse 5′-GGAGTGTCGGTTGTTAAGAACTAGAGCT-3 The PCR cycling profile consisted of an initial denaturation step at 95 °C for 15 min, fol lowed by 35 cycles of 94 °C for 60 s, 58 °C for 60 s, and 72 °C for 60 s. Amplificatio products were run on 1.5% agarose gel soaked in ethidium bromide and visualized unde ultraviolet transillumination. The reference gene for the analysis was Glyceraldehyd 3-phosphate dehydrogenase (GAPDH). For qRT-PCR, forward and reverse primers fo all the genes tested and the internal control gene β-2microglobulin (part n° 4326319E β2M) were purchased from Applied Biosystems (Assays-On-Demand, Applied Biosystems Waltham, MA, USA). The instrument used for amplification was ABI PRISM 7700 sequence detector (Applied Biosystems). The $2^{-\Delta\Delta CT}$ method was used for calculating relative gene expression values in qPCR.

2.7. *Data Evaluation and Sequence Analysis*

mRNA expression was quantified as the average of a set of three independent ex periments, performed by gel image software (Bio-Profil Bio-1D; LTF Labortechnik GmbH Wasserburg, Germany), and the GAPDH-related intensity for each band was expressed as arbitrary units. The identity of each PCR product was confirmed by the size, and the direc sequencing using the gene-specific forward or reverse primers.

2.8. *Western Blot Analysis*

Treated and untreated control SGEC were placed in a homogenization buffer (200 μL containing 1% Triton X-100, 50 mM Tris-HCl (pH 7.4), 1 mM PMSF, 10 μg/mL soybean trypsin inhibitor, and 1 mg/mL leupeptin. After centrifugation, Bradford's protein as say was performed to determine protein concentrations. Electrophoresis on 10% SDS polyacrylamide gels was performed, followed by blotting at 200 mA (constant amperage and 200 V for 110 min. Blots were blocked, washed three times with 0.1% (*v*/*v*) Tween 20-PBS 1× (T-PBS) and membranes were probed with the appropriate primary antibodies listed above. Chemiluminescence was revealed according to the protocol (Santa Cruz Biotechnology). Mouse anti-human β-actin mAb clone AC-15 (1:100, Sigma-Aldrich, St Louis, MO, USA; 0.25 μg/mL) was used as a protein loading control.

2.9. *FSTL1 siRNA Transfection*

The siRNA sequences used for down-regulation of human FSTL1 were designed and synthesized by Thermo Fisher Scientific. An irrelevant siRNA with random nucleotides and no known specificity was used to normalize relative gene inhibition of the target gene Cells were transfected with siRNA for FSTL1 using the siPORT NeoFX transfection agent (Ambion, Austin, TX, USA) accordingly to the manufacturer's manual. A mixture of siRNA duplexes was used to obtain the highest efficiency. GAPDH siRNA primers were used as positive controls (Ambion), and a negative control with no known sequence similarity to human genes was included. Silencing was observed by mRNA quantification by qRT–PCR.

2.10. Statistical Analysis

Statistical analysis was performed by calculation of the mean percentage ± SE of data obtained from a minimum of three experiments. Differences among groups were determined using *t*-test. Statistical significance was set at * $p < 0.05$ and ** $p < 0.01$.

3. Results

3.1. Aberrant Expression of FSTL1 in SS SGs Is Associated with Inflammatory Grade

We examined the expression of FSTL1 by immunohistochemistry (IHC) in pSS biopsy samples, in comparison with healthy subjects. The number and the distribution of lymphocytic foci in the different pSS SGs bioptic specimens were quantified and then classified as I, low; II, intermediate; and III, advanced, respectively. Ten biopsy specimens for each group were analyzed. Anti-human FSTL1 antibody pAb was used to evidence SGs FSTL1 expression (Figure 1). As shown in Figure 1, the staining of FSTL1 protein ranged from weak to strong, and the results showed that FSTL1 positive staining was increased in those biopsies characterized by a higher inflammatory degree. As observed FSTL1 acinar cell expression was weak and, in all glandular specimens, FSTL1 seems to be expressed more in the epithelial cells of the ducts than in those of the acini (panels a and b. In addition, the experimental procedures clearly showed a different intensity of expression between glands of healthy and diseased subjects: the intensity of FSTL1 expression detected at the level of the ducts is much more pronounced in the biopsy of pSS subjects than in healthy control glands (Figure 1a,b). Absorbance measurements performed by ImageJ software (ImageJ, version 1.46c; WS Rasband, National Institutes of Health, Bethesda, MD, USA) (Figure 1b) confirmed this observation and highlights how the intensity of expression increases with the inflammatory degree showing that staining for FSTL1 was significantly darker in pSS glands, grade III, than in the control glands (93.9 ± 2.34 vs. 15.8 ± 1.43, $p < 0.01$).

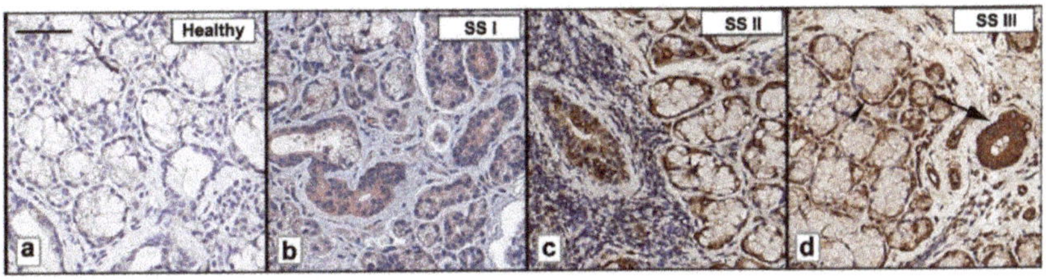

Figure 1. FSTL1 was immunohistochemically evaluated in pSS biopsy samples classified as I, low; II, intermediate; and III (**b–d**). Healthy SGs bioptic specimen was used as control (**a**). As observed, FSTL1 acinar cell expression was weak while FSTL1 staining was more pronounced in ductal epithelium (**b–d**); furthermore, a positive correlation was found between FSTL1 staining and inflammatory degree (**b–d**). Brown staining shows positive immunoreaction; blue staining shows nuclei. Bar = 20 µm. Arrows show FSTL1 distribution in ducts (large arrows) and acini (small arrows).

3.2. TGF-β1 Upregulates FSTL1 Expression in Healthy Salivary Glands Epithelial Cells

Healthy SGEC were treated with 10 ng/mL of TGF-β1 for 24 and 48 h. Figure 2A,B, shows that the TGF-β1 treatment resulted in the upregulation of FSTL1 mRNA expression (detected after a 24-h treatment) ($p < 0.01$) in comparison with untreated cells. These results were confirmed by Real-Time PCR as reported in Figure 2C. Regarding the FSTL1 protein expression, it significantly increased in the healthy SGEC were significantly increased after a 48-h treatment with TGF-β1 ($p < 0.01$) (Figure 2D,E). As a positive control, FSTL1 was also analyzed directly in pSS SGEC, confirming an overexpression of the FSTL1 gene and protein (Figure 2A–E).

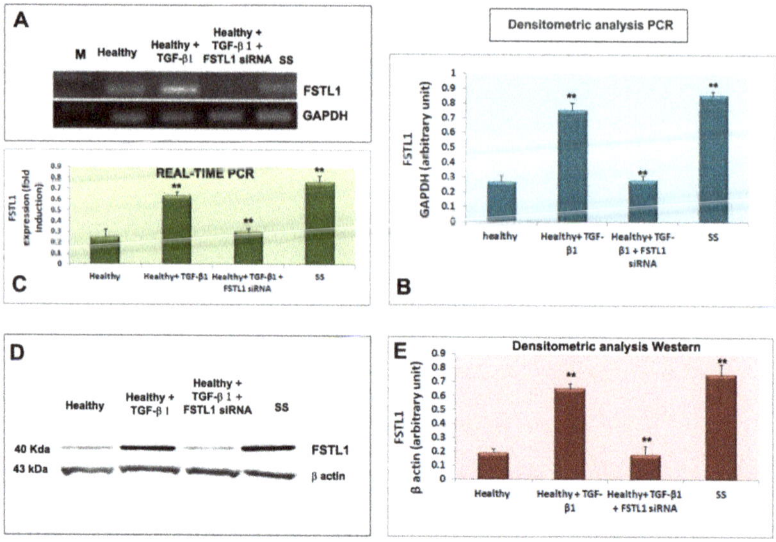

Figure 2. TGF-β1 treatment resulted in the upregulation of FSTL1 expression in healthy SGEC treated with TGF-β1. (**A**,**B**) show that the TGF-β1 treatment resulted in the upregulation of FSTL1 mRNA expression compared to untreated cells, with GAPDH as a reference gene. Quantitative Real-Time PCR confirmed this result (**C**). Normalized gene expression levels were given as the ratio between the mean value for the target gene and that for the β-2 microglobulin. PCR reactions were performed in triplicate and the data were presented as fold changes in gene expression (mean ± SE of three independent experiments). FSTL1 protein expression was significantly induced by TGF-β1 treatment as demonstrated by immunoblotting (**D**,**E**); (** = $p < 0.01$).

3.3. *FSTL1 Neutralization Attenuates EMT-Related Morphological Changes Induces by TGF-β1 Treatment*

As previously demonstrated and microscopically revealed, TGF-β1 has been implicated as a primary inducer of EMT in SS [13]. To evaluate the influence of overexpression of FSTL1 on TGF-β1-induced EMT and examine the impact of FSTL1 expression on TGF-β1-induced morphological changes in SGEC, we decide to transiently silence the expression of the FSTL1 gene with siRNA in healthy SGEC before stimulation with TGF-β1. SGEC cell morphology was microscopically evaluated. Following treatment with TGF-β1 for a maximum of 72 h, primary healthy SGEC exhibited a marked alteration in cell morphology, changing from the characteristic organized 'cobblestone' appearance of differentiated epithelial cell monolayers to a disorganized elongated fibroblast-like phenotype (Figure 3c). In particular, TGF-β1-treated SGEC lost their junctions and, consequently, their polarized epithelial phenotype and acquired elongated mesenchymal traits, becoming dispersed and showing a fibroblast-like morphology with a front/back polarity. FSTL1 siRNA transfection significantly inhibited TGF-β1-induced morphologic changes in SGEC. After FSTL1 gene silencing, these cells maintained the morphologic characteristic of epithelial cells and showed no evidence of a transformation towards mesenchymal phenotype (Figure 3d,e). Based on these phenomena, we speculated that FSTL1 is induced in response to TGF-β1 treatment and is causally involved in driving the EMT program.

3.4. *FSTL1 Moderates EMT-Related Mesenchymal Markers Expression in TGF-β1-Treated SGEC*

We next investigated whether diminished epithelial cell activation in TGF-β1-treated healthy SGEC after the FSTL1 gene knockdown, altered the expression of mesenchymal and epithelial markers, often used in the evaluation of EMT activation. We reasoned that TGF-β1-treated glandular epithelial cells may underwent an EMT program activation through FSTL1 overexpression which may influence epithelial and mesenchymal factors modulation. Healthy SGEC were treated with 10 ng/mL of TGF-β1 after the transfection with FSTL1 siRNA, and the expression of the gene biomarkers of EMT was examined by RT-PCR and quantitative Real-time PCR. As shown in Figure 4A–C, TGF-β1-treated SGEC shows reduced E-cadherin gene expression accompanied by upregulation of gene mesenchymal marker vimentin, but the FSTL1 gene expression inhibition significantly reverses the situation by blocking mesenchymal gene transcription ($p < 0.01$) (Figure 4A–C). We also detected these markers' expression at protein's levels. By Western blot analysis, we found that the level of EMT protein markers significantly changed following 10 ng/mL of TGF-β1 in cells transfected with FSTL1 siRNA for 48 h (Figure 5A,B). In fact, blocking the effect of TGF-β1-dependent release of FSTL1 by the gene silencing technique, the expression of E-cadherin was increased, and vimentin was decreased in a significant manner ($p < 0.01$) (Figure 5A,B). As control in these experiments, we also used SS SGEC treated with FSTL1 siRNA in vitro, which confirm genes and proteins results obtained in TGF-β1-trated healthy SGEC, demonstrating that FSTL1 could promote EMT in SS SGEC.

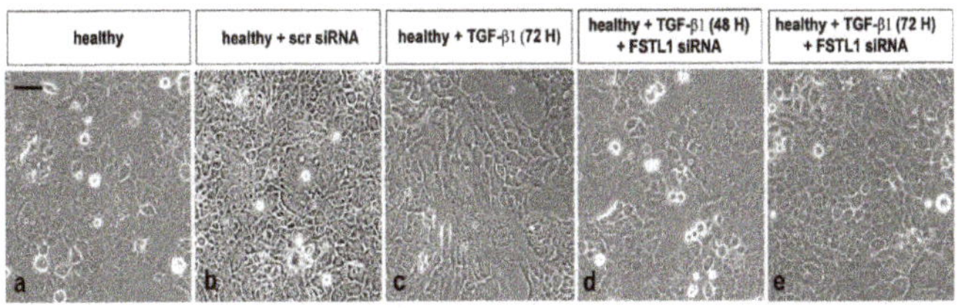

Figure 3. Bright-field micrographs of SGEC treated with TGF-β1 after FSTL1 gene silencing. SGEC cell morphology was microscopically evaluated. FSTL1 gene knockdown significantly inhibited TGF-β1-induced morphologic changes in SGEC (**e**). After transfection with FSTL1 siRNA, SGEC show a more epithelial-like morphology in comparison with SGEC treated with TGF-β1 alone for 48–72 h (**d**,**e**). (**a**): untreated control cells; (**b**): healthy SGEC transfected with scrambled control siRNA; (**c**): TGF-β1 treated SGEC for 72 h.

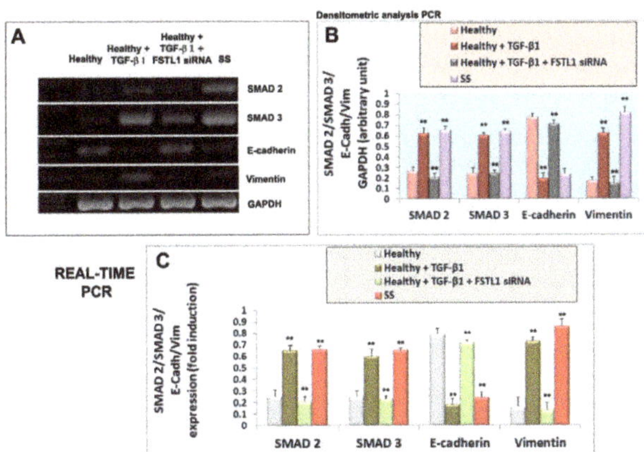

Figure 4. Effect of FSTL1 gene silencing on E-cadherin, vimentin, SMAD2 and SMAD3 gene expression evaluated by RT-PCR (**A**,**B**) and quantitative Real-Time PRC (**C**). (**A**): E-cadherin, vimentin, SMAD2, and SMAD3 gene expression were determined by RT-PCR in healthy SGEC (control, lane 1) cultured for 24 h with 10 ng/mL of TGF-β1 in which FSTL1 gene silencing was induced (lanes 2, 3). SS SGEC mRNA was used as a positive control (lane 4). (**B**) represent the densitometric analysis. Real-time PCR conducted on SGEC submitted to some treatments was shown in (**C**). GAPDH (**A**,**B**) and β-2-microglobulin (**C**) were used as reference genes for mRNA analyses. Values represent the mean ± SE of three independent experiments, with ** = $p < 0.01$.

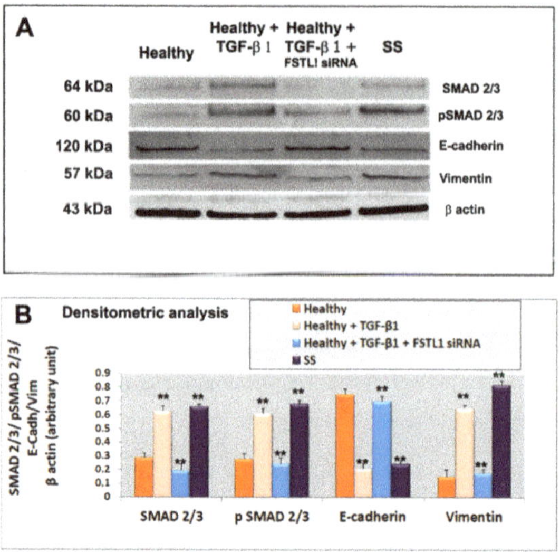

Figure 5. (**A**): representative Western blot analysis of E-cadherin, vimentin, total SMAD2/3 anc P-SMAD2/3 proteins expression in healthy untreated control SGEC (lane 1), healthy SGEC treatec with TGF-β1 for 48 h (lane 2), cells transfected with FSTL1 siRNA and subsequently treated witl TGF-β1 for 48 h (lane 3). SS SGEC protein lysate was used as a positive control. For quantitativ analysis banding densities were compared with test marker β-actin (**B**). Data are expressed a a significant change relative to the untreated control cells. Each bar represents the mean ± SI **, $p < 0.01$. Each experiment was repeated three times.

3.5. FSTL1 Modulates EMT by Facilitating TGF-β1 Signaling through SMAD2/3 Phosphorylation and Activation

To evaluate the roles of FSTL1 in the TGF-β1 signaling cascade, we blocked FSTL1gen expression by FSTL1 siRNA in human SGEC treated with TGF-β1. As already demonstratec activation of the TGF-β1-SMAD2/3 pathway by TGF-β1 treatment resulted in phosphoryla tion and activation of SMAD2 and SMAD3 [13]. Interestingly, we observed that FSTL1 gen silencing severely impaired ($p < 0.01$) SMAD2 and SMAD3 phosphorylation in response tc TGF-β1 stimulation (Figure 5A,B). The inhibition of phosphorylation of SMAD2/3 protein observed after FSTL1 gene expression downregulation, was confirmed also for SMAD2 anc SMAD3 gene analysis performed by RT-PCR and Real-time PCR (Figure 4A–C). These result indicate that FSTL1 is a crucial component of TGF-β1 signaling in SGEC contexts.

4. Discussion

SS is a lifelong chronic inflammatory autoimmune disorder affecting primarily th lachrymal and SGs [22]. In this disease, the glandular secretory activity is reduced resultin in dryness in the eyes, mouth, and throat. In addition, often, SS dysfunction involves othe organs, along with complications such as pain, fatigue, and digestive problems [22]. A targeted and early diagnosis is necessary to develop more effective therapies. The majo obstacle to overcome in order to identify therapeutics is a lack of complete understandin of the molecular mechanisms underlying the pathogenesis of this disease; SS seems, ir fact, multifactorial, but a key role is certainly played by the chronic release of inflamma tory mediators. The findings reported here add new insights into the knowledge of SS pathogenesis and consolidate the hypothesis of the role of FSTL1 in promoting EMT.

EMT is a process of dedifferentiation and transformation of epithelial cells into mes enchymal cells [23]. During EMT, the expression of epithelial markers such as E-cadherir is decreased, while the expression of mesenchymal markers, for example, vimentin, is up-regulated [24]. The EMT program foresees the triggering of a cascade of events in whicl various factors are activated, and among these, the phosphorylation of SMADs represents a crucial event [25,26]. Cells that undergo EMT show a phenotypic switch from epithelial cells to fibroblastic or mesenchymal cells [23].

EMT may drive inflammatory reactions and, in turn, is influenced by the inflammatory microenvironment [27–29]. Based on these characteristics, EMT is a key process in determining the onset of fibrotic phenomena that lead to the loss, or, at least, to the alteration of the functionality of the affected organs [30–32]. Therefore, identifying molecules that can inhibit EMT could help reduce the tendency to evolve toward fibrosis.

In this scenario, the Follistatin Like (FSTL) family of proteins fits well. FSTL proteins are involved in cell migration, proliferation, and cellular differentiation, through the binding to the activin protein of the TGF-β family, which represents key activators of the EMT program [6]. Recently, pioneering studies conducted on human SGEC have led to very intriguing results; they demonstrated that, in SS, TGF-β activates EMT by both the canonical SMAD2/3 pathway and the non-canonical MAPK pathway influenced by the release of pro-inflammatory cytokines in a condition of chronic inflammation. The EMT program includes the activation of Snail, a transcription factor, and determines, consequently, an imbalance in favor of the expression of mesenchymal markers compared to epithelial markers. Interestingly, the activation of the EMT cascade leads to a dramatic evolution toward fibrosis [13,29,32].

In the experimental study reported here, we wanted to analyze the relationship between FSTL1 and EMT in SS, since elevated serum levels of FSTL1 were already detected in the serum of SS patients [17]. For the first time, we detected the expression of FSTL1 in pSS SGs biopsies. IHC analysis showed that the expression of FSTL1 was positively correlated with the inflammatory grade, and, based on the correlation between inflammation and EMT, this led us to evaluate, as a second step, the correlation between FSTL1 and EMT.

Bright field microscopic evaluation demonstrated that by blocking the activity of FSTL1 by its gene knockdown, human healthy SGEC treated with TGF-β1 as an EMT inducer, did not show any morphological changes: on the contrary, cells treated with TGF-β1 alone showed mesenchymal phenotypes, as already demonstrated [13]. Moreover, using healthy SGEC in vitro-treated with TGF-β1 and transfected with FSTL1 siRNA, we demonstrated that the over-expression of FSTL1 down-regulated the expression of E-cadherin and up-regulated the expression of vimentin, confirming that FSTL1 could promote EMT. To further explore our findings of a role for SMAD2/3 activation in the FSTL1-induced EMT process in SS, we examined healthy SGEC treated with TGF-β1 following or not FSTL1 siRNA transfection, demonstrating that cells in which FSTL1 is active show an extremely high expression of p-SMAD2/3 similar to the levels of SMAD2/3 phosphorylation observed in SS SGEC, utilized as a useful positive control. Results obtained identified FSTL1 as a component of the TGF-β-SMAD2/3 pathway that stimulates SMAD2/3 phospho-activation in SS. In conclusion, our observations suggest that interactions between FSTL1 and TGF-β1 signal transduction pathways may determine a cascade of mechanisms activation by which alterations in p-SMAD2/3 expression occur, and neutralization of FSTL1 gene activity had inhibitory effects on the phosphorylation of SMAD2/3 induced by TGF-β1; this effect, consequently, attenuates EMT (Figure 6). Our findings suggest a promising therapeutic approach for SGEC EMT in SS. However, all experimental research in the present study was performed in vitro, and, actually, there were no in vivo data supporting these results. Hence, further research in SS patients or animal models needs to be performed in the future to confirm the therapeutic potential of FSTL1.

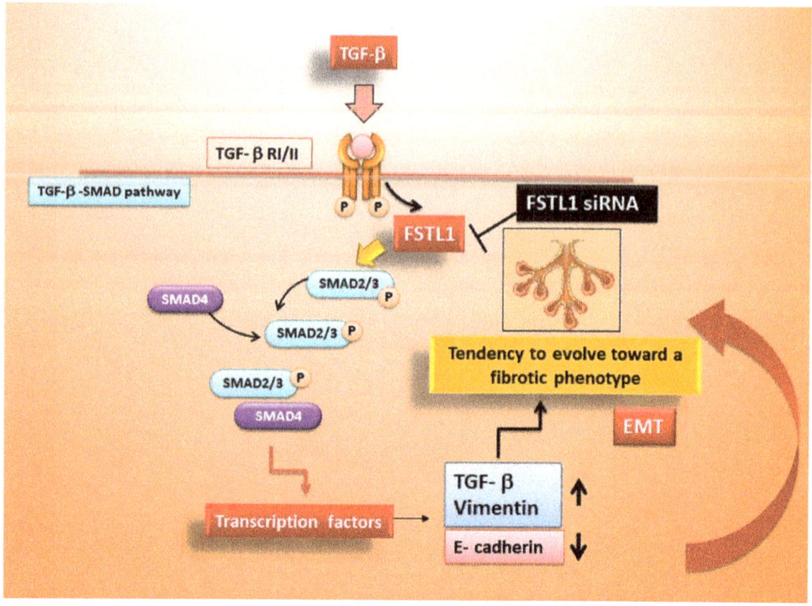

Figure 6. Schematic representation of FSTL1 role in TGF-β1-induced EMT in SS.

Author Contributions: Methodology, M.S., G.I. and S.L.; investigation, M.S., G.I. and S.L.; writing-original draft preparation, M.S. and S.L.; supervision, D.R. All authors have read and agreed to the published version of the manuscript.

Funding: This research received no external funding.

Institutional Review Board Statement: The study was conducted in accordance with the Declaration of Helsinki. Ethical review and approval were waived for this study: Since the study data were collected during routine clinical activity and fully anonymized, a formal institutional review board approval was exempted.

Informed Consent Statement: Oral consent was obtained from all subjects involved in the study.

Data Availability Statement: All relevant data are within the paper.

Conflicts of Interest: The authors declare no conflict of interest.

References

1. Shibanuma, M.; Mashimo, J.; Mita, A.; Kuroki, T.; Nose, K. Cloning from a mouse osteoblastic cell line of a set of transforming-growth-factor-beta 1-regulated genes, one of which seems to encode a follistatin-related polypeptide. *Eur. J. Biochem.* **1993**, *217*, 13–19. [CrossRef] [PubMed]
2. Mattiotti, A.; Prakash, S.; Barnett, P.; van den Hoff, M.J.B. Follistatin-like 1 in development and human diseases. *Cell Mol. Life Sci.* **2018**, *75*, 2339–2354. [CrossRef] [PubMed]
3. Geng, Y.; Dong, Y.; Yu, M.; Zhang, L.; Yan, X.; Sun, J.; Qiao, L.; Geng, H.; Nakajima, M.; Furuichi, T.; et al. Follistatin-like 1 (Fstl1) is a bone morphogenetic protein (BMP) 4 signaling antagonist in controlling mouse lung development. *Proc. Natl. Acad. Sci. USA* **2011**, *108*, 7058–7063. [CrossRef] [PubMed]
4. Li, X.; Li, L.; Chang, Y.; Ning, W.; Liu, X. Structural and functional study of FK domain of Fstl1. *Protein Sci.* **2019**, *28*, 1819–1829. [CrossRef]
5. Oshima, Y.; Ouchi, N.; Sato, K.; Izumiya, Y.; Pimentel, D.R.; Walsh, K. Follistatin-like 1 is an Akt-regulated cardioprotective factor that is secreted by the heart. *Circulation* **2008**, *117*, 3099–3108. [CrossRef]
6. Chaly, Y.; Hostager, B.; Smith, S.; Hirsch, R. Follistatin-like protein 1 and its role in inflammation and inflammatory diseases. *Immunol. Res.* **2014**, *59*, 266–272. [CrossRef]

7. Liu, T.; Liu, Y.; Miller, M.; Cao, L.; Zhao, J.; Wu, J.; Wang, J.; Liu, L.; Li, S.; Zou, M.; et al. Autophagy plays a role in FSTL1-induced epithelial mesenchymal transition and airway remodeling in asthma. *Am. J. Physiol. Lung Cell. Mol. Physiol.* **2017**, *313*, L27–L40. [CrossRef]
8. Kalluri, R.; Weinberg, R.A. The basics of epithelial-mesenchymal transition. *J. Clin. Investig.* **2009**, *119*, 1420–1428. [CrossRef]
9. Dongre, A.; Weinberg, R.A. New insights into the mechanisms of epithelial–mesenchymal transition and implications for cancer. *Nat. Rev. Mol. Cell Biol.* **2019**, *20*, 6984. [CrossRef]
10. Zheng, X.; Qi, C.; Zhang, S.; Fang, Y.; Ning, W. TGF-β1 induces Fstl1 via the Smad3-c-Jun pathway in lung fibroblasts. *Am. J. Physiol. Lung Cell Mol. Physiol.* **2017**, *313*, L240–L251. [CrossRef]
11. Dong, Y.; Geng, Y.; Li, L.; Li, X.; Yan, X.; Fang, Y.; Li, X.; Dong, S.; Liu, X.; Li, X.; et al. Blocking follistatin-like 1 attenuates bleomycin-induced pulmonary fibrosis in mice. *J. Exp. Med.* **2015**, *212*, 235–252. [CrossRef] [PubMed]
12. Lamouille, S.; Xu, J.; Derynck, R. Molecular mechanisms of epithelial–mesenchymal transition. *Nat. Rev. Mol. Cell Biol.* **2014**, *15*, 178–196. [CrossRef] [PubMed]
13. Sisto, M.; Lorusso, L.; Ingravallo, G.; Tamm, A.R.; Ribatti, D.; Lisi, S. The TGF-β1 Signaling Pathway as an Attractive Target in the Fibrosis Pathogenesis of Sjögren's Syndrome. *Mediat. Inflamm.* **2018**, *2018*, 1965935. [CrossRef] [PubMed]
14. Biernacka, A.; Dobaczewski, M.; Frangogiannis, N.G. TGF-β signaling in fibrosis. *Growth Factors* **2011**, *29*, 196–202. [CrossRef]
15. Kim, K.K.; Sheppard, D.; Chapman, H.A. TGF-β1 Signaling and Tissue Fibrosis. *Cold Spring Harb. Perspect. Biol.* **2018**, *10*, a022293. [CrossRef]
16. Li, X.; Fang, Y.; Jiang, D.; Dong, Y.; Liu, Y.; Zhang, S.; Guo, J.; Qi, C.; Zhao, C.; Jiang, F.; et al. Targeting FSTL1 for Multiple Fibrotic and Systemic Autoimmune Diseases. *Mol. Ther.* **2021**, *29*, 347–364. [CrossRef]
17. Li, D.; Wang, Y.; Xu, N.; Wei, Q.; Wu, M.; Li, X.; Zheng, P.; Sun, S.; Jin, Y.; Zhang, G.; et al. Follistatin-like protein 1 is elevated in systemic autoimmune diseases and correlated with disease activity in patients with rheumatoid arthritis. *Arthritis Res. Ther.* **2011**, *13*, R17. [CrossRef]
18. Mariette, X.; Criswell, L.A. Primary Sjögren's syndrome. *N. Engl. J. Med.* **2018**, *378*, 931–939. [CrossRef]
19. Franceschini, F.; Cavazzana, I.; Andreoli, L.; Tincani, A. The 2016 classification criteria for primary Sjogren's syndrome: What's new? *BMC Med.* **2017**, *15*, 69. [CrossRef]
20. Sens, D.A.; Hintz, D.S.; Rudisill, M.T.; Sens, M.A. Spicer SS Explant culture of human submandibular gland epithelial cells: Evidence for ductal origin. *Lab. Investig.* **1985**, *52*, 559–567.
21. Kapsogeorgou, E.K.; Dimitriou, I.D.; Abu-Helu, R.F.; Moutsopoulos, H.M.; Manoussakis, M.N. Activation of epithelial and myoepithelial cells in the salivary glands of patients with Sjögren's syndrome: High expression of intercellular adhesion molecule-1 (ICAM.1) in biopsy specimens and cultured cells. *Clin. Exp. Immunol.* **2001**, *124*, 126–133. [CrossRef] [PubMed]
22. Saraux, A.; Devauchelle-Pensec, V. Primary Sjögren's syndrome: New beginning for evidence-based trials. *Lancet* **2022**, *399*, 121–122. [CrossRef]
23. Huang, Z.; Zhang, Z.; Zhou, C.; Liu, L.; Huang, C. Epithelial-mesenchymal transition: The history, regulatory mechanism, and cancer therapeutic opportunities. *MedComm* **2022**, *3*, e144. [CrossRef]
24. Yang, J.; Antin, P.; Berx, G.; Blanpain, C.; Brabletz, T.; Bronner, M.; Campbell, K.; Cano, A.; Casanova, J.; Christofori, G.; et al. Guidelines and definitions for research on epithelial-mesenchymal transition. *Nat. Rev. Mol. Cell Biol.* **2020**, *21*, 341–352. [CrossRef] [PubMed]
25. Valcourt, U.; Kowanetz, M.; Niimi, H.; Heldin, C.H.; Moustakas, A. TGF-beta and the Smad signaling pathway support transcriptomic reprogramming during epithelial-mesenchymal cell transition. *Mol. Biol. Cell* **2005**, *16*, 1987–2002. [CrossRef]
26. Hua, W.; ten Dijke, P.; Kostidis, S.; Giera, M.; Hornsveld, M. TGFβ-induced metabolic reprogramming during epithelial-to-mesenchymal transition in cancer. *Cell. Mol. Life Sci.* **2020**, *77*, 2103–2123. [CrossRef]
27. Ricciardi, M.; Zanotto, M.; Malpeli, G.; Bassi, G.; Perbellini, O.; Chilosi, M.; Bifari, F.; Krampera, M. Epithelial-to-mesenchymal transition (EMT) induced by inflammatory priming elicits mesenchymal stromal cell-like immune-modulatory properties in cancer cells. *Br. J. Cancer* **2015**, *112*, 1067–1075. [CrossRef]
28. Suarez-Carmona, M.; Lesage, J.; Cataldo, D.; Gilles, C. EMT and inflammation: Inseparable actors of cancer progression. *Mol. Oncol.* **2017**, *11*, 805–823. [CrossRef]
29. Sisto, M.; Lorusso, L.; Tamma, R.; Ingravallo, G.; Ribatti, D.; Lisi, S. Interleukin-17 and -22 synergy linking inflammation and EMT-dependent fibrosis in Sjögren's syndrome. *Clin. Exp. Immunol.* **2019**, *198*, 261–272. [CrossRef]
30. Kalluri, R.; Neilson, E.G. Epithelial-Mesenchymal Transition and Its Implications for Fibrosis. *J. Clin. Investig.* **2003**, *112*, 1776–1784. [CrossRef]
31. López-Novoa, J.M.; Nieto, M.A. Inflammation and EMT: An alliance towards organ fibrosis and cancer progression. *EMBO Mol. Med.* **2009**, *1*, 303–314. [CrossRef] [PubMed]
32. Sisto, M.; Ribatti, D.; Lisi, S. Organ Fibrosis and Autoimmunity: The Role of Inflammation in TGF β-Dependent EMT. *Biomolecules* **2021**, *11*, 310. [CrossRef] [PubMed]

Journal of
Clinical Medicine

MDPI

Article

Imaging Activated-T-Lymphocytes in the Salivary Glands of Patients with Sjögren's Syndrome by ^{99m}Tc-Interleukin-2: Diagnostic and Therapeutic Implications

Giuseppe Campagna [1], Luz Kelly Anzola [2], Michela Varani [1], Chiara Lauri [1], Guido Gentiloni Silveri [1], Lorenzo Chiurchioni [1], Francesca Romana Spinelli [3], Roberta Priori [3], Fabrizio Conti [3] and Alberto Signore [1,*]

1 Nuclear Medicine Unit, Department of Medical-Surgical Sciences and of Translational Medicine, "Sapienza" University, 00161 Rome, Italy; gius.campagna@gmail.com (G.C.); varanimichela@gmail.com (M.V.); chiara.lauri@uniroma1.it (C.L.); guido.gentiloni@hotmail.it (G.G.S.); lorenzo.chiurchioni@gmail.com (L.C.)
2 Nuclear Medicine, Clinica Colsanitas, Bogotà 110221, Colombia; lkanzola@gmail.com
3 Rheumatology Unit, Department of Applied Clinical and Medical Therapy, Faculty of Medicine and Pharmacy, "Sapienza" University, 00161 Rome, Italy; francescaromana.spinelli@uniroma1.it (F.R.S.); roberta.priori@uniroma1.it (R.P.); fabrizio.conti@uniroma1.it (F.C.)
* Correspondence: alberto.signore@uniroma1.it

Abstract: Background: Sjögren's syndrome (SS) is a progressive autoimmune disease characterized by local mononuclear cell infiltration of the salivary and lachrymal glands. Labial biopsy demonstrates local infiltration by Th1 cells that produce pro-inflammatory cytokines, such as interleukin-2 (IL2). The aim of this study was to assess the utility of ^{99m}Tc-labelled-IL2 (^{99m}Tc-IL2) in evaluating in vivo the extent and severity of lympho-mononuclear cell infiltration in the salivary glands of patients with SS. Methods: We investigated 48 patients with primary SS and 27 control subjects using ^{99m}Tc-IL2 scintigraphy. Furthermore, in a subgroup of 30 patients, we also performed ^{99m}Tc-pertechnetate scintigraphy ($^{99m}TcO_4^-$) for evaluation of the salivary gland function. Results: ^{99m}Tc-IL2 uptake in the salivary glands of SS patients was higher than in the control subjects (1.30 ± 0.16 vs. 0.83 ± 0.08 for parotids and 1.36 ± 0.15 vs. 1.16 ± 0.07 for submandibular glands; $p < 0.0001$). The salivary gland uptake of ^{99m}Tc-IL2 in patients with a longer history of disease was lower compared with the recently diagnosed patients. A significant direct correlation was found between the uptake of ^{99m}Tc-IL2 and histology. Conclusions: ^{99m}Tc-IL2 scintigraphy showed that the degree of lymphocytic infiltration of major salivary glands is variable in patients with different disease durations. Patients with a high ^{99m}Tc-IL2 uptake could be efficiently treated with immuno-modulatory drugs and the efficacy of treatment could be followed-up by ^{99m}Tc-IL2 scintigraphy.

Keywords: Sjögren's syndrome; ^{99m}Tc-interleukin-2; activated lymphocytes; salivary glands; inflammation imaging

Citation: Campagna, G.; Anzola, L.K.; Varani, M.; Lauri, C.; Gentiloni Silveri, G.; Chiurchioni, L.; Spinelli, F.R.; Priori, R.; Conti, F.; Signore, A. Imaging Activated-T-Lymphocytes in the Salivary Glands of Patients with Sjögren's Syndrome by ^{99m}Tc-Interleukin-2: Diagnostic and Therapeutic Implications. *J. Clin. Med.* **2022**, *11*, 4368. https://doi.org/10.3390/jcm11154368

Academic Editor: Margherita Sisto

Received: 4 July 2022
Accepted: 25 July 2022
Published: 27 July 2022

Publisher's Note: MDPI stays neutral with regard to jurisdictional claims in published maps and institutional affiliations.

1. Introduction

Sjögren's syndrome (SS) is a chronic inflammatory disease of the lachrymal and salivary glands causing keratoconjunctivitis sicca (KCS) and xerostomia [1]. SS is the second immunological disease in frequency and women are more affected compared with men (9:1) [2]. Nowadays, the diagnosis of SS is based on clinical, serological, and instrumental parameters, such as the presence of KCS, xerostomia, auto-antibodies, and positive sub-labial salivary gland (SSG) biopsy [3,4]. Of these, the most important criteria are the histological findings, including acinar atrophy, fibrosis, ductal changes, and focal lymphocytic infiltrations in the minor salivary glands' tissues [5].

Lymphocytic infiltration is initially characterised by activated T-lymphocytes of the CD4+ phenotype (Th1), which produce a large amount of mRNA for interleukn-2 (IL2), interferon-alpha (IFN-a), and interleukin-10 (IL10) [6]. These cytokines cause tissue damage, ultimately evolving in the fibrosis of salivary glands, and causing complete loss of functionality. This process is signal-mediated through the T-cell receptor that interacts with class II antigens on the epithelial cells of exocrine glands. In particular, T-cells become activated and express a high quantity of IL2 receptors (I2R), which are surface hetero-trimeric proteins that bind IL2. The IL2−IL2R interaction causes the activation, differentiation, and growth of various immunological cells [7,8]. In particular, IL2R has been found on the surface of activated T-cells, but also in some B-cells and macrophages. Therefore, IL2R is considered an early marker of T-lymphocyte activation [9]. In the following phases of disease progression, Th2 and Th17 cells may appear with the production of other cytokines, as well as the so-called follicular helper T-cells that seem to play a protective role [10].

IL2 labelled with ^{123}I (^{123}I-IL2) and ^{99m}Tc (^{99m}Tc-IL2) has been used in vivo to detect activated lymphocytes in different autoimmune diseases, such as Coeliac disease [11], IDDM [12], Hashimoto's thyroiditis, Takayasu's arteritis [13], multiple-autoimmunity [14] and, recently, to detect immune infiltration on cancer [15]. We also demonstrated that ^{99m}Tc-IL2 allows for planning specific immunotherapy in patients with active disease and the non-invasive follow-up of patients [16]. Interestingly, we observed that patients with thyroid autoimmune diseases (i.e., Graves' disease or Hashimoto thyroiditis) may show ^{99m}Tc-IL2 uptake in the salivary glands, predicting the development of a secondary Sjögren's syndrome in the following years [17,18].

The aim of our study was to evaluate the uptake of ^{99m}Tc-IL2 in the salivary glands as an indicator of inflammation. We also studied its relationship with other clinical, serological, histological, and functional parameters, such as salivary gland scintigraphy with ^{99m}Tc-sodium pertechnetate ($^{99m}TcO_4^-$) [19].

2. Materials and Methods

2.1. Study Design

This is a prospective, open study. The study protocol was approved by the ethics committee of the University of Rome, "Sapienza". All patients and normal volunteers gave written informed consent.

2.2. Patients

We studied 48 patients with SS (36 women and 12 men; mean age 50.78 $\pm$ 13.08 years (95% CI 46.59 to 54.96) in whom the disease was diagnosed based on the fulfilment of at least four of the six European Community Study Group's criteria, and by labial salivary gland biopsys [4]. In all patients, we excluded other processes that may have caused sicca syndrome as well as the absence of other systemic autoimmune diseases. We compared our patients with 27 sex and age-matched control oncological subjects (14 women and 13 men; age range 35–83 years), with no evidence of autoimmune diseases, who performed the ^{99m}Tc-IL2 scintigraphy for investigating the presence of T-cell infiltrates in tumor lesions.

2.3. Clinical and Laboratory Assessments

All patients complained about a subjective feeling of ocular or oral dryness (Table 1). Nevertheless, xerophthalmia was objectively assessed by the Schirmer and/or Break Up Time (BUT) tests. Oral involvement was studied by salivary gland scintigraphy with ^{99m}Tc-$^{99m}TcO_4^-$ in 30 patients. Histopathological examination of the labial salivary glands, accepted as the gold standard in primary Sjogren's syndrome [20], was performed in 28 patients. The standard grading criteria [21] ranged from 0 to 4 based on the presence of mononuclear cell infiltration with a periductal distribution. This is a typical finding in patients with primary SS, compared with the perivascular infiltration that occurs mainly in secondary SS.

Table 1. Patient's characteristics and the criteria for clinical diagnosis.

Patient	Sex	Biopsy	Antibodies	Xerophthalmia	Xerostomia	Schirmer's Test or BUT	EF or %Max Uptake
1	F	3	pos	yes	yes	pos	pos
2	F		pos	yes	yes		pos
3	F	4	pos	yes	yes		pos
4	F	0	pos	yes	yes		pos
5	F		neg	yes	yes	pos	pos
6	F	0	pos	yes	yes		pos
7	F	0	pos	yes	yes		pos
8	F	4	pos	yes	yes		pos
9	F		pos	yes	yes		pos
10	F	1	neg	yes	yes		pos
11	F	0	pos	yes	yes	pos	pos
12	F		pos	yes	yes		pos
13	F		pos	yes	yes		pos
14	F		pos	yes	yes		pos
15	F	3	pos	yes	no		pos
16	F	2	pos	yes	yes		pos
17	F		pos	yes	yes		pos
18	F		pos	yes	yes		pos
19	F	1	pos	no	yes		pos
20	F	3	pos	no	yes		pos
21	F		pos	yes	yes		pos
22	F	1	pos	yes	yes		pos
23	F	2	neg	yes	yes		pos
24	F		pos	yes	yes		pos
25	M	4	neg	yes	yes		pos
26	F		pos	yes	yes		pos
27	F	4	pos	yes	yes		pos
28	F		pos	yes	yes		pos
29	F	1	pos	yes	yes		pos
30	M	4	neg	yes	yes		pos
31	M		pos	yes	yes		pos
32	F		pos	yes	yes		pos
33	F		pos	yes	yes		pos
34	M	0	neg	yes	yes	pos	pos
35	F		pos	yes	yes		pos
36	F	1	pos	yes	yes		
37	F	0	pos	yes	yes	pos	
38	F	2	pos	yes	yes		
39	F	2	pos	yes	yes		pos
40	F	3	neg	yes	yes		pos

Table 1. *Cont.*

Patient	Sex	Biopsy	Antibodies	Xerophthalmia	Xerostomia	Schirmer's Test or BUT	EF or %Max Uptake
41	F	2	pos	yes	yes		pos
42	F	3	pos	yes	yes		pos
43	F	1	pos	yes	yes		pos
44	F		pos	yes	yes		pos
45	F		pos	yes	yes	pos	
46	F		pos	yes	yes		pos
47	F		pos	yes	yes		pos
48	M	3	pos	yes	yes		pos

Biopsy score according to Chisholm e Mason classification; antibodies = positivity to either SSA or SSB or both antibodies; EF or %max uptake = reduced ejection fraction or reduced maximum $^{99m}TcO_4^-$ uptake of salivary glands at functional scintigraphy. Empty boxes = not performed.

We also tested the presence of antinuclear antibodies (ANA) and anti-extractable nuclear antigen-antibodies (ENA) by indirect immunofluorescence, and auto-antibodies anti-Ro (SSA) and anti-La (SSB) by immune-electrophoresis [22].

2.4. *Salivary Gland Scintigraphy*

Both ^{99m}Tc-IL2 and $^{99m}TcO_4^-$ scintigraphy were performed in patients at a time interval of 1 to 5 weeks.

2.4.1. ^{99m}Tc-IL2 Scintigraphy

Human recombinant IL2 (Proleukin®, Novartis, Basel, Switzerland) was labelled using the method described by Chianelli et al. [23]. Scintigraphy was performed in all patients and control subjects after i.v. injection of 111–185 MBq of ^{99m}Tc-IL2. Planar anterior images (256 × 256 pixel matrix) of the neck were acquired 45 min after injection. Quantitative analysis of the planar images was carried out by drawing an irregular region of interest (ROI) over the parotid and submandibular glands. The background was calculated with a rectangular ROI drawn below the two submandibular glands and above the thyroid region.

In the control subjects and when the salivary glands were not detectable, a circular ROI was drawn corresponding to the parotid or submandibular region (Figure 1).

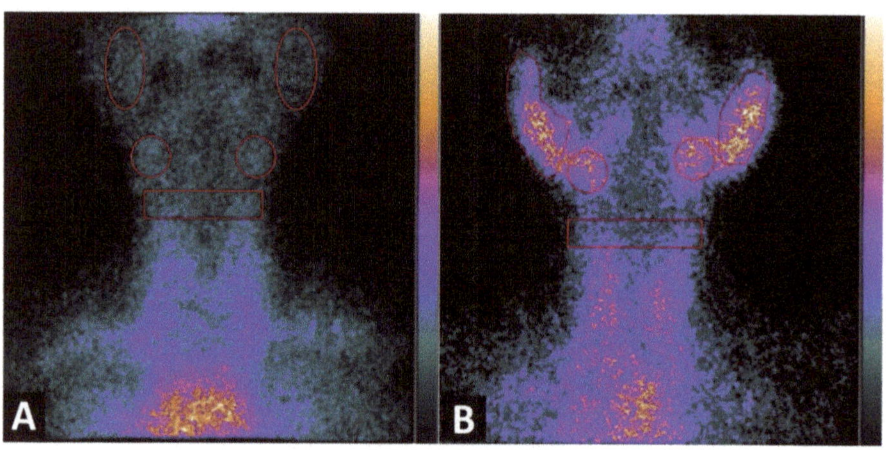

Figure 1. Planar image of the neck obtained 1h after ^{99m}Tc-IL2 injection in a control subject (**A**) and in a patient with Sjögren syndrome at time of diagnosis (**B**). In (**A**) the scan shows no ^{99m}Tc-IL2 uptake

by the salivary glands. In (**B**) an evident accumulation of ^{99m}Tc-IL2 can be observed in both parotids and submandibular glands, indicating the presence of activated lymphocytes. The calculated parotid to background (P/B) ratios are 1.35 and 1.30 in right and left glands, respectively, and the submandibular gland to background (S/B) ratios are 1.57 and 1.64 in right and left glands, respectively.

The results of the quantitative analysis were expressed as the parotid to background (P/B) ratio and submandibular to background (S/B) ratio, after calculating the mean uptake between the two contralateral glands.

2.4.2. $^{99m}TcO_4^-$ Scintigraphy

Dynamic salivary gland scintigraphy was performed in 30 patients, after i.v. injection of 80–150 MBq $^{99m}TcO_4^-$, with a gamma camera equipped with a parallel-hole, low energy, high sensitivity collimator, and 140 keV photopeak for the technetium. Anterior sequential images were acquired at 1 s per frame for 1 min (vascular phase) and 10 s per frame for the next 24 min. Fifteen minutes after the injection, 3 mL of lemon juice was administered orally as a stimulus, as described by Bohulaslavizki et al. [24] and Anjos et al. [25].

Data analysis of the acquired images was performed by drawing irregular ROIs on each parotid and oval-shaped regions over each submandibular gland.

For the background regions, we drew two ROIs on the temporal regions [24].

The quantitative analysis included the evaluation of the ^{99m}Tc-pertechnetate ejection fraction (EF), which was calculated with the following equation:

$$EF(\%) = [(U12\text{-}14\text{-}U18\text{-}20) \times 100]/U12\text{-}14. \quad (1)$$

The maximum $^{99m}TcO_4^-$ uptake was calculated as the percentage of the injected dose (ID), as described by Anjos et al. (Figure 2) [25]. A positive scintigraphy was considered when the EF or maximum uptake was lower than the lower value of the confidence interval of the normal subjects.

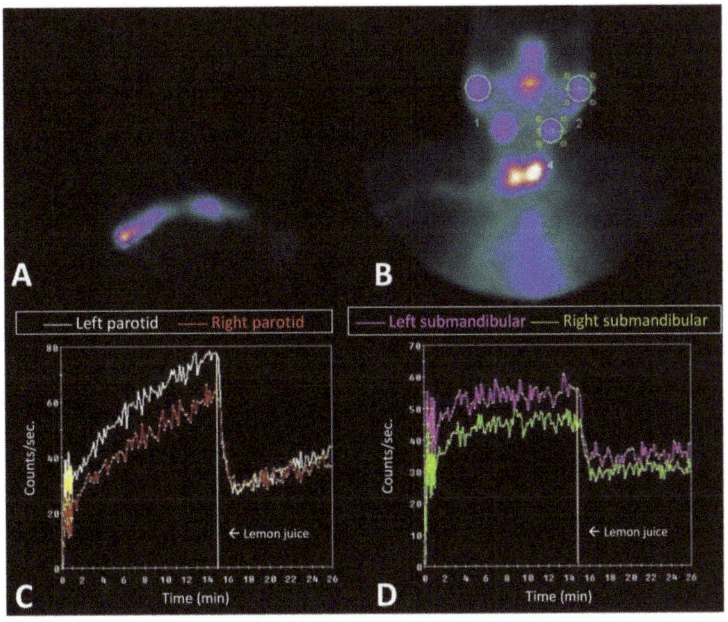

Figure 2. Dynamic study with $^{99m}TcO_4^-$ in patients with Sjögren syndrome 3 years after diagnosis. (**A**,**B**) show the start of dynamic images and the summary of all dynamic images, respectively.

(**C**,**D**) show the quantitative analysis of the parotid and submandibular glands, respectively. A moderate accumulation of $^{99m}TcO_4{}^-$ can be observed in the parotids and, to a lesser extent, in the submandibular glands, indicating the presence of a residual function.

2.5. Statistical Analysis

Continuous variables were shown as mean ± standard deviation with a 95% CI (confidence interval). Categorical variables were expressed as absolute frequencies and percentages, as *n* (%). Comparisons between the control subjects vs. Sjögren's patients of the ^{99m}Tc-IL2 uptake in the parotid glands (mean P/B) and ^{99m}Tc-IL2 uptake in the submandibular glands (mean P/B) were evaluated using the Student's test. The normality of these variables was tested using the Shapiro–Wilk test and checking the Q-Q plot. In the presence of heteroscedasticity, we used the correction of Satterthwaite.

The correlation between disease duration and biopsy vs. ^{99m}Tc-IL2 uptake in parotid glands (mean P/B), and ^{99m}Tc-IL2 uptake in submandibular glands (mean P/B) was evaluated using Kendall's tau-b (τb), because the normality of the continuous variables analysed not was verified and the confidence intervals were determined using the bootstrapping method. Statistical analysis was performed using SAS v.9.4 and JMP PRO v.16 (Institute Inc., Cary, NC, USA). A *p*-value < 0.05 was considered statistically detectable.

3. Results

The characteristics of the patients and the criteria for the diagnosis of SS are summarized in Table 1. Patients with SS differed significantly from the control subjects. The mean ^{99m}Tc-IL2 uptake in parotid glands was 1.30 ± 0.16 (95% CI 1.25 to 1.34) in patients vs. 0.83 ± 0.08 (95% CI 0.80 to 0.86) in the controls, $p < 0.001$ (Figure 3). In the submandibular glands, ^{99m}Tc-IL2 uptake was 1.36 ± 0.15 (95% CI 1.31 to 1.40) in patients vs. 1.16 ± 0.07 (95% CI 1.13 to 1.18) in the controls, $p < 0.001$ (Figure 4).

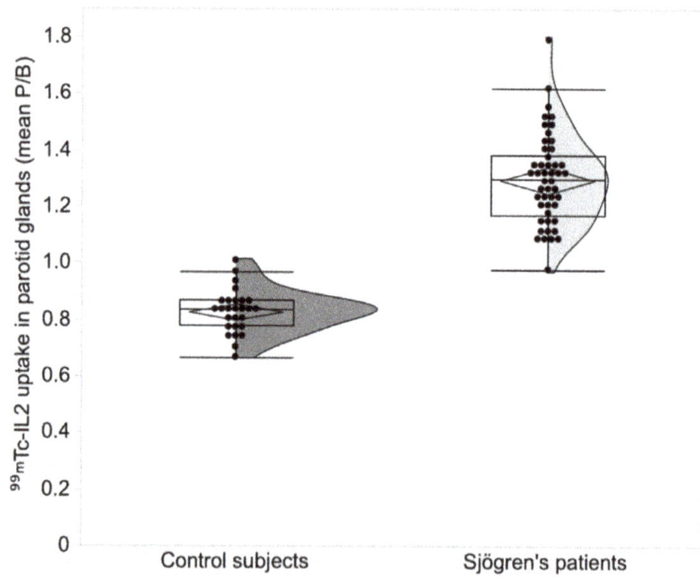

Figure 3. Parotid gland uptake of ^{99m}Tc-IL2 in patients with Sjögren disease compared to control subjects ($p < 0.001$).

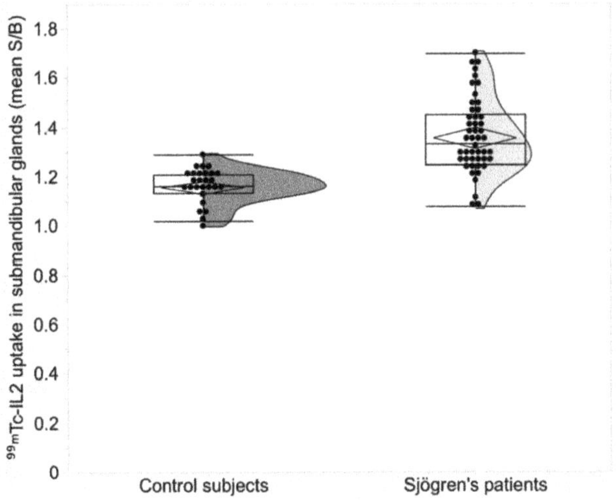

Figure 4. Submandibular gland uptake of ^{99m}Tc-IL2 in patients with Sjögren disease compared to control subjects ($p < 0.001$).

Interestingly, despite the variability of ^{99m}Tc-IL2 uptake in the glands of patients, we found a significant inverse correlation between the mean target/background ratios (P/B and S/B) with disease duration (Figure 5). The correlation coefficient was −0.22 (95% CI −0.43 to −0.02), $p = 0.03$, for the parotids and −0.29 (95% CI −0.47 to −0.09), $p = 0.006$, for the submandibular glands.

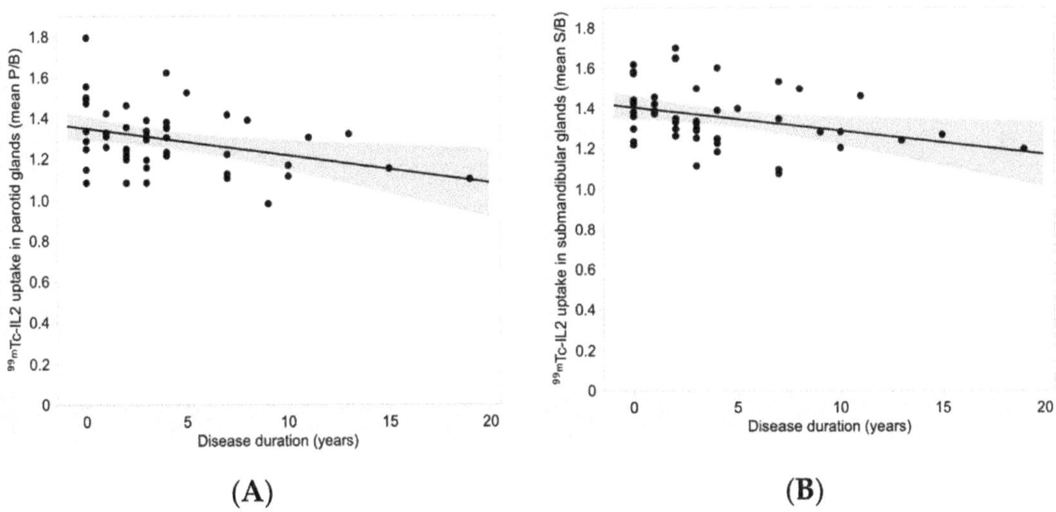

Figure 5. Distribution of the mean ^{99m}Tc-IL2 uptake (P/B) in the parotid glands (**A**) and (S/B) in the submandibular glands (**B**) over the disease duration. A significant inverse correlation can be observed in all glands (correlation coefficient is −0.22 ($p = 0.03$) for the parotids and −0.29 ($p = 0.006$) for the submandibular glands).

3.1. Histopathological Tissue Analysis

The histology examination of the minor salivary glands biopsies showed a typical characteristic of SS according to Chisholm e Mason classification in 22 out of 28 patients. Moreover, positive grading (between 3 and 4) was detected in 11 (39.3%) patients while 17 patients (60.7%) resulted with negative biopsy (between 0 and 2) (Table 1).

Despite this high variability in biopsies, a significant correlation was found between ^{99m}Tc-IL2 uptake and biopsy score, in both parotid and submandibular glands (Figure 6). The correlation coefficient was 0.46 (95% CI 0.18 to 0.68), $p = 0.001$, for the parotids and 0.60 (95% CI 0.35 to 0.76), $p < 0.0001$, for the submandibular glands.

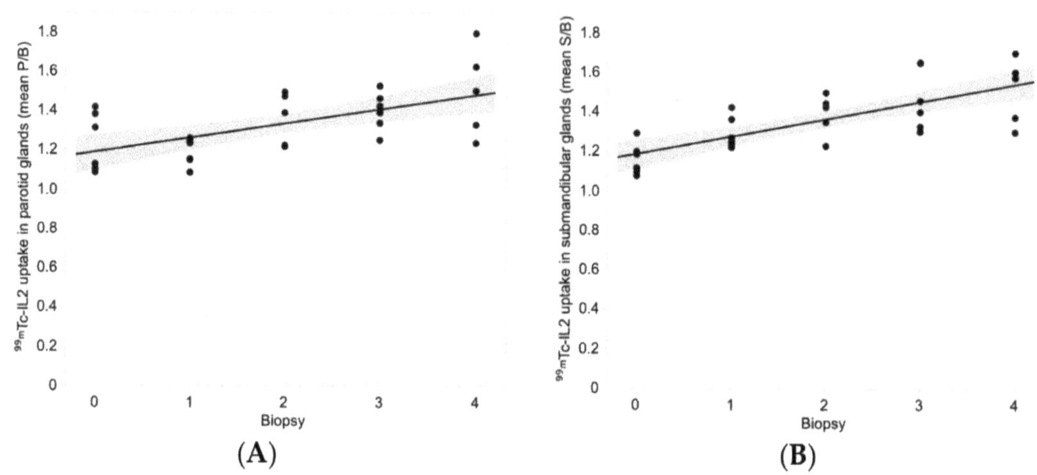

Figure 6. Distribution of the mean ^{99m}Tc-IL2 uptake (P/B) in the parotid glands (**A**) and (S/B) in the submandibular glands (**B**) over the biopsy score. A significant correlation can be observed in all glands (correlation coefficient is 0.46 ($p = 0.001$) for the parotids and 0.60 ($p < 0.0001$) for the submandibular glands).

No correlation was found between the biopsy score and quantitative parameters obtained by $^{99m}TcO_4^-$ scintigraphy or with antibody titres.

3.2. ^{99m}Tc-IL2 Scintigraphy

Through the qualitative analysis, we observed an uptake of ^{99m}Tc-IL2 in at least one gland in all of the patients. The semi-quantitative analysis showed that only one patient had only one gland (parotid) with a T/B higher than the maximum T/B found in the controls. Seventeen patients had at least two glands, 10 patients had three glands, and 20 patients had all four glands with a T/B higher than the maximum T/B found in the controls.

3.3. $^{99m}TcO_4^-$ Scintigraphy

$^{99m}TcO_4^-$ scintigraphy provided two different parameters: the ejection fraction and the maximum uptake of $^{99m}TcO_4^-$ as a percentage of the injected dose. All of the patients had a reduced EF in at least three glands. In contrast, the maximum uptake was reduced in 24/30 patients (80%) when considering at least one functioning gland. We found no correlation between SGS parameters and all of the other variables. In particular, a mild, non-statistically detectable, inverse correlation was found between the SGS parameter and ^{99m}Tc-IL2 uptake in the glands. In particular, the EF and ^{99m}Tc-IL2 uptake in the parotids showed a correlation coefficient of −0.16 (95% CI −0.42 to 0.17), $p = 0.21$. The maximum uptake and ^{99m}Tc-IL2 uptake in the parotids showed a correlation coefficient of −0.10 (95% CI −0.36 to 0.17), p = 0.45. EF and ^{99m}Tc-IL2 uptake in the submandibular glands showed a correlation coefficient of −0.15 (95% CI −0.40 to 0.14), p = 0.24. The maximum uptake and ^{99m}Tc-IL2 uptake in the submandibular glands showed a correlation coefficient of −0.12 (95% CI −0.34 to 0.11), p = 0.36.

4. Discussion

Nowadays, there is no single "gold standard" of oral involvement that is sensitive and specific enough to be the basis for a diagnosis of SS. Moreover, many different diagnostic methods such as sialography, salivary glands scintigraphy with technetium, and lip biopsy have been included into the criteria system of the European Community [3].

Parotid sialography is the most specific (92%–100%) and is accepted as a generally safe method of assessing anatomic changes in SS. However, its usefulness in diagnosis remains questionable for a wide range of sensitivities due to negative results, especially in the early stage of disease [26,27]. Moreover, some technical difficulties and complications related to the procedure have been reported [28]. Some authors have proposed computed tomography (CT) and magnetic resonance imaging (MRI) as alternative accurate methods to detect the parenchymal inhomogeneity characteristic of glands in Sjogren's syndrome, but both of them are expensive and are not able to show the activity of the disease [29,30]. Other studies have been published on ultrasonography (US) as a non-invasive and safe imaging procedure to obtain information about the morphological changes of salivary glands in primary SS [31–33]. More recently, Milic et al. described that patients with primary SS present more frequent pathological changes of the posterior borders, parenchymal inhomogeneity with hypoechogenic areas, and/or hyperechogenic reflections in major salivary glands [34]. Although US is able to follow-up on parenchymal damage, it cannot directly show the grading of inflammation useful in planning treatment.

In the past, salivary glands scintigraphy with ^{99m}Tc-pertechnetate have been proposed to evaluate intact salivary gland parenchyma. Its major advantage, compared with other imaging methods, is its ability to present information on parenchymal damage as well as the excretion function of all glands simultaneously. At present, there is no consensus about which quantitative indices are trustworthy for the diagnosis of SS. However, some reports have described that decreased secretion parameters in parotid glands and decreased accumulation of ^{99m}Tc in the submandibular glands are highly sensitive indicators of SS [35]. Nevertheless, our data do not support the hypothesis that a decreasing salivary function is correlated with the severity of lymphocytic infiltration. Instead, it seems that there is an inverse correlation between these parameters.

Indeed, although quantitative SGS is sensitive enough to detect abnormalities of parenchyma, it reflects only the gland's function in SS. Moreover, these alterations can be found in other diseases, and its rate will increase with age, even in healthy subjects. Therefore, SGS provides an overall sensitivity from 62% to 89% because of the early stage of disease and the low grade of damage in salivary glands [36].

The criteria of the European Community consider the lip biopsy to be the most reliable diagnostic test, and it is still most accurate method for the definitive diagnosis of SS. Nevertheless, in some cases, it is not conclusive. The sensitivity and specificity of the lip biopsy range from 82% to 95% and from 75% to 90%, respectively [37]. It also shows false-negative findings in 18–40% of patients and false-positive in 6–9% of healthy subjects [38]. Moreover, patients with myasthenia gravis, sialolithiasis, and other autoimmune diseases with no syndrome sicca may present lymphocytic infiltration in the salivary glands [26]. Furthermore, the lip biopsy cannot be used as a routine procedure in the follow-up of patients, because it is invasive and is not well accepted. Finally, in some patients, in the early stage of disease, the lip biopsy may not show a lymphocytic infiltration [39], which can become detectable in a second sample repeated after 1 year [40]. In addition, the degree of lymphocytic infiltrate may change over time [41]. Moreover, in major and minor salivary glands, there may be different damage and the degree of epithelial cell damage in a salivary gland biopsy does not always correspond to the salivary flow secretion [42]. Overall, the lip biopsy provides limited information that cannot be applied to all major salivary glands and should not be used to select the most appropriate therapy or to follow-up its efficacy over time.

A non-invasive method to detect lymphocytic infiltration in all major glands is thus desirable [43,44]. Our results suggest that ^{99m}Tc-IL2 scintigraphy could be used to detect and quantify the lymphocytic infiltration in all major salivary glands. Despite finding a positive correlation between the lip biopsy score and ^{99m}Tc-IL2 uptake in major glands, this analysis could be affected by the presence of scores 0–1 and 2 that, indeed, are not related to lymphocytic infiltration. Therefore, larger studies are needed to clearly establish the clinical role of ^{99m}Tc-IL2 and the relation of its uptake in glands with different phases of the diseases.

Most of our patients had a recent diagnosis (within 4 years) and only a few patients had a diagnosis between 5 and 20 years. Furthermore, we did not study the patients over time. This can be a limit of our population, thus not allowing us to conclude on the course of lymphocytic infiltration over time, despite finding an inverse correlation between disease duration and ^{99m}Tc-IL2 uptake in all of the glands. Another limitation of this study is that biopsy was scored in classes from 0 to 4, and this may not reflect the extent of lymphocytic infiltration in salivary glands. Furthermore, as the process is not synchronous in all glands, a biopsy of submandibular and parotid glands would have certainly been more correct, but ethically impossible to perform. Indeed, if we consider only patients within 2−3 years of diagnosis, there would be a high variability in ^{99m}Tc-IL2 uptake in the glands, suggesting that there is a great variability between patients and that the disease is not synchronous in all glands. This finding may have important therapeutic implications.

5. Conclusions

In conclusion, our data suggest ^{99m}Tc-IL2 scintigraphy can be a new tool to assess lymphocytic infiltration in SS. The gland uptake of ^{99m}Tc-IL2 is higher in patients with early diagnosis, from 0 to 1 years of disease, whereas in older diagnoses, the infiltration decreases followed by a fibro-sclerotic process. This scintigraphy could be used to monitor in vivo, non-invasively, the efficacy of immune-modulatory therapies.

Author Contributions: Conceptualization, A.S. and L.K.A.; methodology, G.C.; software, G.C.; validation, A.S., C.L. and M.V.; formal analysis, G.C.; investigation, L.K.A.; resources, A.S., L.K.A., F.R.S. R.P. and F.C.; data curation, L.C. and G.G.S.; writing—original draft preparation, A.S.; writing—review and editing, C.L.; visualization, L.C. and G.C.; supervision, A.S.; project administration, A.S. All authors have read and agreed to the published version of the manuscript.

Funding: This research received no external funding.

Institutional Review Board Statement: The study was conducted in accordance with the Declaration of Helsinki and was approved by the Institutional Ethics Committee of "Sapienza" University of Rome.

Informed Consent Statement: Informed consent was obtained from all of the subjects involved in the study.

Data Availability Statement: All data are available upon request to G.C.

Conflicts of Interest: The authors declare no conflict of interest.

References

1. Fox, R.I. Sjögren's syndrome. *Lancet* **2005**, *366*, 321–331. [CrossRef]
2. Manthorpe, R.; Jacobsson, L.T.; Kirtava, Z.; Theander, E. Epidemiology of Sjögren's syndrome, especially its primary form. *Ann. Med. Interne* **1998**, *149*, 7–11.
3. Vitali, C.; Moutsopoulos, H.M.; Bombardieri, S. The European Community Study Group on diagnostic criteria for Sjogren's syndrome. Sensitivity and specificity of tests for ocular and oral involvement in Sjogren's syndrome. *Ann. Rheum. Dis.* **1994**, *53*, 637–647. [CrossRef] [PubMed]
4. Vitali, C.; Bombardieri, S.; Jonsson, R.; Moutsopoulos, H.M.; Alexander, E.L.; Carsons, S.E.; Daniels, T.E.; Fox, P.C.; Fox, R.I.; Kassan, S.S.; et al. Classification criteria for Sjogren's syndrome: A revised version of the European criteria proposed by the American-European Consensus Group. *Ann. Rheum. Dis.* **2002**, *6*, 554–558. [CrossRef] [PubMed]

5. Daniels, T.E.; Whitcher, J.P. Association of patterns of labial salivary gland inflammation with keratoconjunctivitis sicca. Analysis of 618 patients with suspected Sjogren's syndrome. *Arthritis Reum.* **1994**, *37*, 869–877. [CrossRef] [PubMed]
6. Van Blokland, S.C.A.; Versnel, M.A. Pathogenesis of Sjogren's syndrome: Characteristics of different mouse model for autoimmune exocrinopathy. *Clin. Immun.* **2002**, *103*, 111–124. [CrossRef]
7. Yao, Y.; Ma, J.F.; Chang, C.; Xu, T.; Gao, C.Y.; Gershwin, M.E.; Lian, Z.X. Immunobiology of T Cells in Sjögren's Syndrome. *Clin. Rev. Allergy Immunol.* **2021**, *60*, 111–131. [CrossRef]
8. O'Garra, A. Interleukins and immune system. *Lancet.* **1989**, *1*, 943–947. [CrossRef]
9. Fox, R.I.; Kong, H.I.; Ando, D.; Abrams, J.; Pisa, E. Cytokine mRNA expression in salivary biopsies in Sjögren's syndrome. *J. Immunol.* **1994**, *152*, 5532–5539.
10. Ríos-Ríos, W.J.; Sosa-Luis, S.A.; Torres-Aguilar, H. T Cells Subsets in the Immunopathology and Treatment of Sjogren's Syndrome. *Biomolecules* **2020**, *10*, 1539. [CrossRef]
11. Signore, A.; Chianelli, M.; Annovazzi, A.; Rossi, M.; Maiuri, L.; Greco, M.; Ronga, G.; Britton, K.E.; Picarelli, A. Imaging of active lymphocytic infiltration in coeliac disease with 123I-Interleukin-2 and its response to diet. *Eur. J. Nucl. Med.* **2000**, *27*, 18–24. [CrossRef]
12. Signore, A.; Chianelli, M.; Parisella, M.G.; Capriotti, G.; Giacalone, P.; Di Leve, G.; Barone, R. In vivo imaging of insulitis in autoimmune diabetes. *J. Endocrinol. Investig.* **1999**, *22*, 151–158. [CrossRef] [PubMed]
13. Lucia, P.; Parisella, M.G.; Danese, C.; Bruno, F.; Manetti, L.L.; Capriotti, G.; Martinis, C.D.; Scopinaro, F.; Perego, M.A.; Signore, A. Diagnosis and followup of Takayasu's arteritis by scintigraphy with radiolabelled interleukin 2. *J. Rheumatol.* **2003**, *31*, 1225–1227.
14. Signore, A.; Picarelli, A.; Annovazzi, A.; Britton, K.E.; Grossman, A.B.; Bonanno, E.; Maras, B.; Barra, D.; Pozzilli, P. 123I-Interleukin-2: Biochemical characterization and in vivo use for imaging autoimmune disease. *Nucl. Med. Commun.* **2003**, *24*, 305–316. [CrossRef]
15. Markovic, S.N.; Galli, F.; Suman, V.J.; Nevala, W.K.; Paulsen, A.M.; Hung, J.C.; Gansen, D.N.; Erickson, L.A.; Marchetti, P.; Wiseman, G.A.; et al. Non-invasive visualization of tumor infiltrating lymphocytes in patients with metastatic melanoma undergoing immune checkpoint inhibitor therapy: A pilot study. *Oncotarget* **2018**, *9*, 30268–30278. [CrossRef] [PubMed]
16. Annovazzi, A.; Biancone, L.; Caviglia, R.; Chianelli, M.; Capriotti, G.; Mather, S.J.; Caprilli, R.; Pallone, F.; Scopinaro, F.; Signore, A. 99mTc-interleukin-2 and (99m)Tc-HMPAO granulocyte scintigraphy in patients with inactive Crohn's disease. *Eur. J. Nucl. Med. Mol. Imaging* **2003**, *30*, 374–382. [CrossRef] [PubMed]
17. Signore, A.; Parisella, M.G.; Conti, F.; Chianelli, M.; Spinelli, F.R.; Borseti, G.; D'Ignazio, L.; Mather, S.J.; Valesini, G. 99 m Tc-IL2 scintigraphy detects pre-clinical lymphocytic infiltration of salivary glands in patients with autoimmune disease. *Eur. J. Nucl. Med.* **2000**, *27*, 925.
18. Parisella, M.G.; Conti, F.; D'Alessandria, C.; Spinelli, F.R.; Mather, S.J.; Chianelli, M. Scintigraphy with 99MTc-IL2 in Sjogren syndrome. *Q. J. Nucl. Med.* **2002**, *46*, 18.
19. Markusse, H.M.; Pillay, M.; Cox, P.H. A quantitative inedx derived from 99 m Tc-pertechnetate scintigraphy to assist in the diagnsis of primary Sjogren's Syndrome. *Nucl. Med.* **1992**, *31*, 3–6.
20. Daniels, T.E. Labial salivary gland biopsy in Sjögren's syndrome: Assessment as a diagnostic criterion in 362 suspected cases. *Arthritis Rheum.* **1984**, *24*, 147–156. [CrossRef]
21. Chisholm, D.M.; Waterhouse, J.P.; Mason, D.K. Lymphocytic sialoadenitis in the major and minor salivary glands: A correlation in postmortem subjects. *J. Clin. Path.* **1970**, *23*, 690–694. [CrossRef] [PubMed]
22. Huo, A.P.; Lin, K.C.; Chou, C.T. Predictive and prognostic value of antinuclear antibodies and rheumatoid factor in primary Sjogren's syndrome. *Int. J. Rheum. Dis.* **2010**, *13*, 39–47. [CrossRef] [PubMed]
23. Chianelli, M.; Signore, A.; Fritzberg, A.R.; Mather, S.J. The development of technetium-99m-labelled interleukin-2: A new radiopharmaceutical for the in vivo detection of mononuclear cell infiltrates in immune-mediated diseases. *Nucl. Med. Biol.* **1997**, *24*, 579–586. [CrossRef]
24. Bohuslavizki, K.H.; Brenner, W.; Wolf, H.; Sippel, C.; Tonshoff, G.; Tinnemeyer, S.; Clausen, M.; Henze, E. Value of quantitative salivary gland scintigraphy in the early stage of Sjögren's syndrome. *Nucl. Med. Commun.* **1995**, *16*, 917–922. [CrossRef] [PubMed]
25. Anjos, D.A.; Etchebehere, E.C.; Santos, A.O.; Lima, M.C.; Ramos, C.D.; Paula, R.B.; Camargo, E.E. Normal values of [99mTc]pertechnetate uptake and excretion fraction by major salivary glands. *Nucl. Med. Commun.* **2006**, *27*, 395–403. [CrossRef] [PubMed]
26. Vitali, C.; Tavoni, A.; Simi, U.; Marchetti, G.; Vigorito, P.; d'Ascanio, A.; Neri, R.; Cristofani, R.; Bombardieri, S. Parotid sialography and minor salivary gland biopsy in the diagnosis of Sjögren's Syndrome: A comparative study of 84 patients. *J. Rheumatol.* **1988**, *15*, 262–267. [PubMed]
27. Takashima, S.; Morimoto, S.; Tomiyama, N.; Takeuchi, N.; Ikezoe, J.; Kozuka, T. Sjögren's Syndrome: Comparison of sialography and ultrasonography. *J. Clin. Ultrasound.* **1992**, *20*, 99–109. [CrossRef]
28. Cockrell, D.J.; Rout, P. Adverse reaction following following sialography. *Dentomaxillofac Radiol.* **1993**, *22*, 41–42. [CrossRef]
29. De Clerk, L.S.; Corthous, R.; Francx, L.; Brussaard, C.; de Schepper, A.; Vercruysse, H.A.; Steven, W.J. Ultrasonography and computer tomography of the saliary glands in the evaluation of Sjögren's Syndrome. Comparison with parotid sialography. *J. Rheumatol.* **1988**, *15*, 1777–1781.

30. Valesini, G.; Gualdi, G.F.; Priori, R.; Di Biasi, C.; Polettini, E.; Trasimeni, G.; Filippi, A.; Pezzi, P.P.; Balsano, F. Magnetic Resonance imaging of the parotid glands and lip biopsy in the evaluation of xerostomia in Sjogren's Syndrome. *Scand. J. Rheumatol.* **1994**, *23*, 103–106. [CrossRef]
31. De Vita, S.; Lorenzon, G.; Rossi, G.; Sabella, M.; Fossaluzza, V. Salivary gland echosonography in primari and secondary Sjogren' syndrome. *Clin. Exp. Rheumatol.* **1992**, *10*, 351–356. [PubMed]
32. Ariji, Y.; Ohki, M.; Eguchi, K.; Lzumi, M.; Ariji, E.; Mizokami, A.; Nagataki, S.; Nakamura, T. Texture analysis of sonograpic features of the parotid gland in Sjogren's syndrome. *Am. J. Roentgenol.* **1996**, *166*, 935–941. [CrossRef] [PubMed]
33. Salaffi, F.; Carotti, M.; Iagnocco, A.; Luccioli, F.; Ramonda, R.; Sabatini, E.; Nicola, M.D.; Maggi, M.; Priori, R.; Valesini, G.; et a Ultrasonography of salivary glands in primary Sjogren's syndrome: A comparison with sialography and scintigraphy. *Rheumato* **2008**, *47*, 1244–1249. [CrossRef] [PubMed]
34. Milic, V.D.; Petrovic, R.R.; Boricic, I.V.; Marinkovic-Eric, J.; Radunovic, G.L.; Jeremic, P.D.; Pejnovic, N.N.; Damjanov, N. Diagnostic value of salivary gland ultrasonographic scoring system in primary Sjogren's Syndrome: A comparison with scintigraphy and biopsy. *J. Rheumatol.* **2009**, *36*, 1495–1500. [CrossRef] [PubMed]
35. Makula, E.; Pokorny, G.; Rajtar, M.; Kiss, I.; Kovacs, A.; Kovacs, L. Parotid gland ultrasonography as a diagnostic tool in primary Sjogren's Syndrome. *Br. J. Rheumatol.* **1996**, *35*, 972–977. [CrossRef] [PubMed]
36. Uhmehara, I.; Yamada, I.; Murata, Y.; Takanashi, Y.; Okada, N.; Shibuya, H. Quantitative evaluation of salivary gland scintigraphy in Sjogren Syndrome. *J. Nucl. Med.* **1999**, *40*, 64–69.
37. Sugihara, T.; Yoshimura, Y. Scintigraphic evaluation of the salivary glands in patients with Sjögren's syndrome. *Int. J. Maxillofac Surg.* **1988**, *17*, 71–75. [CrossRef]
38. Soto-Rojas, A.E.; Kraus, A. The oral side of Sjogren Syndrome. Diagnosis and treatment. A review. *Arch. Med. Res.* **2002** *33*, 95–106. [CrossRef]
39. Leroy, J.P.; Pennec, Y.L.; Soulier, C.; Berthelot, J.M.; Letoux, G.; Youinou, P. Follow up study of labial salivary gland lesions in primary Syogren's syndrome. *Ann. Rheum. Dis.* **1992**, *51*, 777–780. [CrossRef]
40. Lindvall, A.M.; Jonsson, R. The salivary gland component of Sjogren's syndrome: An evaluation of diagnostic methods. *Oral Surg. Oral. Med. Oral. Pathol.* **1986**, *62*, 32–42. [CrossRef]
41. Jonson, R.; Kroneld, U.; Backman, K.; Magnusson, B.; Tarkowski, A. A progression of sialoadenitis in Sjogren's syndrome. *Br. J. Rheumatol.* **1993**, *32*, 578–581. [CrossRef] [PubMed]
42. Haga, H.J.; Rygh, T.; Jacobsen, H.; Johannessen, A.C.; Mjanger, O.; Jonsson, R. Sjögren's syndrome. New diagnostic aspects *Tidsskr. Nor. Laegeforen* **1997**, *117*, 2197–2200. [PubMed]
43. Ramos-Casals, M.; Tzioufas, A.G.; Stone, J.H.; Sisò, A.; Bosch, X. Treatment of primary Sjögren's syndrome. *JAMA* **2010** *304*, 452–460. [CrossRef] [PubMed]
44. Fox, R.I.; Fox, C.M.; Gottenberg, J.E.; Dörner, T. Treatment of Sjögren's syndrome: Current therapy and future directions *Rheumatology* **2021**, *60*, 2066–2074. [CrossRef]

Journal of
Clinical Medicine

MDPI

Article

Comparison Benefit between Hydrogen Peroxide and Adrenaline in Tonsillectomy: A Randomized Controlled Study

Cheng-Yu Hsieh [1], Chuan-Jen Hsu [1,2], Hung-Pin Wu [1,2] and Chuan-Hung Sun [1,2,*]

1 Department of Otolaryngology, Head and Neck Surgery, Taichung Tzu Chi Hospital, Buddhist Tzu Chi Medical Foundation, Taichung 427, Taiwan; chengyu384650@gmail.com (C.-Y.H.); cjhsu@ntu.edu.tw (C.-J.H.); hungpin_wu@yahoo.com.tw (H.-P.W.)

2 School of Medicine, Tzu Chi University, Hualien 970, Taiwan

* Correspondence: sunch7297@gmail.com; Tel.: +886-4-3606-0666; Fax: +886-4-3606-5928

Abstract: This study aimed to further evaluate the benefit of topical hemostasis agents in tonsillectomy. We compared the clinical effects of topical application between hydrogen peroxide and adrenaline in tonsillectomy. Overall, 60 patients (120 tonsils) were prospectively enrolled for tonsillectomy between February 2018 and December 2020. The patients were randomly assigned to either the hydrogen peroxide or adrenaline group. Then, tonsillectomy was performed using hydrogen peroxide as a hemostatic agent on the assigned side, while adrenaline was applied to the other side. All procedures were performed by a surgeon who was blinded to the randomization. The outcome measurements of operation time, intraoperative blood loss, postoperative pain, and hemorrhage events were analyzed. The intraoperative blood loss was significantly lower in the hydrogen peroxide group than in the adrenaline group (9.99 ± 4.51 mL vs. 13.87 ± 6.32 mL; $p = 0.0$). The median operation time was also significantly lower in the hydrogen peroxide group (8.02 ± 3.59 min vs. 9.22 ± 3.88 min; $p = 0.019$). Meanwhile, the visual analogue scale (VAS) scores were significantly higher in the hydrogen peroxide group (4.98 ± 1.94 vs. 4.27 ± 1.97; $p = 0.001$). The topical application of hydrogen peroxide as a hemostatic agent effectively decreases the operation time and intraoperative blood loss. Thus, hydrogen peroxide can be used as a routine hemostatic agent for bleeding control in tonsillectomy.

Keywords: hydrogen peroxide; adrenaline; blood loss; tonsillectomy

Citation: Hsieh, C.-Y.; Hsu, C.-J.; Wu, H.-P.; Sun, C.-H. Comparison Benefit between Hydrogen Peroxide and Adrenaline in Tonsillectomy: A Randomized Controlled Study. *J. Clin. Med.* **2022**, *11*, 2723. https://doi.org/10.3390/jcm11102723

Academic Editor: Margherita Sisto

Received: 6 April 2022
Accepted: 9 May 2022
Published: 11 May 2022

Publisher's Note: MDPI stays neutral with regard to jurisdictional claims in published maps and institutional affiliations.

1. Introduction

Tonsillectomy is one of the most common surgical procedures in otolaryngology. Despite improvements in anesthesia and surgical techniques, intraoperative and postoperative hemorrhage remain major concerns in tonsillectomy [1], with primary (<24 h) postoperative bleeding occurring in 0.3–5.4% of patients [2,3]. Primary postoperative bleeding is generally related to surgical techniques and hemostasis strategies, while secondary bleeding is more likely related to surgical site infection or sloughing of the eschar covering the tonsillar fossa.

The blood supply of the tonsils mainly comes from the lingual and tonsillar branches of the facial artery. The pharyngobasilar fascia, which extends into the tonsils, covers the lateral surface of the tonsils. The complexity of the blood supply of the tonsil and the distanced and limited operation field increase the risk of massive intraoperative bleeding during tonsillectomy. Therefore, a rapid-onset hemostasis agent is essential to avoid major surgical complications. Effective hemostasis contributes to a lower operation time, better outcomes, and uneventful wound healing.

Traditional electrocauterization for hemostasis may create thermal injury and result in explosive vaporization, which would lead to severe damage to the surrounding tissue. Topical hemostatic agents help the surgeon to target bleeding sources and reduce tissue damage in non-bleeding regions. In this regard, several topical agents, such as hydrogen peroxide, adrenaline, saline solution, and lidocaine [4–6], have been introduced to minimize blood loss. However, there is still no gold standard for topical hemostasis in tonsillectomy.

Post-tonsillectomy pain is another major problem, as it might lead to poor oral intake, dehydration, sleep disturbance, and prolonged hospitalization. Thus, the effect of pain control should be considered when a hemostasis agent is applied. Many local applications, such as bismuth sulfate, oral rinse, lidocaine spray, fibrin glue, and betadine silver nitrate, have been investigated to control postoperative pain [7].

Hydrogen peroxide is an oxidizing agent that is easily degraded by tissue catalase to form oxygen and water. It is a widely available topical antiseptic and nontoxic hemostasis agent that produces oxidative burst and local oxygen production [8]. In the early stages, the "bubble effect" may provide some chemical burn and mechanical debridement in areas of the wound that are not easily accessible to the surgeon. In addition, the bubble effect caused by erythrocyte catalase degradation of hydrogen peroxide can help the surgeon to localize areas that require cauterization and rapidly reduce hemorrhage [9]. In the late stages, delivering hydrogen peroxide into wounds can kill fibroblasts and promote re-epithelialization [10]. A previous report showed that the topical application of hydrogen peroxide could control hemostasis and greatly reduce operation time in tonsillectomy [5]. Adrenaline has also been demonstrated to be a reasonable hemostatic agent because of its low cost, low risk, powerful vasoconstrictor, and platelet aggregation. Topical use of adrenaline is an effective and reasonable hemostatic agent in tonsillectomy [11].

The advantages of both hydrogen peroxide and adrenaline include rapid onset, acceptable duration, easy accessibility, and cost effectiveness. However, to date, there has been no direct, comparative, randomized controlled trial to achieve consensus on the optimal topical hemostasis agent in tonsillectomy. Therefore, this study aimed to compare the clinical effects of the topical application of hydrogen peroxide and adrenaline in tonsillectomy.

2. Materials and Methods

2.1. Experimental Design

A total of 60 patients aged 8–68 years were prospectively enrolled for tonsillectomy in tertiary referral centers between February 2018 and December 2020. All subjects fulfilled the American Academy of Otolaryngology Head and Neck Surgery criteria for chronic or recurrent tonsillitis, recurrent tonsil hemorrhage, peritonsillar abscess, or tonsillar hypertrophy with obstructive symptoms. Subjects were excluded if they had tonsillar cancer, underwent combination surgeries, had severe underlying diseases, such as cardiovascular disease, or had bleeding tendency disorder.

All surgical procedures were performed via blunt dissection under general anesthesia by the same surgeon. The application of hydrogen peroxide and adrenaline was randomized preoperatively. A local anesthetic injection of 2 cc lidocaine over the peritonsillar area was performed prior to removing each side of the tonsil to reduce pain by blocking peripheral nociceptive excitation. To achieve the best confounding control, we focused on the same subjects, and all patients' tonsils were randomly assigned to either the hydrogen peroxide or adrenaline group. Then, tonsillectomy was performed using hydrogen peroxide as a hemostatic agent on the assigned side, while adrenaline was applied to the other side. All procedures were performed by a "blind" surgeon. During tonsillectomy, cotton balls soaked with 3% hydrogen peroxide were tightly packed into the tonsillar fossa for hemostasis of mucosal bleeding, and 1% adrenaline was applied on the other side of the tonsillar fossa. We rinsed both cotton balls with 2% lidocaine and then packed them into the tonsillar fossa until complete hemostasis was achieved. Bipolar electrocauterization was used for hemostasis if persistent active bleeding was not controlled.

The intraoperative blood loss on each side was measured by weighing the cotton balls and suction bottle before and after the operation. The operation time was calculated as the period between the first incision and the time all bleeding or oozing was secured entirely on the single side, encompassing the time of dissection and hemostasis. We avoided opioid drugs due to nausea and possible respiratory inhibition. In addition, anti-inflammatory drugs, such as non-steroidal anti-inflammatory drugs, were excluded because of their adverse effects on platelet function, which are associated with a tendency to bleed.

Postoperative pain in the first 24 h and 48 h after tonsillectomy was recorded. Postoperative pain was assessed by determining the more painful side during follow-up. Pain intensity was evaluated by a blinded physician using a visual analogue scale, with a score of 0 indicating no pain and 10 indicating maximum pain. All patients were blinded to which technique was applied on each side. Postoperative data about pain score, fever, time to oral intake, and bleeding events were collected. All patients received the same dose of acetaminophen four times daily. In general, the patients were discharged 2 days postoperatively after examination of the uneventful surgical wound without oozing.

2.2. Statistical Analysis

Data on operation time, intraoperative blood loss, postoperative pain, and hemorrhage events were collected and analyzed. Descriptive statistics were presented as the means and standard deviations, and categorical variables were presented as counts and percentages. The 95% confidence intervals (CIs) were determined for the strength of association and intergroup correlation. For the main analysis, the differences in operation time, blood loss and postoperative pain between groups are expressed as means (95% CI). The study had a statistical power of 80% and an effect size of 70%. The paired t test was used to analyze postoperative pain score, intraoperative blood loss, and operation time. All statistical analyses were performed using SPSS 20.0 statistical software. $p < 0.05$ was considered statistically significant.

3. Results

3.1. Patient Characteristics

In total, 60 subjects were enrolled. None of the patients had any hypersensitivity response to the ingredients of the locally applied hydrogen peroxide and adrenaline. No complications or postoperative secondary bleeding were noted after tonsillectomy. The operation time, hemostasis time and intraoperative blood loss for each side are shown in Table 1. The postoperative pain scores in the first 24 h and 48 h after tonsillectomy are shown in Table 2. A comparison of the operation time, hemostasis time and blood loss on each side is shown in Table 3.

Table 1. Between-group comparison of operation time, hemostasis time and blood loss.

Variables	Hydrogen Peroxide Group (n = 60)	Adrenaline Group (n = 60)	Median Difference Mean (95% CI)	p-Value *
Operation time (min)	8.02 ± 3.59	9.22 ± 3.88	−71.62 (−127.70, −15.53)	0.019
Hemostasis time (min)	3.43 ± 2.75	4.49 ± 3.35	−63.83 (−110.91, −16.76)	0.007
Blood loss (mL)	9.99 ± 4.51	13.87 ± 6.32	−3.88 (−5.76, −2.00)	0

Data are presented as the median values and 95% confidence intervals. The paired t test is used for continuous variables. * $p < 0.05$.

Table 2. Between-group comparison of postoperative pain score.

Variables	Hydrogen Peroxide (n = 60)	Adrenaline (n = 60)	Median Difference Mean (95% CI)	p-Value *
VAS, 24 h	4.98 ± 1.94	4.27 ± 1.97	0.72 (0.32, 1.12)	0.001
VAS, 48 h	3.47 ± 1.58	3.23 ± 1.52	0.23 (−0.83, 0.55)	0.147

Data are presented as the median values and 95% confidence intervals. The paired t test is used for continuous variables. * $p < 0.05$.

Table 3. Comparison of operation time, hemostasis time and blood loss by side of application.

Variables	Left (n = 60)	Right (n = 60)	p-Value *
Operation time (min)	8.85 ± 4.04	8.39 ± 3.49	0.458
Hemostasis time (min)	4.04 ± 3.23	3.88 ± 2.99	0.504
Blood loss (mL)	12.55 ± 6.28	11.30 ± 5.26	0.239

The paired t test is used for continuous variables. * $p < 0.05$.

3.2. Outcomes

3.2.1. Intraoperative Blood Loss

The average intraoperative blood loss was significantly higher in the hydrogen perox-ide group than in the adrenaline group (9.99 ± 4.51 mL vs. 13.87 ± 6.32 mL, p = 0; Table 1). The ratio of patients with <10 cc blood loss was also significantly higher in the hydrogen peroxide group (61.6% vs. 36.6%).

3.2.2. Operation Time

The median operation time was 8.02 ± 3.59 min in the hydrogen peroxide group and 9.22 ± 3.88 min in the adrenaline group (Table 1). Apparently, surgery was signif-icantly faster in the hydrogen peroxide group than in the adrenaline group (p = 0.019; Table 1). The hemostasis time was also significantly shorter in the hydrogen peroxide group (3.43 ± 2.75 min vs. 4.49 ± 3.35 min, p = 0.07; Table 1).

3.2.3. Postoperative Pain

The mean 24 h postoperative VAS score was significantly higher in the hydrogen peroxide group than in the adrenaline group (4.98 ± 1.94 vs. 4.27 ± 1.97, p = 0.001; Table 2). However, there was no significant difference in the mean 48 h postoperative VAS score between the two groups (3.47 ± 1.58 vs. 3.23 ± 1.52, p = 0.147; Table 2).

3.2.4. Left versus Right Side Outcomes

The median operation time was 8.85 ± 4.04 min in the left group and 8.39 ± 3.49 min in the right group, with no significant difference (p = 0.458; Table 3). The median hemostasis time was 4.04 ± 3.23 min in the left group and 3.88 ± 2.99 min in the right group. The intraoperative blood loss in the left and right groups were 12.55 ± 6.28 and 11.30 ± 5.26, respectively, with no significant difference (p = 0.239).

4. Discussion

Post-tonsillectomy hemorrhage and pain are the major complications of tonsillectomy; the optimal modality for achieving hemostasis remains unclear. According to our results, both hydrogen peroxide and adrenaline can help to reduce intraoperative blood loss; more-over, the intraoperative blood loss and the median operation time were significantly lower in the hydrogen peroxide group than in the adrenaline group. To the best of our knowledge, this is the first study to compare hydrogen peroxide and adrenaline as hemostatic agents for tonsillectomy.

Unlike other studies that divided the patients into two groups, the distinctive charac-teristic of our study was that we focused on the same subjects; all patients served as their own control because hydrogen peroxide and adrenaline were applied to the opposing sides of the tonsillar fossa. Therefore, confounding factors, such as underlying disease, age, sex and tonsil size, can be excluded. A few outliers may cause a disproportionate effect on the statistical results because of the small amount of intraoperative blood loss in tonsillectomy. For example, the influence of surgeon handedness in tonsillectomy has not been exam-ined in previous reports. To eliminate differences due to handedness, we compared the operation time and intraoperative blood loss on each side and further analyzed by type of agent (hydrogen peroxide and adrenaline) (Tables 4 and 5). Our results revealed that hand preference did not influence the overall outcomes based on operation time and blood loss, as evidenced by the lack of significant differences between the two groups.

Table 4. Intergroup correlation of operation time, hemostasis time and blood loss by side in the hydrogen peroxide group.

Variables	Left (n = 30)	Right (n = 30)	p-Value *
Operation time (min)	9.72 ± 3.99	8.43 ± 3.74	0.201
Hemostasis time (min)	3.56 ± 2.53	3.65 ± 2.50	0.891
Blood loss (mL)	10.62 ± 4.60	9.96 ± 4.91	0.589

The independent t test is used for continuous variables. * $p < 0.05$.

Table 5. Intergroup correlation of operation time, hemostasis time and blood loss by side in the adrenaline group.

Variables	Left (n = 30)	Right (n = 30)	p-Value *
Operation time (min)	7.99 ± 3.98	8.36 ± 3.29	0.696
Hemostasis time (min)	4.51 ± 3.79	4.12 ± 3.45	0.674
Blood loss (mL)	14.48 ± 7.18	12.64 ± 5.33	0.263

The independent t test is used for continuous variables. * $p < 0.05$.

A 2017 meta-analysis revealed that the application of local anesthetic, either by infiltration or the topical method, could provide a modest reduction in post-tonsillectomy pain and hemorrhage [12]. The meta-analysis concluded that a preoperative local anesthetic injection is a valuable method for decreasing blood loss and surgical time. Another meta-analysis suggested that topical local anesthetics on swabs provide similar analgesic effects as preoperative infiltration [13]. Previous studies showed that the general operation time by blunt dissection in tonsillectomy was 24.6–29.1 min [14,15]. Adopting the above-mentioned strategies, including preoperative local anesthetic injection and postoperative topical application of hemostatic agents, reduced the mean operation time to 9.99–13.87 min in our study.

Electrocauterization for hemostasis can significantly decrease the operation time and intraoperative blood loss; however, it can also increase postoperative pain [16,17]. Further, it also results in excessive eschar on the tonsillar fossa, which may cause secondary bleeding [3] and infection. In addition, the time to wound healing and return to a full diet is longer in patients undergoing bipolar cauterization hemostasis [18].

In our study, the intraoperative blood loss was small (median volume < 15 mL) in both the hydrogen peroxide and adrenaline groups. Topical hemostatic agents that have the benefit of rapid onset, easy accessibility, cost effectiveness and analgesic effect are highly beneficial. We performed blunt dissection and applied topical hemostatic agents. Topical application of a hemostatic agent can treat all potential bleeding sites, not only focusing on an active bleeding area, but also on hard-to-access bleeding areas, such as the low pole of the tonsil. Thus, a topical hemostatic agent may be a feasible method to control hemorrhage. Hemostasis with the compression of a cotton ball may also cause lower postoperative pain than bipolar cauterization and ligation [19]. Topical hemostatic agents can also prevent sloughing of the eschar and help control mucosal bleeding across surface areas. No secondary bleeding after tonsillectomy occurred in the present study.

Hydrogen peroxide is widely used for wound irrigation, owing to its hemostatic and antimicrobial effects. Chang et al. and Al-Abbasi et al. reported that the use of hydrogen peroxide significantly reduced the operation time in tonsillectomy by 35% and 31%, respectively [5,20]. In our study, hydrogen peroxide better reduced the operation time by 14.9% and achieved a better hemostatic effect than adrenaline. The decreased operation time in the hydrogen peroxide group could be due to the relatively short hemostasis time, in line with previous findings [5,20].

For intraoperative blood loss, the median volume was significantly lower in the hydrogen peroxide group than in the adrenaline group. We found that both hydrogen peroxide and adrenaline could decrease intraoperative hemorrhage. However, although the effect size of 3.88 mL of intraoperative blood loss may be significantly different, this little change may not have clinical significance. In addition, we also found that the mucosa and soft tissue turned white after hydrogen peroxide was pressed tightly. The chemical burns and bitter taste of hydrogen peroxide might explain the higher 24 h postoperative pain score in the hydrogen peroxide group (4.98 ± 1.94) than in the adrenaline group (4.27 ± 1.97).

There are three main applications of hydrogen peroxide: antiseptic, hemostasis and wound healing. Reactive oxygen species (ROS) defend the host from invading microbes by damaging microbial DNA. When hydrogen peroxide is degraded, reactive oxygen species are released, causing DNA strand breakage by DNA oxidization [21]. ROS induce interferon activation and result in an antiviral state, which limits viral replication. ROS may help promote cytokine production, autophagy and granuloma formation, resulting in an antimycobacterial state. By decreasing the colonization of bacteria and viruses, the severity of infection and pain can be reduced.

In addition to the antiseptic benefit, we also found a decrease in operation time. Further analysis of the decreased operation time in the hydrogen peroxide group showed that the "bubble effect", due to oxidation in the early stage, rapidly turned the bleeding area to white. This helped the surgeon to easily localize the bleeding source requiring cauterization and clarify the visual field. It also shortened the operation time. Applying hydrogen peroxide to the wound at the late stage can kill fibroblasts and promote re-epithelialization [22]. Hydrogen peroxide facilitates hemostasis through several mechanisms, including platelet aggregation, stimulation of platelet-derived growth factor activation, and regulation of the contractility and barrier function of endothelial cells [23].

There are numerous theories regarding the hemostatic effects of hydrogen peroxide, including thermal injury of the vascular ends, oxygen embolization of vessels, and reactive vascular spasms [24]. More recently, it has been suggested that thrombolytic hyperactivity and thrombus formation can trigger hemostatic effects [24]. In addition, when catalase in red blood cells reacts with hydrogen peroxide, the chemical reaction induces the release of oxygen and heat, helping the surgeon to localize the bleeding site.

Currently, hydrogen peroxide is used clinically not only as a hemostatic and antiseptic agent, but also as a wound-healing agent [23]. Hydrogen peroxide may help to clear pathogen debris and promote cytokine secretion, helping tissue regeneration [25]. In our study, 3% hydrogen peroxide appeared to have no negative effect on wound healing. It should be noted that highly concentrated hydrogen peroxide (30%) carries a risk of cardiac arrest and stroke, due to oxygen embolism formation [26]. However, the use of a low concentration of hydrogen peroxide (3%) does not induce serious systemic side effects [9,24,27]. The application time should be limited to prevent tissue damage and limit pain. Collectively, these findings support the fact that 3% hydrogen peroxide is a safe and effective agent for intraoperative hemostasis and wound cleaning.

Hatton et al. reported that topical adrenaline is an effective hemostatic agent in tonsillectomy [11]. The application of bismuth subgallate and adrenaline paste to the tonsillar fossae reduced the operating time by 23% and blood loss by 21% [28]. Epinephrine, a platelet-stimulating agent, can cause aggregation of human platelets through alpha-adrenergic mechanisms [29]. In this study, we found that the topical use of adrenaline is mildly inferior to hydrogen peroxide, with respect to hemostatic function. The vasoconstriction effect of adrenaline on arterioles, capillaries and venules helps to delay intraoperative bleeding initially. However, post-tonsillectomy bleeding may result from a blood vessel that initially spasms and later resumes bleeding if hemostasis is not complete. Importantly, adrenaline takes longer to work in these cases. In the current study, the operation time and intraoperative blood loss were lower, at 14.9% and 38.8% (3.88 cc), respectively, in the hydrogen peroxide group than in the adrenaline group. However, in comparison with hydrogen peroxide, adrenaline was more effective in controlling postoperative pain in the first 24 h, but the pain scores were similar at 48 h postoperatively.

We combined lidocaine and adrenaline in this study because lidocaine could stabilize the neural membrane by inhibiting voltage-gated sodium channels, resulting in the suppression of impulse conduction, affecting local anesthetic action. To prevent the systemic circulation and adverse effects of central nervous system toxicity, tachycardia, convulsion, respiratory obstruction [30] and vocal palsy [31], adrenaline was applied topically. The vasoconstrictor property of adrenaline prolongs anesthesia activity and minimizes the risk of systemic circulation. By stimulating α-adrenergic receptors on the neural vasculature, combining adrenaline with lidocaine can lower the local blood flow, slow the clearance of lidocaine, and extend the duration of peripheral nerve block action. To eliminate differences in the pain control effect of the topical use of lidocaine, cotton balls rinsed with lidocaine were applied on both sides as the final step in the study. However, although rare, toxicity at high doses of lidocaine can influence cardiovascular and central nervous system function in a concentration-dependent manner.

This study has some limitations. The number of subjects enrolled in our study was too small to draw a definite conclusion. In the absence of a control group in this study, where no topical agents are used, it is difficult to interpret the absolute benefit of each other's hemostatic agents. Previous studies measured pain before and after the administration of supplemental analgesia; however, there may still have been some residual analgesic effect on subsequent measurements in the early period. Meanwhile, we assessed the pain score at 24 h postoperatively, when the anesthetic effect may have little residual activity. Furthermore, we found that it was difficult for some patients to precisely discriminate the exact pain score on each side, possibly resulting in bias. Further studies should investigate the effects of hemostatic agents over a longer duration with a larger set of participants.

5. Conclusions

The topical application of hydrogen peroxide is beneficial for reducing the operation time and intraoperative blood loss, with minor complications, in tonsillectomy. Thus, hydrogen peroxide can be used as a routine topical hemostatic agent in tonsillectomy. Meanwhile, the topical application of adrenaline provides significant pain relief on the first day compared to hydrogen peroxide.

Author Contributions: Writing—original draft preparation, C.-Y.H.; analysis and interpretation—C.-J.H., H.-P.W.; supervision and editing—C.-H.S. All authors have read and agreed to the published version of the manuscript.

Funding: This research was funded by Buddhist Tzu Chi Medical Foundation (TCMF-CP 111-09).

Institutional Review Board Statement: The prospective, randomized control study was conducted according to the guidelines of the Declaration of Helsinki and approved by the Research Ethics Committee of Taichung Tzu Chi Hospital (REC 108-01).

Informed Consent Statement: Written informed consent was obtained from all patients prior to enrolment.

Data Availability Statement: The data presented in this study are available on request from the corresponding author. The data are not publicly available due to privacy or research ethics.

Conflicts of Interest: The authors declare no conflict of interest.

References

1. Randall, D.A.; Hoffer, M.E. Complications of tonsillectomy and adenoidectomy. *Otolaryngol. Head Neck Surg.* **1998**, *118*, 61–68. [CrossRef]
2. Wieland, A.; Belden, L.; Cunningham, M. Preoperative coagulation screening for adenotonsillectomy: A review and comparison of current physician practices. *Otolaryngol. Head Neck Surg.* **2009**, *140*, 542–547. [CrossRef] [PubMed]
3. Audit, N.P.T.; van der Meulen, J. Tonsillectomy technique as a risk factor for postoperative haemorrhage. *Lancet* **2004**, *364*, 697–702.
4. Adoga, A.; Okeke, E. Hemostasis during cold dissection tonsillectomy: Comparing the use of adrenaline and normal saline. *J. Clin. Med. Res.* **2011**, *3*, 105–108. [CrossRef]
5. Al-Abbasi, A.M.; Saeed, Z.K. Hydrogen peroxide 3%: Is it beneficial in tonsillectomy? *Sultan Qaboos Univ. Med. J.* **2008**, *8*, 201. [PubMed]
6. Özmen, Ö.A.; Özmen, S. Topical bupivacaine compared to lidocaine with epinephrine for post-tonsillectomy pain relief in children: A randomized controlled study. *Int. J. Pediatric Otorhinolaryngol.* **2011**, *75*, 77–80. [CrossRef]

7. Fedorowicz, Z.; van Zuuren, E.J.; Nasser, M.; Carter, B.; Al Langawi, J.H. Oral rinses, mouthwashes and sprays for improving recovery following tonsillectomy. *Cochrane Database Syst. Rev.* **2013**, CD007806. [CrossRef]
8. Hankin, F.M.; Campbell, S.E.; Goldstein, S.A.; Matthews, L.S. Hydrogen peroxide as a topical hemostatic agent. *Clin. Orthop. Relat. Res.* **1984**, *186*, 244–248. [CrossRef]
9. Potyondy, L.; Lottenberg, L.; Anderson, J.; Mozingo, D.W. The use of hydrogen peroxide for achieving dermal hemostasis after burn excision in a patient with platelet dysfunction. *J. Burn Care Res.* **2006**, *27*, 99–101. [CrossRef] [PubMed]
10. Loo, A.E.K.; Halliwell, B. Effects of hydrogen peroxide in a keratinocyte-fibroblast co-culture model of wound healing. *Biochem. Biophys. Res. Commun.* **2012**, *423*, 253–258. [CrossRef]
11. Hatton, R.C. Bismuth subgallate–epinephrine paste in adenotonsillectomies. *Ann. Pharmacother.* **2000**, *34*, 522–525. [CrossRef]
12. Vlok, R.; Melhuish, T.; Chong, C.; Ryan, T.; White, L.D. Adjuncts to local anaesthetics in tonsillectomy: A systematic review and meta-analysis. *J. Anesth.* **2017**, *31*, 608–616. [CrossRef] [PubMed]
13. Grainger, J.; Saravanappa, N. Local anaesthetic for post-tonsillectomy pain: A systematic review and meta-analysis. *Clin. Otolaryngol.* **2008**, *33*, 411–419. [CrossRef]
14. D'Agostino, R.; Tarantino, V.; Calevo, M.G. Blunt dissection versus electronic molecular resonance bipolar dissection for tonsillectomy: Operative time and intraoperative and postoperative bleeding and pain. *Int. J. Pediatric Otorhinolaryngol.* **2008**, *72*, 1077–1084. [CrossRef] [PubMed]
15. Ericsson, E.; Hultcrantz, E. Tonsil surgery in youths: Good results with a less invasive method. *Laryngoscope* **2007**, *117*, 654–661. [CrossRef] [PubMed]
16. Maini, S.; Waine, E.; Evans, K. Increased post-tonsillectomy secondary haemorrhage with disposable instruments: An audit cycle. *Clin. Otolaryngol. Allied Sci.* **2002**, *27*, 175–178. [CrossRef]
17. Mowatt, G.; Cook, J.; Fraser, C.; McKerrow, W.S.; Burr, J.M. Systematic review of the safety and efficacy of electrosurgery for tonsillectomy. *Clin. Otolaryngol. Off. J. ENT-UK Off. J. Neth. Soc. Otorhino-Laryngol. Cervico-Facial Surg.* **2006**, *31*, 95–102.
18. Ragab, S. Six years of evidence-based adult dissection tonsillectomy with ultrasonic scalpel, bipolar electrocautery, bipolar radiofrequency or 'cold steel'dissection. *J. Laryngol. Otol.* **2012**, *126*, 1056. [CrossRef]
19. Rungby, J.A. Methods of haemostasis in tonsillectomy assessed by pain scores and consultation rates: The roskilde county tonsillectomy study. *Acta Oto-Laryngol.* **2000**, *120*, 209–214. [CrossRef]
20. Chang, H.J.; Baek, S.H.; Choi, C.Y.; Kang, S.N.; Park, J.B.; Lee, W.Y.; Kim, C. Hemostatic efficacy of topical application of cold hydrogen peroxide in adenoidectomy. *Korean J. Otorhinolaryngol.-Head Neck Surg.* **2003**, *46*, 946–949.
21. Krötz, F.; Sohn, H.-Y.; Pohl, U. Reactive oxygen species: Players in the platelet game. *Arterioscler. Thromb. Vasc. Biol.* **2004**, *24*, 1988–1996. [CrossRef] [PubMed]
22. Lineaweaver, W.; Howard, R.; Soucy, D.; McMorris, S.; Freeman, J.; Crain, C.; Robertson, J.; Rumley, T. Topical antimicrobial toxicity. *Arch. Surg.* **1985**, *120*, 267–270. [CrossRef] [PubMed]
23. Zhu, G.; Wang, Q.; Lu, S.; Niu, Y. Hydrogen peroxide: A potential wound therapeutic target. *Med. Princ. Pract.* **2017**, *26*, 301–308. [CrossRef]
24. Urban, M.V.; Rath, T.; Radtke, C. Hydrogen peroxide (H_2O_2): A review of its use in surgery. *Wien. Med. Wochenschr.* **2019**, *169*, 222–225. [CrossRef] [PubMed]
25. Loo, A.E.K.; Wong, Y.T.; Ho, R.; Wasser, M.; Du, T.; Ng, W.T.; Halliwell, B. Effects of hydrogen peroxide on wound healing in mice in relation to oxidative damage. *PLoS ONE* **2012**, *7*, e49215. [CrossRef]
26. Beattie, C.; Harry, L.; Hamilton, S.; Burke, D. Cardiac arrest following hydrogen peroxide irrigation of a breast wound. *J. Plast. Reconstr. Aesthetic Surg.* **2010**, *63*, e253–e254. [CrossRef]
27. Hossainian, N.; Slot, D.; Afennich, F.; Van der Weijden, G. The effects of hydrogen peroxide mouthwashes on the prevention of plaque and gingival inflammation: A systematic review. *Int. J. Dent. Hyg.* **2011**, *9*, 171–181. [CrossRef]
28. Sharma, K.; Kumar, D.; Sheemar, S. Evaluation of bismuth subgallate and adrenaline paste as haemostat in tonsillectomy bleeding. *Indian J. Otolaryngol. Head Neck Surg.* **2007**, *59*, 300–302. [CrossRef]
29. Zhou, L.; Schmaier, A.H. Platelet aggregation testing in platelet-rich plasma: Description of procedures with the aim to develop standards in the field. *Am. J. Clin. Pathol.* **2005**, *123*, 172–183. [CrossRef]
30. Carr, A.; Elliot, D. Otorhinolaryngology: Anesthesic considerations. In *Pediatric Anesthesia Basic Principles-State of Art-Future*; People's Medical Publishing House: Shelton, CT, USA, 2011; p. 1707.
31. Weksler, N.; Nash, M.; Rozentsveig, V.; Schwartz, J.; Schily, M.; Gurman, G. Vocal cord paralysis as a consequence of peritonsillar infiltration with bupivacaine. *Acta Anaesthesiol. Scand.* **2001**, *45*, 1042–1044. [CrossRef]

Journal of
Clinical Medicine

MDPI

Article

Epitope Mapping of Pathogenic Autoantigens on Sjögren's Syndrome-Susceptible Human Leukocyte Antigens Using In Silico Techniques

Shivai Gupta [1], Danmeng Li [2], David A. Ostrov [2] and Cuong Q. Nguyen [1,3,4,*]

1 Department of Infectious Diseases and Immunology, College of Veterinary Medicine, University of Florida, Gainesville, FL 32611, USA; shivai.gupta@ufl.edu
2 Department of Pathology, Immunology & Laboratory Medicine, College of Medicine, University of Florida, Gainesville, FL 32610, USA; danmeng1986@ufl.edu (D.L.); ostroda@pathology.ufl.edu (D.A.O.)
3 Department of Oral Biology, College of Dentistry, University of Florida, Gainesville, FL 32610, USA
4 Center of Orphaned Autoimmune Diseases, University of Florida, Gainesville, FL 32611, USA
* Correspondence: nguyenc@ufl.edu; Tel.: +1-352-294-4180; Fax: +1-352-392-9704

Abstract: Sjögren's syndrome (SjS) is characterized by lymphocytic infiltration and the dysfunction of the salivary and lacrimal glands. The autoimmune response is driven by the effector T cells and their cytokines. The activation of the effector helper T cells is mediated by autoantigen presentation by human leukocyte antigen (HLA) class II molecules of antigen-presenting cells. Studies using familial aggregation, animal models, and genome-wide association demonstrate a significant genetic correlation between specific risk HLAs and SjS. One of the key HLA alleles is HLA-DRB1*0301; it is one of the most influential associations with primary SjS, having the highest odds ratio and occurrence across different ethnic groups. The specific autoantigens attributed to SjS remain elusive, especially the specific antigenic epitopes presented by HLA-DRB1*0301. This study applied a high throughput in silico mapping technique to identify antigenic epitopes of known SjS autoantigens presented by high-risk HLAs. Furthermore, we identified specific binding HLA-DRB1*0301 epitopes using structural modeling tools such as Immune Epitope Database and Analysis Resource IEDB, AutoDock Vina, and COOT. By deciphering the critical epitopes of autoantigens presented by HLA-DRB1*0301, we gain a better understanding of the origin of the antigens, determine the T cell receptor function, learn the mechanism of disease progression, and develop therapeutic applications.

Keywords: major histocompatibility complex (MHC); human leukocyte antigen (HLA); autoantigens; T cells

Citation: Gupta, S.; Li, D.; Ostrov, D.A.; Nguyen, C.Q. Epitope Mapping of Pathogenic Autoantigens on Sjögren's Syndrome-Susceptible Human Leukocyte Antigens Using In Silico Techniques. *J. Clin. Med.* **2022**, *11*, 1690. https://doi.org/10.3390/jcm11061690

Academic Editor: Margherita Sisto

Received: 2 February 2022
Accepted: 8 March 2022
Published: 18 March 2022

1. Introduction

Sjögren's syndrome (SjS) is a chronic, systemic autoimmune disease that affects the exocrine glands of the body (salivary and lacrimal glands), which may occur in conjunction with another autoimmune disease [1]. It is estimated that approximately 4 million Americans are affected, making SjS the second most common autoimmune disease after rheumatoid arthritis (RA) [2–4]. SjS is a multifactorial disease related to genetic, hormonal, and environmental factors. Based on animal models and candidate gene association studies, susceptibility to developing SjS has been strongly associated with human leukocyte antigen (HLA) class II genes, particularly the HLA-DR and DQ alleles [5]. As with most autoimmune diseases, associations of HLA class II loci with SjS have been described and vary in different ethnic groups [6–10]. In most studies, when an HLA association with primary (p)SjS was demonstrable, a stronger association between HLAs and autoantibody titers could be found to the anti-Ro/SSA and anti-La/SB autoantibody responses. The HLA-DR3 haplotype is associated with SjS and exists within a region with extended linkage disequilibrium not observed in other places in the genome [8]. It is important to note that specific HLA-DR and -DQ alleles have been observed to present autoantigens in SjS (i.e., M3R, α-fodrin, Ro (SSA), and La (SSB)) in different ethnic populations [7,11,12].

The structural determination of disease-relevant peptide–HLA and HLA–peptide–TCR complexes is crucial for the elucidation of the molecular mechanisms responsible for the development of T cell reactivity that promotes autoimmune disease [13]. The HLA-peptide–T cell receptor (TCR) interactions that determine self and non-self-discrimination are guided by a set of rules that malfunction in immunopathology in autoimmunity [14]. There are certain principles that govern HLA restriction and TCR docking geometry with a variety of molecular mechanisms that could affect HLA–peptide–TCR interactions [15] Autoreactive T cells are directly generated and activated by the mechanisms such as atypical HLA–peptide–TCR binding orientation, low-affinity peptide binding that facilitate thymic escape, TCR-mediated stabilization of weak peptide–HLA interaction, and presentation of peptides in a different binding register [13,16–19]. The peptide binding register refers to the ∼9-mer window of a peptide that sits directly within the peptide-binding groove at a given time. Alterations in this register, whereby the same peptide binds a peptide-binding groove utilizing a different 9-mer window, have an altered impact on the generation of autoreactive T cells [20]. Further, autoreactive TCRs can bind self-peptide–HLA complexes with a conventional binding topology and a high affinity as seen in type 1 diabetes and multiple sclerosis, thus highlighting the potential role of the peptide binding register in increasing the risk of autoimmune disease [21].

The first HLA class II associations in SjS described were at the DR3 [22,23] and DR2 [23,24] loci in Caucasian populations [25]. Together these two HLA sub-types were shown to account for up to 90% of the MHC association in patients who had SjS, which have been further confirmed in the majority of subsequent studies evaluating northern European cohorts [24]. In 2005, Anaya and colleagues [26] demonstrated that the HLA-DRB1*0301-DQB1*0201 haplotype was associated with pSjS in Latin Americans. The HLA-DR3 allele is one of the predominant alleles in SjS. The purpose of this study was to use a high-throughput in-silico mapping technique to identify antigenic epitopes binding to known risk HLAs of SjS, with significant emphasis on HLA-DR3 allele. Additionally, we sought to investigate the molecular mimicry of the antigenic epitopes by determining the homology to viral and bacterial pathogens that can bind structurally to individual HLAs.

2. Materials and Methods

2.1. In Silico Binding Affinities of Peptides for HLA-DR3 and Other Risk Alleles

The Immune Epitope Database (IEDB)—La Jolla Institute for Allergy and Immunology (LIAI), La Jolla, CA, USA—hosts a series of machine learning (ML) based tools, each trained on specific datasets of an experimental peptide-MHC binding affinity matrix. These tools encompass the common approaches of ML, namely, linear regression (LR) and utilization of artificial neural networks (ANN). The SMM-align methodology predicted the peptide-MHC binding affinity by fitting a weight matrix that relates peptide sequence to end-point binding affinity value. The datasets used for the IEDB prediction tool SMM-align included complete UniProt protein sequences of human Ro52, Ro60, La, M3R and α-fodrin. Quantitative measurements were selected by choosing the binding assay of identifying the IC50 value, and this was validated by the ΔG measurement values indicating the best possible position the peptide would fit in when being presented to the T cell. The human HLA type II alleles were predicted to bind to 15-mer peptides with a core peptide region of 10 amino acids. Finally, the result sets were analyzed, and the top predicted binders were identified.

2.2. PDB Structures of HLA-DR3 and Predicted Peptide Docking

The 1A6A HLA-DR3 MHC II-peptide binding complex was extracted from the Protein Data Bank and was used as a template for the crystal structure in COOT, and geometry regularization in PHENIX modeling (Figures 1–5). The peptides were mutated using COOT [27] with rotamers that represent a local energy minimum of torsional angles. The geometry of the resulting complex was regularized in PHENIX. Autodock Vina was used for molecular docking after water, and other atoms were removed, with no presence of peptide [28]. Then, the positions of the peptides with the lowest binding energy (ΔG) were complexed using PHENIX. PyMOL (https://pymol.org/2/) accessed on 15 November 2021 v1.7.2 was used to generate molecular graphic images. The site for docking was prepared by removing all water molecules, and the protonation of HLA-DR3 residues was carried out with the SYBYL-X software. Sets of spheres were used to describe potential binding pockets on the molecular surface of HLA-DR3. The four pockets that were determined for molecular docking were determined using the SPHGEN program [28]. This program generated a grid of points that reflected the shape of the selected site, which were filtered through another program called CLUSTER [29]. CLUSTER grouped the selected spheres to define the points used by the following software called DOCK [29]. DOCK was able to match potential ligand atoms with spheres [28]. The next step used the intermolecular van der Waals and columbic AMBER energy scoring coupled with contact scoring and bump filtering. These additional characteristics were applied to the DOCK program algorithm. Atomic coordinates for all predicted peptides positioned in the selected structural pocket in 1000 different orientations were scored, and based on predicted polar (H bond) and nonpolar (van der Waals) interactions, the best images were obtained. PYMOL was used to generate molecular graphic images.

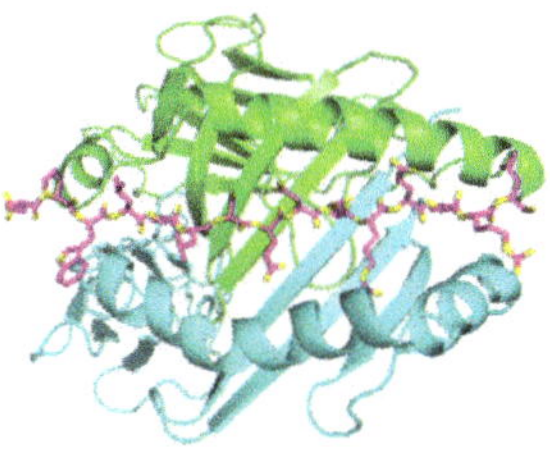

(A)

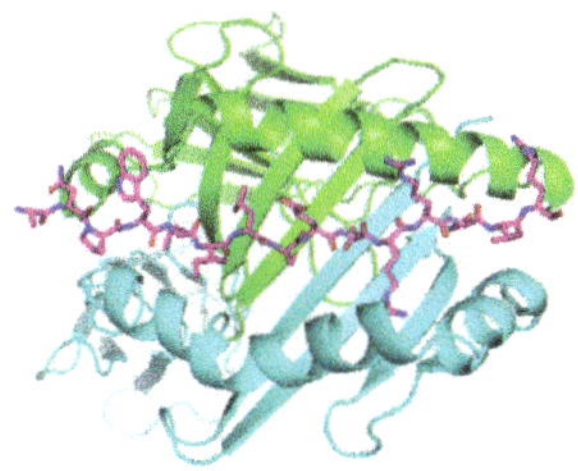

(B)

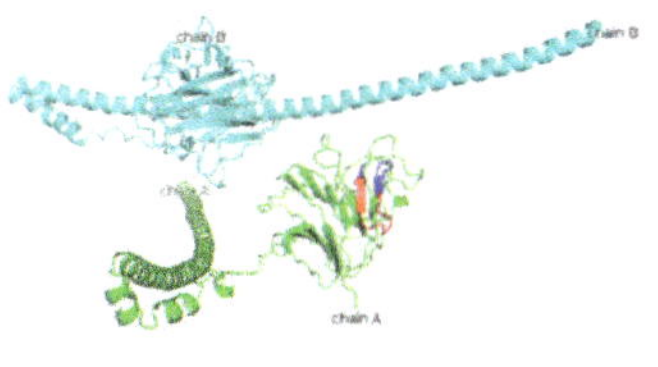

(C)

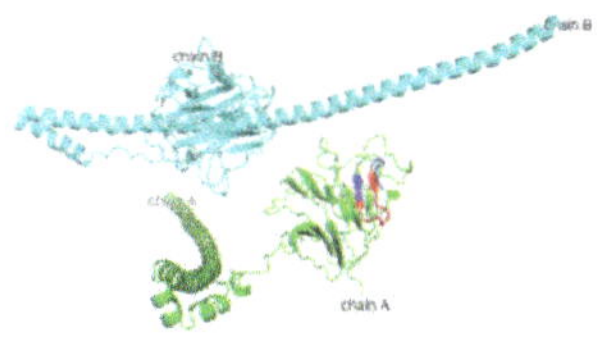

(D)

Figure 1. Predicted Ro52 peptide binders docked on HLA-DRB1*0103. (**A**,**B**) Based on the prediction by SMM-align (stabilization matrix alignment) using IEDB, the top two peptides with IC50 values of 28 and 29 were docked onto the crystal structure of HLA-DRB1*0103 PDB structure 1A6A, and the most optimum predicted position of docking is indicated for both peptides-NPWLILSEDRRQVRL and ANPWLILSEDRRQVR with the core sequence of LSEDRRQVR and LILSEDRRQ, respectively. (**C**,**D**) The highlighted region indicates the presence of the peptides in the three-dimensional structure of the Ro52 protein.

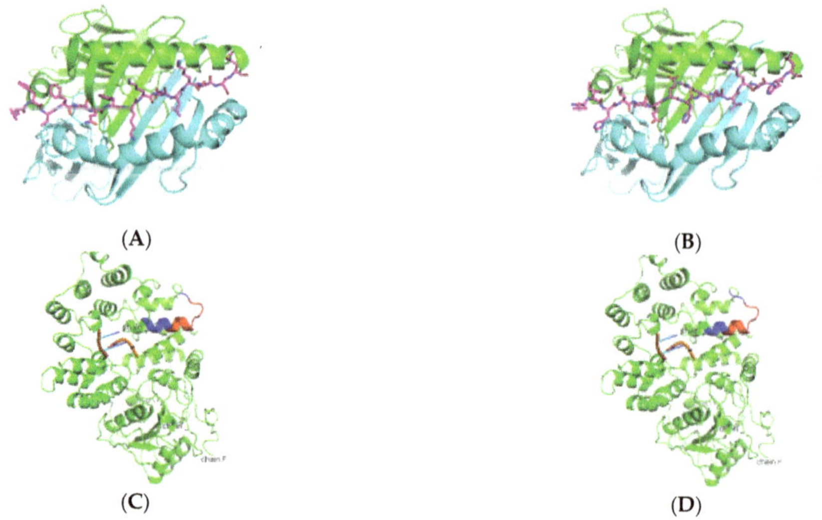

Figure 2. Predicted Ro60 peptide binders docked on HLA-DRB1*0103. (**A**,**B**) SMM-align predicted to two peptides FTFIQFKKDLKESMK and TFIQFKKDLKESMKC with IC50 values of 75 were docke onto the crystal structure of HLA-DRB1*0103 PDB structure 1A6A, and the most optimum predicte position of docking is indicated. Both predicted peptides have the same core sequence FKKDLKESM (**C**,**D**) The highlighted region indicates the presence of the peptides in the three-dimensional structur of the Ro60 protein.

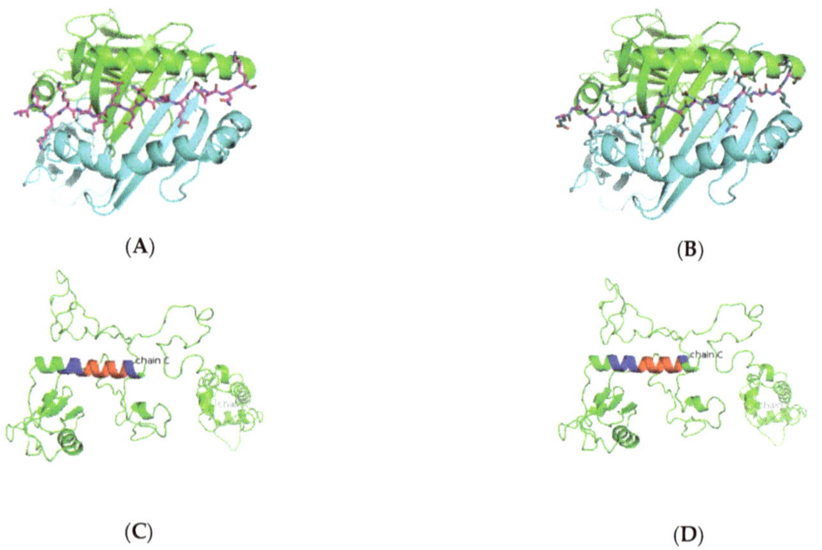

Figure 3. Predicted La peptide binders docked on HLA-DRB1*0103. (**A**,**B**) SMM-align predicte top two peptides ALKKIIEDQQESLNK and EALKKIIEDQQESLN with IC50 values of 49 and 5 were docked onto the crystal structure of HLA-DRB1*0103 PDB structure 1A6A, and the mos optimum predicted position of docking is indicated. Both predicted peptides have the same cor sequence IIEDQQESL. (**C**,**D**) The highlighted region indicates the presence of the peptide in th three-dimensional structure of the La protein.

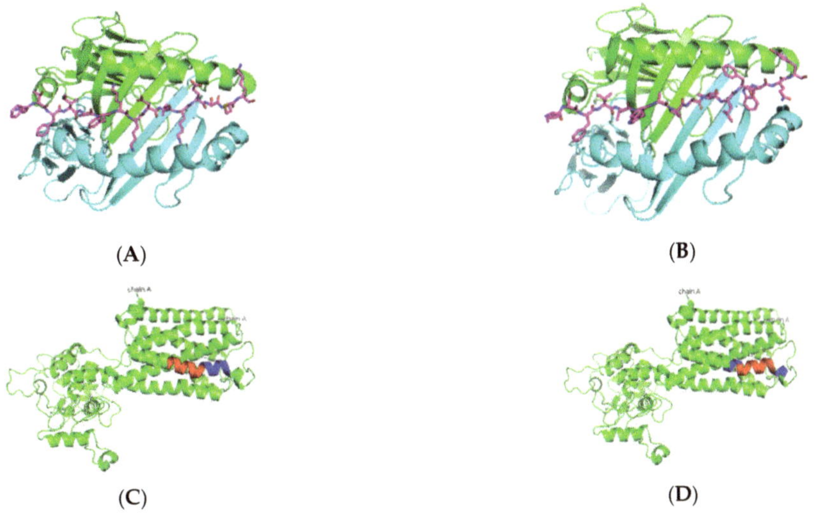

Figure 4. Predicted M3R peptide binders docked on HLA-DRB1*0103. (**A**,**B**) Based on the prediction by SMM-align using IEDB the top two peptides with IC50 values of 120 and 121 were docked onto the crystal structure of HLA-DRB1*0103 PDB structure 1A6A, and the most optimum predicted position of docking is indicated for both peptides AWVISFVLWAPAILF and ISFVLWAPAILFWQY with the core sequence of AWVISFVLW and VLWAPAILF, respectively. (**C**,**D**) The highlighted region indicates the presence of the peptides in the three-dimensional structure of the M3R protein.

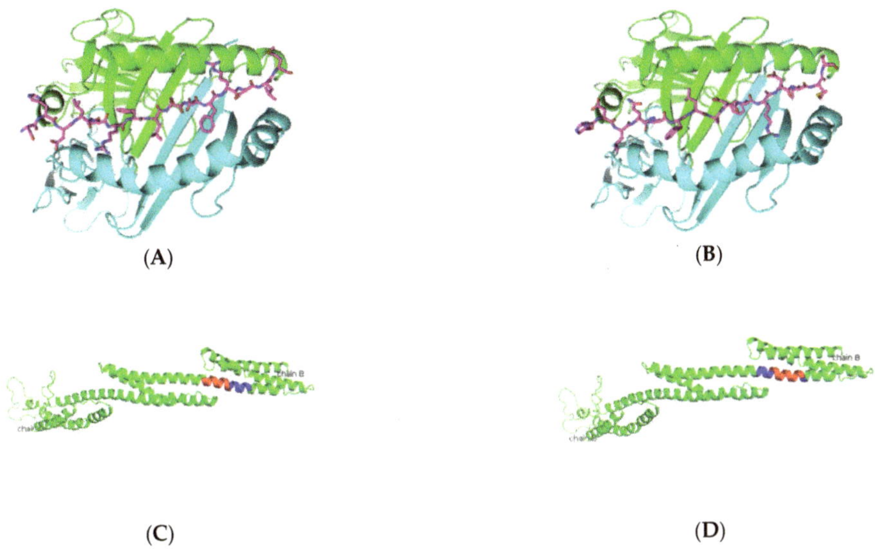

Figure 5. Predicted α-fodrin peptide binders docked on HLA-DRB1*0103. (**A**,**B**) Based on the prediction by SMM-align using IEDB, the top two peptides with IC50 values of 12 were docked onto the crystal structure of HLA-DRB1*0103 PDB structure 1A6A, and the most optimum predicted position of docking is indicated for both peptides SHDLQRFLSDFRDLM and HDLQRFLSDFRDLMS with the core sequence of SHDLQRFLS and FLSDFRDLM, respectively. (**C**,**D**) The highlighted region indicates the presence of the peptides in the three-dimensional structure of the α-fodrin protein.

2.3. Homology Determination for Viral and Bacterial Peptides

The software UniProt—Basic Local Alignment Search Tool (https://www.uniprot.org/blast/, accessed on 15 November 2021) was used to find regions of local similarity between sequences with an E-threshold of 10 amino acids in the viral and bacterial databases of UniProt. The top-scoring homology results were verified by the PubMed database (https://blast.ncbi.nlm.nih.gov/Blast.cgi, accessed on 15 November 2021), recorded, and are presented in Tables 14–17.

3. Results

3.1. In Silico Antigenic Mapping of High-Risk Autoantigens Presented on HLA-DR3

HLA class II alleles play an important role in the regulation of the immune responses against the Ro and La ribonucleoproteins. The generation of these autoantibodies has been correlated with the alleles DRB1*03:01, DQA1*05:01, and DQB1*02:01 in SjS patients [30,31] As indicated in Table 1, among all the risk alleles that have been identified in SjS, the DRB1*03:01 allele was found to be a significant risk factor in many ethnicities [32]. According to the European League Against Rheumatism (EULAR) classification criteria for pSjS, the Ro60 antibodies are one of the leading indicators of the onset of disease in patients. DRB1*03:01 haplotype is found to associate with DPB1*02:01 allele and TNF- α2 alleles in SjS patients [33]. Different HLA alleles can also be protective in nature for varied autoimmune diseases, as presented in Table 2. In DR3 transgenic mice, Ro60 has been shown to induce a strong T and B cell response [34]. Using DRB1*03:01 as the model allele for this study, we sought to map the antigenic epitopes of the five most dominant antigens associated with SjS, which include Ro52, Ro60, La, muscarinic receptor type III (M3R), and α-fodrin as indicated in Table 3. We conducted the mapping using the artificial neural networks of NetMHCIIpan from the Immune Epitope Database and Analysis Resource (IEDB) as a predictive method to identify the 15-amino acid peptides that could potentially be presented by DRB1*03:01. As indicated in Tables 4–8, predicted peptides with the lowest IC50 values, an indicator of half the maximal inhibitory concentration that characterizes the effectiveness of a peptide in substituting a high-affinity molecule for binding to MHC class II represents the binding affinity of that peptide. The lower the IC50 values, the stronger the binding to DRB1*03:01 by the predicted peptides. IEDB primarily uses the threshold of IC50 to select the strong peptide binders respective to the MHC. Peptide binding to MHC class II protein is based on the discrete anchor residues at pockets 1, 4, 6/7, and 9 [35] and these anchor peptide-binding motifs can be used to predict the specific T cell response.

As presented in Table 4 and Figure 1, predicted Ro52 peptides on HLA-DR3 showed the core peptide with an anchor hydrophobic residue leucine at position 1, followed by a negatively charged residue at position 4 with the top-scoring aspartic acid residue and arginine residue at positions 6 and 9. The predicted Ro60 peptides showed a similar trend, in which lysine or phenylalanine (being predominantly a hydrophobic amino acid) was predicted at position 1 followed by a negatively charged residue at position 4, positively charged histidine, lysine, or arginine at position 6, and a positively charged residue at position 9 (Table 5 and Figure 2). The La predicted peptides also indicate the same pattern with isoleucine being present at position 1, followed by a positively charged or uncharged side chain amino acid (e.g., aspartic acid) at position 4 and a polar uncharged side chain at position 6 with a hydrophobic side chain at position 9 (Table 6 and Figure 3). The M3R predicted amino acid 9-mers indicate predominantly hydrophobic side-chained amino acids throughout the entire structure at positions 1, 4, 6, and 9 (Table 7 and Figure 4). Being a 240 KDa protein, α-fodrin showed a similar motif to Ro52, Ro60, and La with a hydrophobic amino acid at position 1 and predominantly charged amino acids at position 4 (predominantly negative) and 6 (predominantly positive), with a hydrophobic amino acid (i.e., lysine) at position 9, as shown in Table 8 and Figure 5.

Table 1. Identifying high-risk human leukocyte antigen (HLA) alleles in Sjögren's syndrome (SjS).

Country of Origin/Population	HLA Alleles Connotation	Auto-Antibodies Identified	References
U.S.A./American Caucasian	HLA-B8	ND *	[36]
U.S.A./American Caucasian	HLA-Dw3	ND *	[22]
U.S.A./American Caucasian	HLA-Dw3-HLA-B8	ND *	[12]
U.S.A./American Caucasian	HLA-DRw3-HLA-B8	Antinuclear antibodies Ro60	[37]
U.S.A./American Caucasian	HLA-DRw3-HLA-B8	Ro52	[18]
U.S.A./American Caucasian	HLA-DRw52	SS-A	[38]
Japan/Japanese population	HLA-DRB1*0301 HLA-DRB3*0101 HLA-DQA1*0501/DQB1*0201	SS-A and SS-B	[39]
Japan/Japanese population	HLA-DRB1*0405 HLA-DRB4*0101 HLA-DQA1*0301/DQB1*0401	SS-A and SS-B	[39]
Japan/Japanese population	HLA-DRw53	Ro/SS-A and La/SS-B	[40]
Japan/Japanese population	HLA-DRB1*8032/DQA1*0103/DQB1*0601 HLA-DRB1*8032 HLA-DRB1*0405-DRB4*0101 HLA-DQA1*0301 HLA-DQB1*0401	Ro/SS-A and La/SS-B	[39,41]
China/Chinese population	HLA-DRB1*0803 HLA-DQA1*0103/DQB1*0601	SS-A and SS-B	[39]
Mexico/Mexican population	HLA-DRB1*01:01 HLA-B*35:01	Ro/SS-A and La/SS-B	[42]
Colombia/Mestizo Colombian population	HLA-DRB1*0301 HLA-DQB1*0201	Ro/SS-A and La/SS-B	[26,32,43]
Israel/Israeli Jewish/Greek	HLA-DQA1*001 HLA-DQA1*0201/DQB1*0501-Jewish HLA-DQA1*0501-Greek	SS-A, and SS-B	[44]
Greece/Greek population	HLA-DRB1*0301	Ro/SSA and anti-La/SSB	[45]
Spain/Spanish population	HLA-Cw7 HLA- DRB1*0301 HLA-DR11	Ro/SSA and anti-La/SSB	[46]

Table 1. *Cont.*

Country of Origin/Population	HLA Alleles Connotation	Auto-Antibodies Identified	References
France/French population	HLA-DRB1*1501 HLA- DRB1*0301 HLA-DQB1*0201 HLA-DQB1*0602	ND *	[33]
France/French population	HLA-DRB1*0301 HLA-DQB1*02	anti-SSA and/or anti-SSB	[31]
Italy/Italian population	HLA-DRB1*0301	anti-Ro/SSA	[47]
Denmark/Danish population	HLA-Dw2	ND *	[23]
Denmark/Danish population	HLA-DQA1*0501 HLA-DQB1*0201 HLA-DQA1*0301	anti-SSA and/or anti-SSB	[48]
Finland/Finnish population	HLA-DRB1*0301 HLA-DQA1*0501 HLA-DQB1*0201	anti-SS-A/Ro and anti-SS-B/La	[49]
Norway/Norwegian Caucasian population	HLA-DRB1*0301	Ro/SSA and La/SSB	[50]
Norway/Norwegian Caucasian population	HLA-DRB1*0301 HLA-DQB1*02 HLA-DQA1*0501	anti-La/SSB strong positive association with DQA1*0501 anti-Ro/SSA and anti-La/SSB autoantibody response was positively associated with DRB1*03, DQB1*02 and DRB1*03/DRB1*15-DQB1*02/DQB1*0602	[19]
United Kingdom/British Caucasian population	HLA-DRB1*0301 HLA-DRw52	Ro/SSA and La/SSB	[51]
Australia/Australian population	HLA-DRB1*0301 HLA-DQA1*0501 HLA-DQB1*02	Ro/SSA and La/SSB	[16]
Tunisian population	HLA-DQB1 CAR1/CAR2	ND *	[52]
European and African American population	HLA-DQB1*0201 HLA-DQA1*0101	SSA	[53]

ND *—not determined.

Table 2. Identifying protective HLA alleles in different autoimmune diseases.

Disease	Protective HLA Class II Allele	References
Graves' disease	HLA-DRB1*07 HLA-DQB1*02 HLA-DQA1*02	[54]
Hashimoto's thyroiditis	HLA-DRB1*07 HLA-DQB1*02 HLA-DQA1*02	[55]
Rheumatoid arthritis	HLA-DRB1*0103 HLA-DRB1*07 HLA-DRB1*1201 HLA-DRB1*1301 HLA-DRB1*1501	[56]
Multiple sclerosis	DRB1*14-DQB1*06-DQA1*0102	[9]
Type 1 diabetes	DRB1*14-DQB1*06-DQA1*0102 DRB1*15-DQB1*06-DQA1*01	[57]
Systemic lupus erythematosus	DR4 DR5 DR11 DR14	[58]

Table 3. Peptides for SjS that have been tested in vivo.

Peptide	Amino Acids	Amino Acid Sequence	In Vivo Confirmation	References	HLA-DR3	IC50
M3R	205–237	LFWQYFVGKRTVPPGECFIQFLSEPTITFGTAI	NOD/LtJ mice	[59]	GECFIQFLSEPTITF	473
	208–227	QYFVGKRTVPPGECFIQFLS Part of second extracellular loop	Immunization of young female NOD/LtJ mice on autoimmune response	[60]	QYFVGKRTVPPGECF	8607
	213–228	KRTVPPGECFIQFLSE	BALB/c	[61]	KRTVPPGECFIQFLS	50,000
	514–527	NTFCDSCIPKTFWN	BALB/c	[61]	NTFCDSCIPKTFWNL	6549
		MTLHSNSTTSPLFPNISSSWVHSPSEAGLP, N1 VHSPSEAGLPLGTVSQLDSYNISGTSGNFS, N2 NISQTSGNFSSNDTSSDPLGGHTIWQV, N3 FTTYIIMNRWALGNLACDLW, Extracellular loop 1 QYFVGKRTVPPGECFIQFLSEP, Extracellular loop 2 VLVNTFCDSCIPKTYWNLGY, Extracellular loop 3	C57BL/6j (B6) mice (M3R+/+) M3R−/− mice Rag1−/− mice	[62]	PNISSSWVHSPSEAG LPLGTVSQLDSYNIS TSGNFSSNDTSSDPL FTTYIIMNRWALGNL QYFVGKRTVPPGECF VLVNTFCDSCIPKTY	4760 6028 6471 955 8607 5219
	H 441–465	PAGGTDCSLPMIWAQKTNTPADVFI	SJL/L (H-2s) A/J(H-2a)	[63]	TDCSLPMIWAQKTNT	2068
	H 316–335	KARIHPFHILIALETYKTGH	SJL/L (H-2s) BALB/c (H-2d) A/J(H-2a)	[63]	IHPFHILIALETYKT	1485
	H 306–325	EKLCNEKLLKKARIHPFHIL	SJL/L (H-2s)	[63]	EKLLKKARIHPFHIL	1721
	H 26–45	QVTDMNRLHRFLCFGSEGGT	SJL/L (H-2s)	[63]	QVTDMNRLHRFLCFG	2266
	H 401–425	MVVTREKDSYVVAFSDEMVPCPVT	SJL/L (H-2s) A/J(H-2a)	[63]	REKDSYVVAFSDEMV	2879
	H 481–505	IALREYRKKMDIPAKLIVCGMSTNG	SJL/L (H-2s)	[63]	REYRKKMDIPAKLIV	622
	H 201–225	YITKGWKEVHELYKEKALSVETEKL	BALB/c (H-2d)	[63]	VHELYKEKALSVETE	2191
	H 241–265	ELEVIHLIEEHRLLTNHLKS	BALB/c (H-2d) A/J(H-2a)	[63]	VIHLIEEHRLLTNHL	130
Ro52	Full peptide	Full protein	New Zealand Mixed Mice (NZMZ) 2758	[64]	NPWLILSEDRRQVRL	28
Ro60	480–494	AIALREYRKKMDIPA	Animals were immunized with peptide Ro480–494	[65,66]	AIALREYRKKMDIPA	1876
	274–290	QEMPLTALLRNLGKMT	Animals were immunized with peptide Ro274–290	[65,66]	EMPLTALLRNLGKMT	1598

Table 3. *Cont.*

Peptide	Amino Acids	Amino Acid Sequence	In Vivo Confirmation	References	HLA-DR3	IC50
	274–290	Human QEMPLTALLRNLGKMT Mouse QEMPLTALLRNLGKMT	Amino acid sequences of the human 60-kd Ro peptides used for immunization of BALB/c mice	[67]	EMPLTALLRNLGKMT	1598
	413–428	Human VAFSDEMVPCPVTTDM Mouse VAFACDMVPFPVTTDM Rabbit VAFSDEMVPCPLTTDM			VAFSDEMVPCPVTTD	20,917
	480–495	Human AIALREYRKKMDIPA Mouse AVALREYRKKMDIPA			AIALREYRKKMDIPA	1876
La	1–107	GYVDISLLVSFNKMKKLTTDGKLI ARALKSSSVVELDLEGTRIRRKKP LGERPKDEEERTVYVELLPKNVTH KAKKRAQKDGVGQAASEVSKESRDL		[68]	MKKLTTDGKLIARAL	136
	243–345	EFCSTEEEKETDRKGDSLSKVKRK HK KKHKERHKMGEEVIPLRVLSKTEW MDLKKEYLALQKASMASLKKTISQ EQAAKAIEFLNNPPEEAPRK			SKTEWMDLKKEYLAL	922
	111–242	PGIFPKTVKNKPIPSLRVAEEKKKKKKKG RIKKEESVQAKESAVDSSSSGVCKATKRPR TASEGSEAETPEAPKQPAKKKKKRDKVEA SSLPEARAGKRERCSAEDEDCL			SSSGVCKATKRPRTA	561

Table 4. HLA-DR3 allele with predicted peptides of human Ro52.

Allele	Start	End	Length	Core Sequence	Peptide Sequence	IC50	Percentile Rank	Adjusted Rank
HLA-DRB1*03:01	297	311	15	LSEDRRQVR	NPWLILSEDRRQVRL	28.00	0.10	0.10
HLA-DRB1*03:01	296	310	15	LILSEDRRQ	ANPWLILSEDRRQVR	29.00	0.11	0.11
HLA-DRB1*03:01	298	312	15	LSEDRRQVR	PWLILSEDRRQVRLG	29.00	0.11	0.11
HLA-DRB1*03:01	299	313	15	LSEDRRQVR	WLILSEDRRQVRLGD	29.00	0.11	0.11
HLA-DRB1*03:01	300	314	15	LSEDRRQVR	LILSEDRRQVRLGDT	29.00	0.11	0.11
HLA-DRB1*03:01	301	315	15	LSEDRRQVR	ILSEDRRQVRLGDTQ	90.00	0.91	0.91
HLA-DRB1*03:01	302	316	15	LSEDRRQVR	LSEDRRQVRLGDTQQ	93.00	0.95	0.95

Table 5. HLA-DR3 allele with predicted peptides of human Ro60.

Allele	Start	End	Length	Core Sequence	Peptide Sequence	IC50	Percentile Rank	Adjusted Rank
HLA-DRB1*03:01	197	211	15	LEKDEREQL	LQELEKDEREQLRIL	129.00	1.60	1.60
HLA-DRB1*03:01	196	210	15	LEKDEREQL	QLQELEKDEREQLRI	137.00	1.60	1.60
HLA-DRB1*03:01	198	212	15	LEKDEREQL	QELEKDEREQLRILG	137.00	1.60	1.60
HLA-DRB1*03:01	126	140	15	FKKDLKESM	FTFIQFKKDLKESMK	75.00	0.70	0.70
HLA-DRB1*03:01	127	141	15	FKKDLKESM	TFIQFKKDLKESMKC	75.00	0.70	0.70
HLA-DRB1*03:01	125	139	15	LFTFIQFKK	LFTFIQFKKDLKESM	76.00	0.74	0.74
HLA-DRB1*03:01	244	258	15	LIEEHRLVR	VIHLIEEHRLVREHL	78.00	0.76	0.76
HLA-DRB1*03:01	128	142	15	FKKDLKESM	FIQFKKDLKESMKCG	79.00	0.77	0.77
HLA-DRB1*03:01	245	259	15	LIEEHRLVR	IHLIEEHRLVREHLL	80.00	0.77	0.77
HLA-DRB1*03:01	129	143	15	FKKDLKESM	IQFKKDLKESMKCGM	81.00	0.79	0.79
HLA-DRB1*03:01	242	256	15	LIEEHRLVR	LEVIHLIEEHRLVRE	82.00	0.82	0.82
HLA-DRB1*03:01	243	257	15	LIEEHRLVR	EVIHLIEEHRLVREH	82.00	0.82	0.82
HLA-DRB1*03:01	241	255	15	ELEVIHLIE	ELEVIHLIEEHRLVR	83.00	0.83	0.83

Table 6. HLA-DR3 allele with predicted peptides of human La.

Allele	Start	End	Length	Core Sequence	Peptide Sequence	IC50	Percentile Rank	Adjusted Rank
HLA-DRB1*03:01	328	15	15	IIEDQQESL	ALKKIIEDQQESLNK	49.00	0.36	0.36
HLA-DRB1*03:01	327	15	15	IIEDQQESL	EALKKIIEDQQESLN	50.00	0.37	0.37
HLA-DRB1*03:01	326	15	15	KEALKKIIE	KEALKKIIEDQQESL	51.00	0.38	0.38
HLA-DRB1*03:01	329	15	15	IIEDQQESL	LKKIIEDQQESLNKW	51.00	0.38	0.38
HLA-DRB1*03:01	330	15	15	IIEDQQESL	KKIIEDQQESLNKWK	54.00	0.40	0.40
HLA-DRB1*03:01	91	15	15	ISEDKTKIR	AELMEISEDKTKIRR	131.00	1.60	1.60

Table 7. HLA-DR3 allele with predicted peptides of human M3R.

Allele	Start	End	Length	Core Sequence	Peptide Sequence	IC50	Percentile Rank	Adjusted Rank
HLA-DRB1*03:01	192	206	15	AWVISFVLW	AWVISFVLWAPAILF	120.00	1.40	1.40
HLA-DRB1*03:01	195	209	15	VLWAPAILF	ISFVLWAPAILFWQY	121.00	1.40	1.40
HLA-DRB1*03:01	193	207	15	VLWAPAILF	WVISFVLWAPAILFW	123.00	1.50	1.50
HLA-DRB1*03:01	194	208	15	VLWAPAILF	VISFVLWAPAILFWQ	123.00	1.50	1.50
HLA-DRB1*03:01	196	210	15	VLWAPAILF	SFVLWAPAILFWQYF	125.00	1.50	1.50
HLA-DRB1*03:01	375	389	15	ILNSTKLPS	STILNSTKLPSSDNL	169.00	2.30	2.30
HLA-DRB1*03:01	374	388	15	ILNSTKLPS	HSTILNSTKLPSSDN	170.00	2.30	2.30
HLA-DRB1*03:01	371	385	15	LPGHSTILN	LPGHSTILNSTKLPS	171.00	2.30	2.30
HLA-DRB1*03:01	372	386	15	ILNSTKLPS	PGHSTILNSTKLPSS	171.00	2.30	2.30
HLA-DRB1*03:01	373	387	15	ILNSTKLPS	GHSTILNSTKLPSSD	171.00	2.30	2.30
HLA-DRB1*03:01	548	562	15	FRTTFKMLL	NKTFRTTFKMLLLCQ	198.00	2.70	2.70
HLA-DRB1*03:01	546	560	15	FRTTFKMLL	LCNKTFRTTFKMLLL	199.00	2.70	2.70
HLA-DRB1*03:01	549	563	15	FRTTFKMLL	KTFRTTFKMLLLCQC	199.00	2.70	2.70
HLA-DRB1*03:01	547	561	15	FRTTFKMLL	CNKTFRTTFKMLLLC	200.00	2.70	2.70

Table 8. HLA-DR3 allele with predicted peptides of human α-fodrin.

Allele	Start	End	Length	Core Sequence	Peptide Sequence	IC50	Percentile Rank	Adjusted Rank
HLA-DRB1*03:01	1318	1332	15	SHDLQRFLS	SHDLQRFLSDFRDLM	12.00	0.01	0.01
HLA-DRB1*03:01	1319	1333	15	FLSDFRDLM	HDLQRFLSDFRDLMS	12.00	0.01	0.01
HLA-DRB1*03:01	1320	1334	15	FLSDFRDLM	DLQRFLSDFRDLMSW	12.00	0.01	0.01
HLA-DRB1*03:01	1322	1336	15	FLSDFRDLM	QRFLSDFRDLMSWIN	12.00	0.01	0.01
HLA-DRB1*03:01	363	377	15	FLADFRDLT	LQRFLADFRDLTSWV	26.00	0.06	0.06
HLA-DRB1*03:01	360	374	15	SYRLQRFLA	SYRLQRFLADFRDLT	27.00	0.07	0.07
HLA-DRB1*03:01	361	375	15	FLADFRDLT	YRLQRFLADFRDLTS	27.00	0.07	0.07
HLA-DRB1*03:01	362	376	15	FLADFRDLT	RLQRFLADFRDLTSW	27.00	0.07	0.07
HLA-DRB1*03:01	364	378	15	FLADFRDLT	QRFLADFRDLTSWVT	28.00	0.10	0.10
HLA-DRB1*03:01	1323	1337	15	FLSDFRDLM	RFLSDFRDLMSWING	36.00	0.16	0.16
HLA-DRB1*03:01	1324	1338	15	FLSDFRDLM	FLSDFRDLMSWINGI	37.00	0.17	0.17
HLA-DRB1*03:01	365	379	15	FLADFRDLT	RFLADFRDLTSWVTE	83.00	0.83	0.83
HLA-DRB1*03:01	366	380	15	FLADFRDLT	FLADFRDLTSWVTEM	85.00	0.83	0.83

In summary, in silico antigenic epitope mapping of DRB1*03:01 allele with Ro52, Ro60, La, M3R, and α-fodrin showed that the general trend of all peptides predicted to bind have a backbone structure with position 1 being occupied by a hydrophobic residue, position 4 favors charged amino acids, position 6 favors negatively charged amino acids, and position 9 (especially for Ro52, Ro60) having a positively charged amino acid; α-fodrin was an anomaly preferring a hydrophobic residue at this position. La and M3R mostly indicate hydrophobic residues and amino acids with polar uncharged side chains. This also predicts the nature of the pockets in HLA DRB1*03:01, with positions 1 and 4 being rigid, whereas flexibility in the presentation of amino acids on positions 6 and 9 with either charged or hydrophobic amino acids.

3.2. Elucidating the Nature of Predicted Peptides Presented on Other Risk Alleles

As presented in Table 1, in addition to the HLA-DRB1*03:01 allele, there are other pertinent risk HLA alleles that were shown to associate with SjS. To further characterize the antigenic epitopes, we selected five different predominant alleles, specifically HLA-DRB1*01:01, HLA-DRB1*15:01, HLA DRB1*04:05, HLA-DRB4*01:01, and HLA-DRB3*01:01. As indicated in Table 9, Ro52 with the same trend of hydrophobic and charged peptides indicates a strong predictive binding by the NetMHCIIPan for the HLA-DRB1*01:01 and HLA DRB1*04:05 alleles with IC50 values that are lower than 50 nM. Most Ro60 potential binders showed higher IC50 predicted scores for most peptides identifying them to be poor binders (Table 10). La predicted peptides point toward having a slightly different amino acid composition for predicted peptides, with the second anchor position being primarily hydrophobic instead of negatively charged (Table 11). M3R peptides showed a wide disparity in predicted peptide binding for some alleles, suggesting that M3R antigens may be selectively processed and presented based on the presence of alleles such as HLA DRB1*04:05, HLA- DRB1*15:01, and HLA-DRB1*01:01 (Table 12). Lastly, α-fodrin peptide analysis indicates a slightly different sequence of peptides on most risk alleles, as indicated in Table 13. Following a similar pattern to the peptide composition presented with slight deviations in HLA-DRB3*01:01 and HLA DRB1*04:05, it was observed that HLA-DRB1*01:01 and HLA- DRB1*15:01 had similar peptide presentation patterns to HLA-DRB1*03:01, indicating the higher probability of these alleles presenting the same peptides. In summary, in silico antigenic epitope mapping of HLA-DRB1*01:01, HLA-DRB1*15:01, HLA DRB1*04:05, HLA-DRB4*01:01, and HLA-DRB3*01:01 alleles with Ro52, Ro60, La, M3R, and α-fodrin showed that a similar trend of positions 1 and 4 having hydrophobic and positively charged residues but positions 6 and 9 being fluid to present either a charged or a hydrophobic amino acid for most predicted peptides.

Table 9. Predicted peptides on risk alleles for human Ro52.

Allele	Core Sequence	Peptide Sequence	IC50
HLA-DRB1*01:01	LKNLRPNRQ	RFLLKNLRPNRQLAN	44.00
	RFLLKNLRP	CRQRFLLKNLRPNRQ	52.00
HLA-DRB1*15:01	TGPLRPFFS	CAFTGPLRPFFSPGF	122.00
	LRPFFSPGF	AFTGPLRPFFSPGFN	123.00
HLA -DRB1*04:05	EAGMVSFYN	LDYEAGMVSFYNITD	39.00
	MVSFYNITD	DYEAGMVSFYNITDH	39.00
HLA-DRB4*01:01	LKNLRPNRQ	RFLLKNLRPNRQLAN	102.00
	RFLLKNLRP	CRQRFLLKNLRPNRQ	110.00
HLA-DRB3*01:01	KRADWKEVI	IAIKRADWKEVIIVL	229.00
	EVEIAIKRA	EVEIAIKRADWKEVI	247.00

Table 10. Predicted peptides on risk alleles for human Ro60.

Allele	Core Sequence	Peptide Sequence	IC50
HLA-DRB1*01:01	LFTFIQFKK	LFTFIQFKKDLKESM	286.00
	FKKDLKESM	FTFIQFKKDLKESMK	289.00
HLA-DRB1*15:01	IQEIKSFSQ	CEVIQEIKSFSQEGR	238.00
	VIQEIKSFS	GRGCEVIQEIKSFSQ	251.00
HLA-DRB1*04:05	LRLSHLKPS	HKDLLRLSHLKPSSE	75.00
	LSHLKPSSE	DLLRLSHLKPSSEGK	75.00
HLA-DRB4*01:01	TYYIKEQKL	EGGTYYIKEQKLGLE	228.00
	KDLLRLSHL	SHKDLLRLSHLKPSS	237.00
HLA-DRB3*01:01	LFTFIQFKK	LFTFIQFKKDLKESM	286.00
	FKKDLKESM	FTFIQFKKDLKESMK	289.00

Table 11. Predicted peptides on risk alleles for human La.

Allele	Core Sequence	Peptide Sequence	IC50
HLA-DRB1*01:01	FNVIVEALS	TDFNVIVEALSKSKA	52.00
	DFNVIVEAL	NRLTTDFNVIVEALS	60.00
HLA- DRB1*15:01	LHILFSNHG	REDLHILFSNHGEIK	34.00
	DLHILFSNH	QTCREDLHILFSNHG	37.00
HLA-DRB1*04:05	FNVIVEALS	LTTDFNVIVEALSKS	66.00
	NRLTTDFNV	NRLTTDFNVIVEALS	67.00
HLA-DRB4*01:01	EIMIKFNRL	VPLEIMIKFNRLNRL	75.00
	IKFNRLNRL	PLEIMIKFNRLNRLT	77.00
HLA-DRB3*01:01	DLDDQTCRE	DLDDQTCREDLHILF	142.00
	CREDLHILF	LDDQTCREDLHILFS	143.00

Table 12. Predicted peptides on risk alleles for human M3R.

Allele	Core Sequence	Peptide Sequence	IC50
HLA-DRB1*01:01	IAFLTGILA	VVFIAFLTGILALVT	9.00
	LTGILALVT	FIAFLTGILALVTII	12.00
HLA- DRB1*15:01	IIGNILVIV	VTIIGNILVIVSFKV	14.00
	ILVIVSFKV	IIGNILVIVSFKVNK	14.00
HLA-DRB1*04:05	VPPGECFIQ	VPPGECFIQFLSEPT	7.00
	FIQFLSEPT	PPGECFIQFLSEPTI	7.00
HLA-DRB4*01:01	LVTIIGNIL	GILALVTIIGNILVI	88.00
	IGVISMNLF	ADLIIGVISMNLFTT	98.00
HLA-DRB3*01:01	GECFIQFLS	GECFIQFLSEPTITF	124.00
	FLSEPTITF	ECFIQFLSEPTITFG	127.00

Table 13. Predicted peptides on risk alleles for human α-fodrin.

Allele	Core Sequence	Peptide Sequence	IC50
HLA-DRB1*01:01	FQKIKSMAA	NGRFQKIKSMAASRR	3.00
	IKLLQAQKL	MREKGIKLLQAQKLV	5.00
HLA- DRB1*15:01	WRRLKAQMI	LDRWRRLKAQMIEKR	68.00
	EVLDRWRRL	NEVLDRWRRLKAQMI	71.00
HLA-DRB1*04:05	FRSSLSSAQ	HDAFRSSLSSAQADF	38.00
	HDAFRSSLS	REAHDAFRSSLSSAQ	39.00
HLA-DRB4*01:01	KMREKGIKL	KMREKGIKLLQAQKL	5.00
	IKLLQAQKL	MREKGIKLLQAQKLV	5.00
HLA-DRB3*01:01	IQETRTYLL	IQETRTYLLDGSCMV	25.00
	YLLDGSCMV	QETRTYLLDGSCMVE	25.00

*3.3. Homology of Predicted Peptides Binding to HLA-DRB1*03:01 to Viral and Bacterial Proteins*

Molecular mimicry is one of the main mechanisms by which infections might trigger autoimmune disease [69]. Several viruses and bacteria have been implicated as potential etiological agents in human patients, and specific viruses were determined to cause various clinical signs of SjS in animal models. However, there is still little information about the causative role in disease initiation and progression [70]. As presented, we have identified specific antigenic epitopes of the DRB1*03:01 allele with Ro52, Ro60, La, M3R, and α-fodrin proteins in silico. To determine whether these antigenic epitopes mimic viral and bacterial proteins, we utilized the BLAST tool to identify the amino acid homology between the SjS-associated antigenic epitopes of HLA-DRB1*03:01 and all known viral proteins in the Uniprot databases. As presented in Table 14, Ro52 peptides showed similarities between bat viruses such as *Miniopterus schreibersii* polyomavirus, and other plant-based pathogens. Ro60 peptides showed 100% homology between *Botrytis* (gray mold) viruses which have been stipulated to infect *Botrytis* (a major agricultural hazard) [71]. M3R peptides showed 88.9% homology between a variety of plant-based viral pathogens and affected the growth of agriculture and horticulture-based fungi (pests). La and human/mouse α-fodrin peptides indicate a similarity between *Helenium* virus and *Caudovirales* phages that belong to the family of multiple *Carlaviruses* that infect various ornamental plants [72]. As presented in Table 15 for bacterial proteins, Ro52 predicted core peptides showed 100% homology to *Stigmatella aurantiaca* and *Cystobacter fuscus* that are naturally occurring and a promising source for the discovery of new biologically active natural products [73,74]. Ro60 peptides did not indicate homology to any known bacterial peptides as represented. M3R peptides present a likeness with *Desulfobacterales bacterium* that has a sulfur-based metabolism [75]. La peptides showed 100% similarity between *Pseudomonas* species which is known to cause pneumonia and infections in blood [76], while α-fodrin peptides are homologous to certain aquatic and terrestrial bacteria with an 88.9% similarity. In summary, the results suggest that several environmental factors may be involved in the pathogenesis of SjS, with the main role being played by infectious agents for animals or plants, with molecular homologs acting as triggers that may contribute to disease progression in the existence of a predisposing genetic background.

Table 14. Homology of predicted peptides binding to HLA-DRB1*03:01 to viral proteins.

Protein	Predicted Peptide	Virus	Protein	Homology with Sequence (Percentage)
Human Ro52	LEKDEREQL	*Miniopterus schreibersii* polyomavirus 1	Large T antigen	88.9%
		Micromonas pusilla virus PL1	Uncharacterized	77.8%
		Miniopterus schreibersii polyomavirus 1	Small T antigen	88.9%
Mouse Ro52	MEMDLTMQR		*Wiseana iridescent* virus (WIV) (Insect iridescent virus type 9)	70%
Mouse Ro52	KELAEKMEM	*Mimivirus* LCMiAC02	Uncharacterized	77.8%
Mouse Ro60	LFTFIQFKK	*Botrytis* virus X (isolate *Botrytis cinerea*/New Zealand/Howitt/2006) (BOTV-X)	RNA replication	100%
Human Ro60	LFTFIQFKK	*Botrytis* virus X (isolate *Botrytis cinerea*/New Zealand/Howitt/2006) (BOTV-X)B19:B22	RNA replication protein	100%
Human M3R	AWVISFVLW	*Pseudomonas* phage PaMx74	Putative membrane protein	75%
Human M3R	LPGHSTILN	Pepper mild mottle virus (strain Spain) (PMMV-S)	Replicase large subunit	88.9%
		Odontoglossum ringspot virus (isolate Korean Cy) (ORSV-Cy)	Replicase large	88.9%
		Tobacco mild green mosaic virus (TMGMV) (TMV strain U2)	Replicase large subunit	88.9%
		Turnip vein-clearing virus (TVCV)	Replicase large subunit	88.9%
		Youcai mosaic virus (YoMV)	Replicase large subunit	88.9%
		Hoya necrotic spot virus	Methyltransferase/RNA helicase	88.9%
		Odontoglossum ringspot virus	Methyltransferase/RNA helicase	88.9%
		Virgaviridae sp.	Replication-associated protein	88.9%
		Tobacco mild green mosaic virus (TMGMV) (TMV strain U2)	Replicase large subunit	88.9%
		Brugmansia mild mottle virus	Methyltransferase/RNA helicase	88.9%
		Streptocarpus flower break virus	Methyltransferase/RNA helicase	88.9%
		Ribgrass mosaic virus (RMV)	Methyltransferase/RNA helicase	88.9%
		Wasabi mottle virus	Methyltransferase/RNA helicase	88.9%
		Piper chlorosis virus	Replicase large subunit	88.9%
Human La	KEALKKIIE	*Helenium* virus S (HelVS)	Helicase	88.9%
		Arthrobacter phage Boersma	DNA polymerase I	100%
Human/Mouse α-fodrin	SYRLQRFLA	Uncultured Caudovirales phage	Uncharacterized protein	88.9%

Table 15. Homology of predicted peptides binding to HLA-DRB1*03:01 to bacterial proteins.

Human Ro52	LSEDRRQVR	*Stigmatella aurantiaca* (strain DW4/3-1)	Peptidase, M20 family	100%
		Cystobacter fuscus DSM 2262	Acetylornithine deacetylase	100%
		Stigmatella aurantiaca (strain DW4/3-1)	Peptidase, M20/M25/M40 family	100%
Human Ro52	LEKDEREQL	*Geobacter* sp. (strain M21)	Endopeptidase La	100%
		Seonamhaeicola marinus	RNA polymerase sigma factor	100%
Mouse Ro52	MEMDLTMQR	*Sulfuriferula nivalis*	Phytoene synthase	88.9%
		Corallococcus exercitus	Phytoene/squalene synthase	88.9%
		Corallococcus aberystwythensis	Phytoene/squalene synthase	88.9%
		Corallococcus sp. CA047B	Phytoene/squalene synthase	88.9%
		Corallococcus exercitus	Phytoene/squalene synthase	88.9%
Mouse Ro52	KELAEKMEM	*Arenicella xantha*	RNA pol sigma factor	100%
		Gamma proteobacterium SS-5	RNA pol sigma factor	100%
		Granulosicoccus antarcticus	RNA pol sigma factor	100%
		Gammaproteobacteria bacterium	RNA pol sigma factor	100%
		Granulosicoccus sp.	RNA pol sigma factor	100%
		Candidatus Methyloumidiphilum	RNA pol sigma factor	100%
		Gammaproteobacteria bacterium	Fumarate flavoprotein	100%
		Tindallia magadiensis	RNA pol sigma factor	100%
		Oceanospirillales bacterium	RNA pol sigma factor	100%
		Cyanobacterium sp. IPPAS	RNA pol sigma factor	100%
		Cyanobacterium sp. HL-69	RNA pol sigma factor	100%
		Culicoidibacter larvae	RNA pol sigma factor	100%
		Chromobacterium violaceum	RNA pol sigma factor	100%
		Cyanobacterium stanieri	RNA pol sigma factor	100%
		Clostridium cellulovorans	RNA pol sigma factor	100%
		Anaerolineaceae bacterium	RNA pol sigma factor	100%
		Pseudobythopirellula maris	RNA pol sigma factor	100%
		Bacteroidetes bacterium	RNA pol sigma factor	100%
		Epulopiscium sp.	RNA pol sigma factor	100%
		Betaproteobacteria bacterium	RNA pol sigma factor	100%
		Fulvivirga imtechensis AK7		100%
Human M3R	AWVISFVLW	*Planctomycetes bacterium*	Uncharacterized protein	88.9%
Mouse M3R	VLWAPAILF	*Desulfobacterales bacterium*	Site-2 protease family protein	88.9%
Human La	KEALKKIIE	*Candidatus Dojkabacteria* bacterium	Uncharacterized protein	100%
		Hydrogenimonas sp.	Anthranilate phosphoribosyltransferase	100%
		candidate division WOR-3 bacterium	Uncharacterized protein	100%
Mouse La	QRYWQKILV	*Planctomycetes bacterium* SM23_25	Uncharacterized protein	88.9%
Mouse La	ILVDRQAKL	*Pseudomonas* sp. NFR16	Uncharacterized	100.0%
		Pseudomonas sp. Bc-h	Uncharacterized	100.0%
		Pseudomonas sp. GV021	Uncharacterized	100.0%
		Pseudomonas abietaniphila	Uncharacterized	100.0%
		Pseudomonas graminis	DUF2914 family	100.0%
		Pseudomonas graminis	Uncharacterized	100.0%
		Pseudomonas graminis	Uncharacterized	100.0%
		Pseudomonas graminis	DUF2914 domain	100.0%
		Pseudomonas graminis	Uncharacterized	100.0%
		Pseudomonas sp.	DUF2914 domain	100.0%
		Pseudomonas sp. NFACC02	Uncharacterized	100.0%
		Pseudomonas sp. LP_7_YM	DUF2914 domain	100.0%
		Pseudomonas sp. M47T1	Uncharacterized	100.0%
		Pseudomonas eucalypticola	DUF2914 domain	100.0%
		Pseudomonas sp. K1S02-6	DUF2914 domain	100.0%
Human/Mouse α-fodrin	FLSDFRDLM	*Cocleimonas flava*	Uncharacterized	88.9%
		Verrucomicrobiales bacterium	Uncharacterized	88.9%
		Planctomycetaceae bacterium	SH3 domain	88.9%

3.4. Homology of Predicted Peptides Binding to Other Risk HLA Alleles to Viral and Bacterial Proteins

As indicated previously, we have also identified antigenic epitopes of HLA-DRB1*01:01, HLA-DRB1*15:01, HLA-DRB1*04:05, HLA-DRB4*01:01, and HLA-DRB3*01:01 alleles with Ro52, Ro60, La, M3R, and α-fodrin. To further determine if these antigenic epitopes mimic any known viral or bacterial proteins, we compared these peptide sequences using the Uniprot databases. As presented in Table 16, Ro60 predicted peptides of HLA-DRB1*01:01 showed homology with the RNA replication protein of *Botrytis* virus X. *Salmonella* phage SPFM12 showed a similarity to La peptides. In contrast, the M3R peptides indicated a 100% similarity with the *Bacillus* phage. While the α-fodrin peptides for this allele did not indicate a homology with any viral proteins, they were very similar to naturally occurring bacteria that are responsible for fermentation, such as *Candidatus pseudoramibacter* [77] and *Eubacteriaceae bacterium,* which is a pathogen that has been recently found to contribute to colorectal cancer initiation via promoting colitis [78]. HLA- DRB1*15:01 exhibited a homology for either bacteria or viruses for Ro52, Ro6,0, and La. Still, it yielded a 100% homology to the viral protein u (Vpu) protein of the human immunodeficiency virus 1 (HIV-1) to the M3R peptide (IIGNILVIV). Furthermore, HLA- DRB1*15:01 allele is predicted to present peptide EVLDRWRRL, which is very similar to many proteins found in *Streptomyces* and *Saccharopolyspora* species which have been investigated extensively for their bioactive natural pharmacological products [79]. The allele HLA-DRB4*01:01 was shown to present RFLLKNLRP peptide of Ro52. This specific peptide showed a 100% homology between the glycoprotein 120 (gp120) of HIV-1. The RFLLKNLRP peptide of Ro52 also showed homology with many phages and other viruses. Lastly, TYYIKEQKL peptide of Ro60 showed a similarity between the Ro-like RNA binding protein for the *Streptomyces* phage.

Compared to the bacterial proteins (Table 17), we found that *Helicobacter* sp. showed a 100% homology with the Ro60 peptide IKLLQAQKL. *Helicobacter* sp. has been found to cause chronic gastritis and plays an important role in peptic ulcer disease, gastric carcinoma, and gastric lymphoma. In addition, the homology between Ro60 peptide TYYIKEQKL of HLA-DRB4*01:01 and *Fusobacterium necrophorum*, a rare causative agent of otitis and sinusitis, indicates the linkage of an oral biology homologue [80]. HLA-DRB3*01:01 for both Ro52 and La peptides showed *Virgibacillus massiliensis* and *Oscillospiraceae* bacterium, which have been isolated from the human stool and may form a part of the microbiome, had a 100% homology with CREDLHILF (La) and KRADWKEVI (Ro52) [81,82]. The α-fodrin peptide IKLLQAQKL was indicated to be 100% similar to the glycosyltransferase protein of both *Eubacteriaceae bacterium* and *Candidatus pseudoramibacter* [83], which are microbes that have been observed in the gut [77]. Alterations in the gut and oral microbiota composition have previously been suggested as possible environmental factors in the etiology of pSjS and SLE [84]. In summary, the results suggest that different species in Table 17 belong to *Bacteriodes, Actinomyces,* and *Lactobacillus* that have been found in patients of both pSjS and SLE [85–88]. In conclusion to the results observed for bacterial homology, it is known that pSjS patients have less diversity in their gut microbiome with less abundant beneficial bacteria and more abundant opportunistic bacteria with pro-inflammatory activity compared with healthy individuals. Out of the primary homologs observed, most of them indicate a 100% homology to the three main bacterial species found in the gut, indicating the gut microbiome contribution in disease progression by molecular mimicry on a genetically predisposed background.

Table 16. Homology of predicted peptides binding to HLA alleles to viral proteins.

Allele	SjS Protein	Core Sequence	Virus	Viral Protein	Homology
HLA-DRB4*01:01	Ro52	RFLLKNLRP	Human Immunodeficiency Virus	Glycoprotein 120	100.0%
			Serratia phage 2050H2	Uncharacterized	87.5%
			Klebsiella phage 31	Endopeptidase Rz	87.5%
			Escherichia phage ECA2	Endopeptidase	87.5%
			Leclercia phage 10164RH	Uncharacterized	87.5%
			Citrobacter phage SH1	Endopeptidase	87.5%
			Citrobacter phage phiCFP-1	Uncharacterized	87.5%
			Serratia phage SALSA	Endopeptidase	87.5%
			Citrobacter phage SH2	Endopeptidase Rz	87.5%
			Klebsiella phage KPP-5	Endopeptidase	87.5%
			Leclercia phage 10164-302	Uncharacterized	87.5%
			Enterobacter phage E-2	Endopeptidase	87.5%
			Klebsiella phage NL_ZS_3	Endopeptidase Rz	87.5%
			Serratia phage SM9-3Y	I-spanin	87.5%
			Escherichia phage LL2	I-spanin	87.5%
			Salmonella phage phiSG-JL2	Gp18.5	87.5%
			Yersinia phage phiYeO3-12	Endopeptidase	87.5%
			Enterobacter phage E-4	Endopeptidase Rz	87.5%
			Enterobacter phage E-3	Endopeptidase	87.5%
			Yersinia phage phiYe-F10	Uncharacterized	87.5%
			Klebsiella phage	endopeptidase	87.5%
HLA-DRB1*01:01	Ro60	LFTFIQFKK	*Botrytis* virus X	RNA replication protein	
100%	Ro60	TYYIKEQKL	*Streptomyces* phage	Ro-like RNA binding protein	88.9%
			Streptomyces phage	Ro-like RNA binding protein	88.9%
			Streptomyces phage Beuffert	Ro-like RNA binding protein	88.9%
			Pyramimonas orientalis virus	Uncharacterized protein	69.2%
		KDLLRLSHL	*Botrytis* virus X	RNA replication	100%
HLA-DRB1*01:01	La	DFNVIVEAL	*Salmonella* phage SPFM12	Uncharacterized	88.9%
HLA-DRB3*01:01	La	DLDDQTCRE	*Leviviridae* sp.	RNA replicase beta chain	64.3%
HLA-DRB1*01:01	M3R	IAFLTGILA	*Bacillus* phage 031MP004	Uncharacterized	100%
			Bacillus phage 055SW001	Uncharacterized	100%
			Bacillus phage 022DV001	Uncharacterized	100%
			Bacillus phage 031MP002	Uncharacterized	100%
			Bacillus phage 031MP003	Uncharacterized	100%
HLA-DRB1*15:01	M3R	IIGNILVIV	Human immunodeficiency virus 1	Protein Vpu	100%

Table 17. Homology of predicted peptides binding to HLA alleles to bacterial proteins.

Allele	SjS Protein	Core Sequence	Bacteria	Bacterial Protein	Homology
HLA -DRB1*04:05	Ro52	EAGMVSFYN	*Legionella moravica*	Ankyrin	88.9%
			Legionella sp. Km535	Ankyrin repeat domain-containing protein	88.9%
	Ro52	MVSFYNITD	*Legionella moravica*	Ankyrin	88.9%
			Legionella sp. Km535	Ankyrin repeat domain-containing protein	88.9%
HLA-DRB4*01:01	Ro60	TYYIKEQKL	*Helicobacter* sp. 11S03491-1	Protoporphyrinogen oxidase	100%
			Fusobacterium	Uncharacterized	100%
			Fusobacterium	Uncharacterized	100%
HLA-DRB3*01:01	La	CREDLHILF	*Virgibacillus massiliensis*	Uncharacterized	100%
HLA-DRB4*01:01	M3R	LVTIIGNIL	Uncultured	Uncharacterized	88.9%
HLA-DRB1*01:01	Alpha Fodrin	IKLLQAQKL	*Eubacteriaceae*	Glycosyltransferase	100.0%
			Candidatus Pseudoramibacter	Glycosyltransferase	100.0%
HLA- DRB1*15:01	Alpha Fodrin	EVLDRWRRL	*Desulfonatronum sp.*	Thioredoxin	88.9%
			Thermoleophilaceae bacterium	Proline RNA ligase	88.9%
			Thermoleophilaceae bacterium	Proline tRNA ligase	88.9%
			Nonomuraea nitratireducens	DUF885 family protein	88.9%
			Nonomuraea phyllanthi	DUF885 domain-containing protein	88.9%
			Firmicutes bacterium	Biotin protein ligase	88.9%
			Firmicutes bacterium	Biotin protein ligase	88.9%
			Streptomyces malaysiensis	Putative non-ribosomal peptide synthetase	100.0%
			Streptomyces malaysiensis	Non-ribosomal peptide synthetase	100.0%
			Streptomyces malaysiensis	Carrier domain-containing protein	100.0%
			Aquisphaera giovannonii	Phosphomannomutase/phosphoglucomutase	100.0%
			Streptomycetaceae bacterium	Uncharacterized protein	88.9%
			Curtobacterium sp. MCPF17_047	Uncharacterized protein	100.0%
			Nitriliruptorales bacterium	DUF1932 domain-containing protein	100.0%
			Paracoccus homiensis	Acetyltransferase (GNAT) family protein	100.0%
			Actinophytocola xanthii	SnoaL-like domain-containing protein	100.0%
			Frigoribacterium sp. PhB160	S-DNA-T family DNA segregation ATPase	100.0%
			Frigoribacterium sp. PhB107	S-DNA-T family DNA segregation ATPase	100.0%
			Frigoribacterium sp. ACAM 257	Cell division protein FtsK	100.0%
			Geodermatophilus sp. DF01_2	Peptidase_M16_C domain-containing protein	100.0%
			Acidobacteria bacterium	Uncharacterized protein	100.0%
			Nitrosococcus oceani C-27	Transposase	88.9%
			Nitrosococcus oceani (strain)	Y1_Tnp domain-containing protein	88.9%
			Dietzia sp. MeA6-2017	Uncharacterized protein	100.0%
			Firmicutes bacterium	Bifunctional ligase/repressor BirA	100.0%
			Dietzia sp. oral taxon 368	Uncharacterized protein	100.0%
			Saccharopolyspora sp. ASAGF58	Uncharacterized protein	100.0%
			Saccharopolyspora spinosa	Uncharacterized protein	100.0%
			Chloroflexi bacterium	Biotin [acetyl-CoA-carboxylase] ligase	100.0%
			Actinobacteria bacterium 13	Biotin [acetyl-CoA-carboxylase] ligase	100.0%
			Pelagibaca abyssi	Uncharacterized protein	100.0%
			Candidatus Kentron sp. LFY	Type III restriction enzyme	88.9%
			Planctomycetes bacterium	Diguanylate cyclase	88.9%
			Candidatus Kentron sp. LFY	Type III restriction enzyme, res subunit	88.9%
			Candidatus Solibacter sp.	3-isopropylmalate dehydratase large subunit	88.9%
			Hyalangium minutum	Uncharacterized protein	88.9%
			Actinokineospora terrae	AraC-type DNA-binding protein	88.9%
			Actinokineospora cianjurensis	AraC-like DNA-binding protein	88.9%
HLA-DRB4*01:01	Alpha Fodrin	IKLLQAQKL	*Eubacteriaceae*	Glycosyltransferase	100.0%
			Candidatus Pseudoramibacter	Glycosyltransferase	100.0%

4. Discussion

HLA genes are the best documented genetic risk factors for the development of autoimmune diseases and could be directly involved in SjS [89]. This study shows the presence of a similar pattern of amino acids that may be presented by the HLAs based on their structure. The similarity and overlap in the peptides presented on different risk alleles suggest that the same antigenic peptides may be responsible for presenting different autoantigens and thereby initiating the autoimmune cascade. In addition, the results provide insight towards not only the genetic predisposition but also environmental and biological factors that contribute to the onset and progression of the disease. The peptide homology represents similarities in peptides presented to the immune system that shows homology to viral pathogens and bacteria that are both environmental triggers. Bacteria form part of the microbiome of an individual.

Different amino acids present at specific positions in the biochemical structure may confer protection in the peptides presented. It has been shown in previous studies that, consistent with our results, the requirements of peptides for binding to HLA-DR3 vary among differer DR3 binding peptides [90]. Similar to our results, the anchor peptides at different positions 4, 6 and 9 indicate the absence of an anchor or the presence of only a weak anchor residue a either position 4 can be compensated for by the presence of a strong, positively charged anchc residue at position 6 in case of both viral antigens and autoimmune peptides [90,91]. Simila to the predicted peptide trend indicated, Verhagen et al. [92] showed that most insulin an pro-insulin peptides presented in type 1 diabetes also show a similar trend of hydrophobi residues at key anchor positions with a mix of charged residues preferred at other anchc locations. In Graves' disease, arginine (a positively charged amino acid) has previously bee reported to confer a high risk if present at a specific position (in the case of the processe peptide presentation), highlighting the importance of specific residues being present at specifi positions for the onset of disease [93,94].

Additionally, we examined certain HLA alleles' protective role that reduces the proba bility of specific antigen presentation. HLA-DRB1*01 allele has been proven to be negativel associated with pSjS, a result consistent with the Hungarian population in the study carrie out by Kovacs et al. [95]. The protective role of the DRB1*01 allele was confirmed by meta-analysis in which serological groups DR1 and DR7 were negatively associated wit pSjS. However, further research is required in the area [32].

Investigating the cross-presentation of the autoantigen epitopes with bacteria o viruses can provide an important insight into a potential mechanism of disease initiatio The results showed predicted peptides of the five autoantigens exhibiting 100% homolog to various reported gut commensal and oral bacteria. Additionally, viral infectious agent that may mimic SjS include hepatitis A, B or C, parvovirus B19, dengue, Epstein Bar virus (EBV), and HIV. Certain viruses express tropism for salivary and lacrimal glandula tissue, especially the herpesvirudae family, which is a large family of DNA viruses tha includes cytomegalovirus (CMV), EBV, and human herpesvirus (HHV)-6,7,8. Several line of epidemiological, serological, and experimental evidence implicate retroviral infections– especially human T-lymphotropic virus type (HTLV)-1, HIVs, human intracisternal A-typ retroviral particle (HIAP)-I, and human rhinoviruses (HRV)-5—as triggering factors fo the development of SjS. The gut is the most abundant site for bacteria, with nearly 100 species having microbes that belong to four major phyla: Firmicutes, Bacteroidetes, Act nobacteria, and Proteobacteria. Bacteroidetes, along with Firmicutes, represent more thar 90% of the entire plethora of microbes in the gut. Based on our findings, the bifunctiona ligase/repressor protein of *Firmicutes bacterium* indicated a 100% homology for a peptid from α-fodrin for the allele HLA- DRB1*15:01. *Eubacteriaceae bacterium, Pseudoramibacte* and other Firmicutes bacteria's glycosyltransferases are indicated to have perfect homolog to a predicted α-fodrin peptide for the allele HLA-DRB4*01:01. There are indications o multiple *Candidatus* bacterial species, which all belong to the *Firmicutes* phylum for multipl predicted peptides in different alleles, as observed in Tables 15 and 17. Most indicated bac teria in the data presented had been found to be from three phyla (*Firmicutes, Bacteroidetes Actinobacteria*) mentioned above that indicate the probability of bacterial peptides being similar to predicted salivary and lacrimal gland-based proteins that are presented on HLA's and result in inflammation.

In this study, we were able to predict antigenic epitopes or pathogenic peptides tha may be presented in SjS based on a structure-based approach for the HLA cell surface protein. The finding may refine the etiology of the autoimmune process. As simplified in Figure 6, the disease progression is initiated by an environmental trigger like a vira infection on a genetically susceptible individual with a specific HLA allele. Salivary gland epithelial cells experience increased apoptosis and act as sources of pro-inflammatory cytokines such as IFN-γ. Macrophages are attracted to the region and act as the main agent for phagocytosis by participating in tissue destruction. Presentation of viral/bacteria antigens by MHC molecules on antigen-presenting cells leads to priming CD4^{+} T cells With the help of T cells, B cells can form lymphocytic infiltrates or participate in ectopic germinal center formation where they can undergo class switching, affinity maturation and differentiation into plasma cells that secrete high levels of antibodies. These antibodies may be cross-reactive against autoantigens such as Ro52, Ro60, La, α-fodrin, and M3R. The autoantibodies can form immune complexes by binding autoantigens and fixing complement or engaging Fc-γ receptors, further facilitating apoptosis. This process results in inflammation and tissue destruction through the recruitment of inflammatory cells and phagocytes to tissues. Apoptotic cells from damaged tissues can be taken up by phagocytes, which present novel autoantigens, supporting further priming and autoreactivity. Therefore, in order to understand the etiology and designing therapies, it is imperative that we understand the genetic factors and the environmental agents working together to create a suitable setting to initiate the autoimmune cascade.

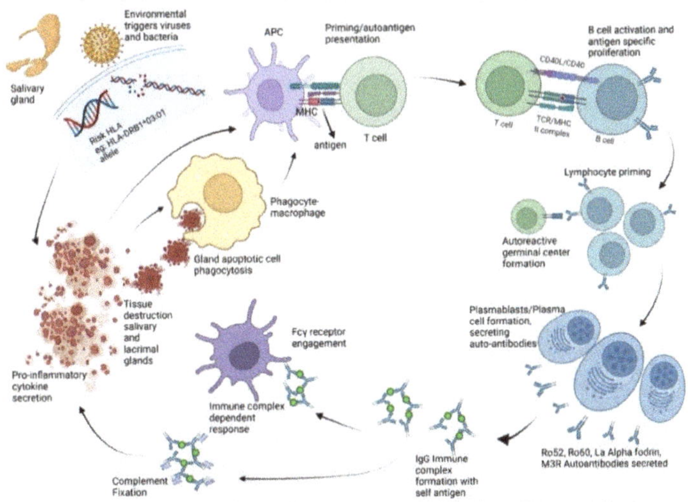

Figure 6. Disease progression for individuals with genetic predisposition (specific HLA) and microbial trigger.

The apparent limitation of the study is that the peptide prediction is strictly based in silico. Since this is an in silico study, the results presented are theoretical and should be subjected to many of the same limitations implicit in the MHC binding affinity prediction tool(s) upon which it is based. Regardless, this is the first study that provides a comprehensive mapping of the antigenic epitopes based on the HLA structure. The advantage of this approach that we describe to map peptides will facilitate in identifying drugs and therapies specific and targeted to disease-susceptible HLA. As listed, many autoimmune diseases are associated with specific HLA alleles and high-resolution crystal structures exist for almost all MHC class II molecules. Strategies for the selection of HLA allele-specific peptides presented and testing their activity in experimental systems can be implemented. Further, this research will aid the ability to identify HLA allele-specific drugs based on the structure that will have applicability for treating autoimmune diseases and other HLA-associated conditions.

Author Contributions: S.G., C.Q.N., D.A.O. and D.L. designed the workflow of all the data generated. D.L. performed the in-silico modeling and docking on HLA-DR3.The authors analyzed all predicted data and prepared the manuscript. All authors have read and agreed to the published version of the manuscript.

Funding: This research was funded by the National Institute of Dental and Craniofacial Research grant number DE028544 and DE028544-02S1.

Institutional Review Board Statement: Not applicable.

Informed Consent Statement: Not applicable.

Acknowledgments: C.Q.N. is supported financially in part by PHS grants DE028544 and DE028544-02S1 from the National Institute of Dental and Craniofacial Research. The content is solely the responsibility of the authors and does not necessarily represent the official views of the National Institutes of Health.

Conflicts of Interest: The authors declare no conflict of interest.

References

1. Nguyen, C.Q.; Sharma, A.; Lee, B.H.; She, J.X.; McIndoe, R.A.; Peck, A.B. Differential gene expression in the salivary gland during development and onset of xerostomia in Sjogren's syndrome-like disease of the C57BL/6.NOD-Aec1Aec2 mouse. *Arthritis Res. Ther.* **2009**, *11*, R56. [CrossRef] [PubMed]
2. Helmick, C.G.; Felson, D.; Lawrence, R.C.; Gabriel, S.; Hirsch, R.; Kwoh, C.K.; Liang, M.H.; Kremers, H.M.; Mayes, M.D.; Merkel, P.A.; et al. Estimates of the prevalence of arthritis and other rheumatic conditions in the United States: Part I. *Arthritis Care Res.* **2007**, *58*, 15–25. [CrossRef]
3. Vivino, F.B.; Bunya, V.Y.; Massaro-Giordano, G.; Johr, C.R.; Giattino, S.L.; Schorpion, A.; Shafer, B.; Peck, A.; Sivils, K.; Rasmussen, A.; et al. Sjogren's syndrome: An update on disease pathogenesis, clinical manifestations and treatment. *Clin. Immunol.* **2019**, *203*, 81–121. [CrossRef]
4. Thomas, E.; Hay, E.M.; Hajeer, A.; Silman, A.J. Sjogren's syndrome: A community-based study of prevalence and impact. *Rheumatology* **1998**, *37*, 1069–1076. [CrossRef]
5. Burbelo, P.D.; Ambatipudi, K.; Alevizos, I. Genome-wide association studies in Sjögren's syndrome: What do the genes tell us about disease pathogenesis? *Autoimmun. Rev.* **2014**, *13*, 756–761. [CrossRef] [PubMed]
6. Haugen, A.J.; Peen, E.; Hultén, B.; Johannessen, A.C.; Brun, J.G.; Halse, A.K.; Haga, H. Estimation of the prevalence of primary Sjögren's syndrome in two age-different community-based populations using two sets of classification criteria: The Hordaland Health Study. *Scand. J. Rheumatol.* **2008**, *37*, 30–34. [CrossRef] [PubMed]
7. Teos, L.Y.; Alevizos, I. Genetics of Sjögren's syndrome. *Clin. Immunol.* **2017**, *182*, 41–47. [CrossRef]
8. Ice, J.A.; Li, H.; Adrianto, I.; Lin, P.C.; Kelly, J.; Montgomery, C.; Lessard, C.J.; Moser, K.L. Genetics of Sjögren's syndrome in the genome-wide association era. *J. Autoimmun.* **2012**, *39*, 57–63. [CrossRef]
9. the International Multiple Sclerosis Genetics Consortium Class II HLA interactions modulate genetic risk for multiple sclerosis. *Nat. Genet.* **2015**, *47*, 1107–1113. [CrossRef]
10. Fernando, M.M.A.; Stevens, C.R.; Walsh, E.C.; De Jager, P.L.; Goyette, P.; Plenge, R.M.; Vyse, T.J.; Rioux, J.D. Defining the Role of the MHC in Autoimmunity: A Review and Pooled Analysis. *PLoS Genet.* **2008**, *4*, e1000024. [CrossRef]
11. Cobb, B.L.; Lessard, C.J.; Harley, J.B.; Moser, K.L. Genes and Sjögren's Syndrome. *Rheum. Dis. Clin. N. Am.* **2008**, *34*, 847–868. [CrossRef] [PubMed]
12. Fye, K.H.; Terasaki, P.I.; Daniels, T.E.; Opelz, G.; Talal, N. Relationship of Hla-Dw3 and Hla-B8 to Sjögren'S Syndrome. *Arthritis Care Res.* **1978**, *21*, 337–342. [CrossRef] [PubMed]
13. Dendrou, C.A.; Petersen, J.; Rossjohn, J.; Fugger, L. HLA variation and disease. *Nat. Rev. Immunol.* **2018**, *18*, 325–339. [CrossRef]
14. Rudolph, M.G.; Stanfield, R.L.; Wilson, I.A. How Tcrs Bind Mhcs, Peptides, and Coreceptors. *Annu. Rev. Immunol.* **2006**, *24*, 419–466. [CrossRef]
15. Muraro, P.; Robins, H.; Malhotra, S.; Howell, M.; Phippard, D.; Desmarais, C.; Sousa, A.D.P.A.; Griffith, L.M.; Lim, N.; Nash, R.A.; et al. T cell repertoire following autologous stem cell transplantation for multiple sclerosis. *J. Clin. Investig.* **2014**, *124*, 1168–1172. [CrossRef]
16. Gebe, J.; Swanson, E.; Kwok, W.W. HLA Class II peptide-binding and autoimmunity. *Tissue Antigens* **2002**, *59*, 78–87. [CrossRef] [PubMed]
17. Rischmueller, M.; Lester, S.; Chen, Z.; Champion, G.; Berg, R.V.D.; Beer, R.; Coates, T.; Mccluskey, J.; Gordon, T. HLA class II phenotype controls diversification of the autoantibody response in primary Sjögren's syndrome (pSS). *Clin. Exp. Immunol.* **1998**, *111*, 365–371. [CrossRef]
18. Mann, D.L.; Moutsopoulos, H.M. HLA DR alloantigens in different subsets of patients with Sjogren's syndrome and in family members. *Ann. Rheum. Dis.* **1983**, *42*, 533–536. [CrossRef]
19. Bolstad, A.I.; Wassmuth, R.; Haga, H.J.; Jonsson, R. HLA markers and clinical characteristics in Caucasians with primary Sjögren's syndrome. *J. Rheumatol.* **2001**, *28*, 1554–1562.
20. Varela-Calvino, R.; Calviño-Sampedro, C.; Gomez-Touriño, I.; Cordero, O.J. Apportioning Blame: Autoreactive CD4+ and CD8+ T Cells in Type 1 Diabetes. *Arch. Immunol. Ther. Exp.* **2017**, *65*, 275–284. [CrossRef]
21. Hahn, M.; Nicholson, M.J.; Pyrdol, J.; Wucherpfennig, K.W. Unconventional topology of self peptide-major histocompatibility complex binding by a human autoimmune T cell receptor. *Nat. Immunol.* **2005**, *6*, 490–496. [CrossRef] [PubMed]
22. Chused, T.M.; Kassan, S.S.; Opelz, G.; Moutsopoulos, H.M.; Terasaki, P.I. Sjögren's Syndrome Associated with HLA-Dw3. *N. Engl. J. Med.* **1977**, *296*, 895–897. [CrossRef] [PubMed]
23. Manthorpe, R.; Morling, N.; Platz, P.; Ryder, L.P.; Svejgaard, A.; Thomsen, M. Hla-D Antigen Frequencies in Sjögren's Syndrome: Differences between the primary and secondary form. *Scand. J. Rheumatol.* **1981**, *10*, 124–128. [CrossRef] [PubMed]

4. Reveille, J.D.; Wilson, R.W.; Provost, T.T.; Bias, W.B.; Arnett, F.C. Primary Sjögren's Syndrome and Other Autoimmune Diseases in Families. *Ann. Intern. Med.* **1984**, *101*, 748–756. [CrossRef]
5. Brito-Zerón, P.; Baldini, C.; Bootsma, H.; Bowman, S.J.; Jonsson, R.; Mariette, X.; Sivils, K.; Theander, E.; Tzioufas, A.; Ramos-Casals, M. Sjögren syndrome. *Nat. Rev. Dis. Prim.* **2016**, *2*, 16047. [CrossRef]
6. Anaya, J.-M.; Mantilla, R.D.; Correa, P.A. Immunogenetics of primary Sjögren's syndrome in Colombians. *Semin. Arthritis Rheum.* **2005**, *34*, 735–743. [CrossRef]
7. Emsley, P.; Lohkamp, B.; Scott, W.G.; Cowtan, K. Features and development of Coot. *Acta Crystallogr. Sect. D Biol. Crystallogr.* **2010**, *66*, 486–501. [CrossRef]
8. Ferrara, P.; Gohlke, H.; Price, D.J.; Klebe, G.; Brooks, C.L. Assessing Scoring Functions for Protein−Ligand Interactions. *J. Med. Chem.* **2004**, *47*, 3032–3047. [CrossRef]
9. Ewing, T.J.; Makino, S.; Skillman, A.G.; Kuntz, I.D. DOCK 4.0: Search strategies for automated molecular docking of flexible molecule databases. *J. Comput. Aided Mol. Des.* **2001**, *15*, 411–428. [CrossRef]
0. Harley, J.B.; Reichlin, M.; Arnett, F.C.; Alexander, E.L.; Bias, W.B.; Provost, T.T. Gene Interaction at HLA-DQ Enhances Autoantibody Production in Primary Sjögren's Syndrome. *Science* **1986**, *232*, 1145–1147. [CrossRef]
1. Gottenberg, J.-E.; Busson, M.; Loiseau, P.; Cohen-Solal, J.; Lepage, V.; Charron, D.; Sibilia, J.; Mariette, X. In primary Sjögren's syndrome, HLA class II is associated exclusively with autoantibody production and spreading of the autoimmune response. *Arthritis Care Res.* **2003**, *48*, 2240–2245. [CrossRef] [PubMed]
2. Cruz-Tapias, P.; Rojas-Villarraga, A.; Maier-Moore, S.; Anaya, J.-M. HLA and Sjögren's syndrome susceptibility. A meta-analysis of worldwide studies. *Autoimmun. Rev.* **2012**, *11*, 281–287. [CrossRef] [PubMed]
3. Jean, S.; Quelvennec, E.; Alizadeh, M.; Guggenbuhl, P.; Birebent, B.; Perdriger, A.; Grosbois, B.; Pawlotsky, P.Y.; Semana, G. DRB1*15 and DRB1*03 extended haplotype interaction in primary Sjögren's syndrome genetic susceptibility. *Clin. Exp. Rheumatol.* **1998**, *16*, 725–728.
4. Paisansinsup, T.; Deshmukh, U.S.; Chowdhary, V.R.; Luthra, H.S.; Fu, S.M.; David, C.S. HLA class II influences the immune response and antibody diversification to Ro60/Sjögren's syndrome-A: Heightened antibody responses and epitope spreading in mice expressing HLA-DR molecules. *J. Immunol.* **2002**, *168*, 5876–5884. [CrossRef] [PubMed]
5. James, E.A.; Moustakas, A.K.; Bui, J.; Nouv, R.; Papadopoulos, G.K.; Kwok, W.W. The Binding of Antigenic Peptides to HLA-DR Is Influenced by Interactions between Pocket 6 and Pocket 9. *J. Immunol.* **2009**, *183*, 3249–3258. [CrossRef] [PubMed]
6. Gershwin, M.E.; Terasaki, P.I.; Graw, R.; Chused, T.M. Increased Frequency of HL-A8 in Sjogren's Syndrome. *Tissue Antigens* **1975**, *6*, 342–346. [CrossRef]
7. Moutsopoulos, H.M.; Mann, D.L.; Johnson, A.H.; Chused, T.M. Genetic Differences between Primary and Secondary Sicca Syndrome. *N. Engl. J. Med.* **1979**, *301*, 761–763. [CrossRef]
8. Molina, R.; Provost, T.T.; Arnett, F.C.; Bias, W.B.; Hochberg, M.C.; Wilson, R.W.; Alexander, E.L. Primary Sjögren's syndrome in men. *Am. J. Med.* **1986**, *80*, 23–31. [CrossRef]
9. Kang, H.I.; Fei, H.M.; Saito, I.; Sawada, S.; Chen, S.L.; Yi, D.; Chan, E.; Peebles, C.; Bugawan, T.L.; Erlich, H.A. Comparison of HLA class II genes in Caucasoid, Chinese, and Japanese patients with primary Sjögren's syndrome. *J. Immunol.* **1993**, *150*, 3615–3623.
0. Moriuchi, J.; Ichikawa, Y.; Takaya, M.; Shimizu, H.; Uchiyama, M.; Sato, K.; Tsuji, K.; Arimori, S. Familial Sjögren's syndrome in the Japanese: Immunogenetic and serological studies. *Clin. Exp. Rheumatol.* **1986**, *4*, 237–241.
1. Miyagawa, S.; Shinohara, K.; Nakajima, M.; Kidoguchi, K.-I.; Fujita, T.; Fukumoto, T.; Yoshioka, A.; Dohi, K.; Shirai, T. Polymorphisms of HLA class II genes and autoimmune responses to Ro/SS-A-La/SS-B among Japanese subjects. *Arthritis Care Res.* **1998**, *41*, 927–934. [CrossRef]
2. Hernández-Molina, G.; Vargas-Alarcón, G.; Rodríguez-Pérez, J.M.; Martínez-Rodríguez, N.; Lima, G.; Sánchez-Guerrero, J. High-resolution HLA analysis of primary and secondary Sjögren's syndrome: A common immunogenetic background in Mexican patients. *Rheumatol. Int.* **2014**, *35*, 643–649. [CrossRef] [PubMed]
3. Anaya, J.-M.; Correa, P.; Mantilla, R.D.; Arcos-Burgos, M. TAP, HLA-DQB1, and HLA-DRB1 polymorphism in Colombian patients with primary Sjögren's syndrome. *Semin. Arthritis Rheum.* **2002**, *31*, 396–405. [CrossRef] [PubMed]
4. Roitberg-Tambur, A.; Friedmann, A.; Safirman, C.; Markitziu, A.; Ben-Chetrit, E.; Rubinow, A.; Moutsopoulos, H.M.; Stavropoulos, E.; Skopouli, F.N.; Margalit, H.; et al. Molecular analysis of HLA class II genes in primary sjo¨gren's syndrome: A study of Israeli Jewish and Greek Non-Jewish patients. *Hum. Immunol.* **1993**, *36*, 235–242. [CrossRef]
5. Manoussakis, M.N.; Georgopoulou, C.; Zintzaras, E.; Spyropoulou, M.; Stavropoulou, A.; Skopouli, F.N.; Moutsopoulos, H.M. Sjögren's syndrome associated with systemic lupus erythematosus: Clinical and laboratory profiles and comparison with primary Sjögren's syndrome. *Arthritis Care Res.* **2004**, *50*, 882–891. [CrossRef] [PubMed]
6. Lope, B.; García, M.T.C.; de Ramón Garrido, E. Immunogenetics of the Sjogren's syndrome in southern Spain. *An. Med. Interna* **1994**, *11*, 56–61.
7. Vitali, C.; Tavoni, A.; Rizzo, G.; Neri, R.; D'Ascanio, A.; Cristofani, R.; Bombardieri, S. HLA antigens in Italian patients with primary Sjogren's syndrome. *Ann. Rheum. Dis.* **1986**, *45*, 412–416. [CrossRef] [PubMed]
8. Morling, N.; Andersen, V.; Fugger, L.; Georgsen, J.; Halberg, P.; Oxholm, P.; Odum, N.; Svejgaard, A. Immunogenetics of rheumatoid arthritis and primary Sjögren's syndrome: DNA polymorphism of HLA class II genes. *Dis. Markers* **1991**, *9*, 289–296.

49. Kerttula, T.O.; Collin, P.; Polvi, A.; Korpela, M.; Partanen, J.; Mäki, M. Distinct immunologic features of finnish Sjögren's syndrom patients with HLA alleles DRB1*0301, DQA1*0501, and DQB1*0201. Alterations in circulating T cell receptor γ/δ subsets. *Arthrit Care Res.* **1996**, *39*, 1733–1739. [CrossRef]
50. Nakken, B.; Jonsson, R.; Brokstad, K.A.; Omholt, K.; Nerland, A.H.; Haga, H.J.; Halse, A.-K. Associations of MHC Class II Allele in Norwegian Primary Sjögren's Syndrome Patients: Implications for Development of Autoantibodies to the Ro52 Autoantige *Scand. J. Immunol.* **2001**, *54*, 428–433. [CrossRef]
51. Pease, C.T.; Shattles, W.; Charles, P.J.; Venables, P.J.; Maini, R.N. Clinical, serological, and HLA phenotype subsets in Sjögren syndrome. *Clin. Exp. Rheumatol.* **1989**, *7*, 185–190. [PubMed]
52. Kacem, H.H.; Kaddour, N.; Adyel, F.; Bahloul, Z.; Ayadi, H. HLA-DQB1 CAR1/CAR2, TNFa IR2/IR4 and CTLA-4 polymorphism in Tunisian patients with rheumatoid arthritis and Sjogren's syndrome. *Rheumatology* **2001**, *40*, 1370–1374. [CrossRef] [PubMed]
53. Scofield, R.; Frank, M.B.; Neas, B.R.; Horowitz, R.M.; Hardgrave, K.L.; Fujisaku, A.; McArthur, R.; Harley, J.B. Cooperativ Association of T Cell β Receptor and HLA-DQ Alleles in the Production of Anti-Ro in Systemic Lupus Erythematosus. *Cli Immunol. Immunopathol.* **1994**, *72*, 335–341. [CrossRef] [PubMed]
54. Chen, Q.-Y.; Huang, W.; She, J.-X.; Baxter, F.; Volpe, R.; MacLaren, N.K. HLA-DRB1108, DRB1103/DRB310101, and DRB31020 Are Susceptibility Genes for Graves' Disease in North American Caucasians, Whereas DRB1107 Is Protective1. *J. Clin. Endocrino Metab.* **1999**, *84*, 3182–3186. [CrossRef] [PubMed]
55. Zeitlin, A.A.; Heward, J.M.; Newby, P.R.; Carr-Smith, J.D.; Franklyn, J.A.; Gough, S.C.L.; Simmonds, M. Analysis of HLA class I genes in Hashimoto's thyroiditis reveals differences compared to Graves' disease. *Genes Immun.* **2008**, *9*, 358–363. [CrossRef]
56. Castro-Santos, P.; Olloquequi, J.; Verdugo, R.A.; Gutiérrez, M.A.; Pinochet, C.; Quiñones, L.A.; Díaz-Peña, R. *HLA-DRB1*07:01* an **08:02* Alleles Confer a Protective Effect Against ACPA-Positive Rheumatoid Arthritis in a Latin American Admixed Populatio *Biology* **2020**, *9*, 467. [CrossRef]
57. Jacobi, T.; Massier, L.; Klöting, N.; Horn, K.; Schuch, A.; Ahnert, P.; Engel, C.; Löffler, M.; Burkhardt, R.; Thiery, J.; et al. HL Class II Allele Analyses Implicate Common Genetic Components in Type 1 and Non–Insulin-Treated Type 2 Diabetes. *J. Cli Endocrinol. Metab.* **2020**, *105*, e245–e254. [CrossRef]
58. De Holanda, M.I.; Klumb, E.; Imada, A.; Lima, L.A.; Alcântara, I.; Gregório, F.; Christiani, L.F.; Martins, C.O.; Timoner, B.E Motta, J.; et al. The prevalence of HLA alleles in a lupus nephritis population. *Transpl. Immunol.* **2018**, *47*, 37–43. [CrossRef]
59. Dawson, L.; Tobin, A.; Smith, P.; Gordon, T. Antimuscarinic antibodies in Sjögren's syndrome: Where are we, and where are w going? *Arthritis Care Res.* **2005**, *52*, 2984–2995. [CrossRef]
60. Yang, L.; Ju, J.; Zhang, W.; Lv, F.; Pang, C.; Yang, G.; Wang, Y. Effects of Muscarinic Acetylcholine 3 Receptor208-227Peptid Immunization on Autoimmune Response in Nonobese Diabetic Mice. *Clin. Dev. Immunol.* **2013**, *2013*, 485213. [CrossRef]
61. Kurien, B.T.; Dsouza, A.; Igoe, A.; Lee, Y.J.; Maier-Moore, J.S.; Gordon, T.; Jackson, M.; Scofield, R.H. Immunization with 60 kD R peptide produces different stages of preclinical autoimmunity in a Sjögren's syndrome model among multiple strains of inbre mice. *Clin. Exp. Immunol.* **2013**, *173*, 67–75. [CrossRef]
62. Espinosa, A.; Zhou, W.; Ek, M.; Hedlund, M.; Brauner, S.; Popovic, K.; Horvath, L.; Wallerskog, T.; Oukka, M.; Nyberg, F.; et a The Sjögren's Syndrome-Associated Autoantigen Ro52 Is an E3 Ligase That Regulates Proliferation and Cell Death. *J. Immuno* **2006**, *176*, 6277–6285. [CrossRef] [PubMed]
63. Deshmukh, U.S.; Lewis, J.E.; Gaskin, F.; Kannapell, C.C.; Waters, S.T.; Lou, Y.-H.; Tung, K.S.K.; Fu, S.M. Immune Responses t Ro60 and Its Peptides in Mice. I. The Nature of the Immunogen and Endogenous Autoantigen Determine the Specificities of th Induced Autoantibodies. *J. Exp. Med.* **1999**, *189*, 531–540. [CrossRef] [PubMed]
64. Szczerba, B.M.; Kaplonek, P.; Wolska, N.; Podsiadlowska, A.; Rybakowska, P.; Dey, P.; Rasmussen, A.; Grundahl, K.; Hefner, K.S Stone, D.U.; et al. Interaction between innate immunity and Ro52-induced antibody causes Sjögren's syndrome-like disorder i mice. *Ann. Rheum. Dis.* **2015**, *75*, 617–622. [CrossRef]
65. Scofield, R.H.; Asfa, S.; Obeso, D.; Jonsson, R.; Kurien, B.T. Immunization with Short Peptides from the 60-kDa Ro Antige Recapitulates the Serological and Pathological Findings as well as the Salivary Gland Dysfunction of Sjögren's Syndrom *J. Immunol.* **2005**, *175*, 8409–8414. [CrossRef] [PubMed]
66. Scofield, R.H.; Pierce, P.G.; James, J.A.; Kaufman, K.M.; Kurien, B.T. Immunization with Peptides from 60 kDa Ro in Divers Mouse Strains. *Scand. J. Immunol.* **2002**, *56*, 477–483. [CrossRef] [PubMed]
67. Scofield, R.H.; Kaufman, K.M.; Baber, U.; James, J.A.; Harley, J.B.; Kurien, B.T. Immunization of mice with human 60-kd R peptides results in epitope spreading if the peptides are highly homologous between human and mouse. *Arthritis Rheum.* **199** *42*, 1017–1024. [CrossRef]
68. Topfer, F.; Gordon, T.; McCluskey, J. Intra- and intermolecular spreading of autoimmunity involving the nuclear self-antigens L (SS-B) and Ro (SS-A). *Proc. Natl. Acad. Sci. USA* **1995**, *92*, 875–879. [CrossRef]
69. Igoe, A.; Scofield, R.H. Autoimmunity and infection in Sjögren's syndrome. *Curr. Opin. Rheumatol.* **2013**, *25*, 480–487. [CrossRef]
70. Witas, R.; Gupta, S.; Nguyen, C.Q. Contributions of Major Cell Populations to Sjögren's Syndrome. *J. Clin. Med.* **2020**, *9*, 305 [CrossRef]
71. Pearson, M.N.; Bailey, A.M. Viruses of Botrytis. *Adv. Virus Res.* **2013**, *86*, 249–272. [CrossRef]
72. Hammond, J.; Reinsel, M.; Grinstead, S.; Lockhart, B.; Jordan, R.; Mollov, D. A Mixed Infection of Helenium Virus S with Tw Distinct Isolates of Butterbur Mosaic Virus, One of Which Has a Major Deletion in an Essential Gene. *Front. Microbiol.* **202** *11*, 612936. [CrossRef] [PubMed]

73. Gulder, T.A.M.; Neff, S.; Schüz, T.; Winkler, T.; Gees, R.; Böhlendorf, B. The myxocoumarins A and B from Stigmatella aurantiaca strain MYX-030. *Beilstein J. Org. Chem.* **2013**, *9*, 2579–2585. [CrossRef] [PubMed]
74. Kunze, B.; Reichenbach, H.; Augustiniak, H.; Höfle, G. Isolation and identification of althiomycin from *Cystobacter fuscus* (Myxobacterales). *J. Antibiot.* **1982**, *35*, 635–636. [CrossRef] [PubMed]
75. Dyksma, S.; Pjevac, P.; Ovanesov, K.; Mussmann, M. Evidence for H2consumption by unculturedDesulfobacteralesin coastal sediments. *Environ. Microbiol.* **2017**, *20*, 450–461. [CrossRef] [PubMed]
76. Palleroni, N.J. The Pseudomonas Story. *Environ. Microbiol.* **2010**, *12*, 1377–1383. [CrossRef] [PubMed]
77. Scarborough, M.J.; Myers, K.S.; Donohue, T.J.; Noguera, D.R. Medium-Chain Fatty Acid Synthesis by "*Candidatus* Weimeria bifida" gen. nov., sp. nov., and "*Candidatus* Pseudoramibacter fermentans" sp. nov. *Appl. Environ. Microbiol.* **2020**, *86*, e02242-19. [CrossRef] [PubMed]
78. Wang, Y.; Wan, X.; Wu, X.; Zhang, C.; Liu, J.; Hou, S. Eubacterium rectale contributes to colorectal cancer initiation via promoting colitis. *Gut Pathog.* **2021**, *13*, 1–11. [CrossRef] [PubMed]
79. Sayed, A.M.; Abdel-Wahab, N.M.; Hassan, H.M.; Abdelmohsen, U.R. Saccharopolyspora: An underexplored source for bioactive natural products. *J. Appl. Microbiol.* **2019**, *128*, 314–329. [CrossRef] [PubMed]
80. Creemers-Schild, D.; Gronthoud, F.; Spanjaard, L.; Visser, L.; Brouwer, C.; Kuijper, E. Fusobacterium necrophorum, an emerging pathogen of otogenic and paranasal infections? *New Microbes New Infect.* **2014**, *2*, 52–57. [CrossRef] [PubMed]
81. Khelaifia, S.; Croce, O.; Lagier, J.-C.; Robert, C.; Couderc, C.; Di Pinto, F.; Davoust, B.; Djossou, F.; Raoult, D.; Fournier, P.-E. Noncontiguous finished genome sequence and description of Virgibacillus massiliensis sp. nov., a moderately halophilic bacterium isolated from human gut. *New Microbes New Infect.* **2015**, *8*, 78–88. [CrossRef] [PubMed]
82. Valentini, F.; Evangelisti, M.; Arpinelli, M.; Di Nardo, G.; Borro, M.; Simmaco, M.; Villa, M.P. Gut microbiota composition in children with obstructive sleep apnoea syndrome: A pilot study. *Sleep Med.* **2020**, *76*, 140–147. [CrossRef] [PubMed]
83. Barandouzi, Z.A.; Starkweather, A.R.; Henderson, W.; Gyamfi, A.; Cong, X.S. Altered Composition of Gut Microbiota in Depression: A Systematic Review. *Front. Psychiatry* **2020**, *11*, 541. [CrossRef] [PubMed]
84. van der Meulen, T.A.; Harmsen, H.J.; Vila, A.V.; Kurilshikov, A.; Liefers, S.C.; Zhernakova, A.; Fu, J.; Wijmenga, C.; Weersma, R.K.; de Leeuw, K.; et al. Shared gut, but distinct oral microbiota composition in primary Sjögren's syndrome and systemic lupus erythematosus. *J. Autoimmun.* **2018**, *97*, 77–87. [CrossRef] [PubMed]
85. Szymula, A.; Rosenthal, J.; Szczerba, B.M.; Bagavant, H.; Fu, S.M.; Deshmukh, U.S. T cell epitope mimicry between Sjögren's syndrome Antigen A (SSA)/Ro60 and oral, gut, skin and vaginal bacteria. *Clin. Immunol.* **2014**, *152*, 1–9. [CrossRef] [PubMed]
86. Corrêa, J.D.; Calderaro, D.C.; Ferreira, G.A.; Mendonça, S.M.S.; Fernandes, G.R.; Xiao, E.; Teixeira, A.L.; Leys, E.J.; Graves, D.T.; Silva, T.A. Subgingival microbiota dysbiosis in systemic lupus erythematosus: Association with periodontal status. *Microbiome* **2017**, *5*, 1–13. [CrossRef]
87. Mandl, T.; Marsal, J.; Olsson, P.; Ohlsson, B.; Andréasson, K. Severe intestinal dysbiosis is prevalent in primary Sjögren's syndrome and is associated with systemic disease activity. *Arthritis Res. Ther.* **2017**, *19*, 237. [CrossRef]
88. De Paiva, C.S.; Jones, D.B.; Stern, M.E.; Bian, F.; Moore, Q.L.; Corbiere, S.; Streckfus, C.F.; Hutchinson, D.S.; Ajami, N.J.; Petrosino, J.F.; et al. Altered Mucosal Microbiome Diversity and Disease Severity in Sjögren Syndrome. *Sci. Rep.* **2016**, *6*, 23561. [CrossRef] [PubMed]
89. Tsunawaki, S.; Nakamura, S.; Ohyama, Y.; Sasaki, M.; Ikebe-Hiroki, A.; Hiraki, A.; Kadena, T.; Kawamura, E.; Kumamaru, W.; Shinohara, M.; et al. Possible function of salivary gland epithelial cells as nonprofessional antigen-presenting cells in the de-velopment of Sjögren's syndrome. *J. Rheumatol.* **2002**, *29*, 1884–1896.
90. Geluk, A.; Van Meijgaarden, K.E.; Southwood, S.; Oseroff, C.; Drijfhout, J.W.; De Vries, R.R.; Ottenhoff, T.H.; Sette, A. HLA-DR3 molecules can bind peptides carrying two alternative specific submotifs. *J. Immunol.* **1994**, *152*, 5742–5748.
91. Becerra-Artiles, A.; Cruz, J.; Leszyk, J.D.; Sidney, J.; Sette, A.; Shaffer, S.A.; Stern, L.J. Naturally processed HLA-DR3-restricted HHV-6B peptides are recognized broadly with polyfunctional and cytotoxic CD4 T-cell responses. *Eur. J. Immunol.* **2019**, *49*, 1167–1185. [CrossRef] [PubMed]
92. Verhagen, J.; Yusuf, N.; Smith, E.L.; Whettlock, E.M.; Naran, K.; Arif, S.; Peakman, M. Proinsulin peptide promotes autoimmune diabetes in a novel HLA-DR3-DQ2-transgenic murine model of spontaneous disease. *Diabetologia* **2019**, *62*, 2252–2261. [CrossRef] [PubMed]
93. Li, C.W.; Osman, R.; Menconi, F.; Concepcion, E.; Tomer, Y. Cepharanthine blocks TSH receptor peptide presentation by HLA-DR3: Therapeutic implications to Graves' disease. *J. Autoimmun.* **2020**, *108*, 102402. [CrossRef] [PubMed]
94. Li, C.W.; Menconi, F.; Osman, R.; Mezei, M.; Jacobson, E.M.; Concepcion, E.; David, C.S.; Kastrinsky, D.B.; Ohlmeyer, M.; Tomer, Y. Identifying a Small Molecule Blocking Antigen Presentation in Autoimmune Thyroiditis. *J. Biol. Chem.* **2016**, *291*, 4079–4090. [CrossRef] [PubMed]
95. Kovacs, A.; Endreffy, E.; Petri, I.; Kovacs, L.; Pokorny, G. HLA class II allele polymorphism in Hungarian patients with primary Sjögren's syndrome. *Scand. J. Rheumatol.* **2006**, *35*, 75–76. [CrossRef] [PubMed]

Journal of
Clinical Medicine

MDPI

rticle

A Computational Text Mining-Guided Meta-Analysis Approach to Identify Potential Xerostomia Drug Targets

Micaela F. Beckman, Elizabeth J. Brennan, Chika K. Igba, Michael T. Brennan, Farah B. Mougeot * and Jean-Luc C. Mougeot *

Department of Oral Medicine, Carolinas Medical Center, Atrium Health, Charlotte, NC 28203, USA; micaela.beckman@atriumhealth.org (M.F.B.); liz.brennan.3@gmail.com (E.J.B.); chikaigba7@gmail.com (C.K.I.); mike.brennan@atriumhealth.org (M.T.B.)

* Correspondence: farah.mougeot@atriumhealth.org (F.B.M.); jean-luc.mougeot@atriumhealth.org (J.-L.C.M.)

Abstract: Xerostomia (subjective complaint of dry mouth) is commonly associated with salivary gland hypofunction. Molecular mechanisms associated with xerostomia pathobiology are poorly understood, thus hampering drug development. Our objectives were to (i) use text-mining tools to investigate xerostomia and dry mouth concepts, (ii) identify associated molecular interactions involving genes as candidate drug targets, and (iii) determine how drugs currently used in clinical trials may impact these genes and associated pathways. PubMed and PubMed Central were used to identify search terms associated with xerostomia and/or dry mouth. Search terms were queried in pubmed2ensembl. Protein–protein interaction (PPI) networks were determined using the gene/protein network visualization program search tool for recurring instances of neighboring genes (STRING). A similar program, Cytoscape, was used to determine PPIs of overlapping gene sets. The drug–gene interaction database (DGIdb) and the clinicaltrials.gov database were used to identify potential drug targets from the xerostomia/dry mouth PPI gene set. We identified 64 search terms in common between xerostomia and dry mouth. STRING confirmed PPIs between identified genes (CL = 0.90). Cytoscape analysis determined 58 shared genes, with cytokine–cytokine receptor interaction representing the most significant pathway ($p = 1.29 \times 10^{-23}$) found in the Kyoto encyclopedia of genes and genomes (KEGG). Fifty-four genes in common had drug interactions, per DGIdb analysis. Eighteen drugs, targeting the xerostomia/dry mouth PPI network, have been evaluated for xerostomia, head and neck cancer oral complications, and Sjögren's Syndrome. The PPI network genes IL6R, EGFR, NFKB1, MPO, and TNFSF13B constitute a possible biomarker signature of xerostomia. Validation of the candidate biomarkers is necessary to better stratify patients at the genetic and molecular levels to facilitate drug development or to monitor response to treatment.

Keywords: xerostomia; dry mouth; protein–protein interaction; drug target; head and neck cancer; Sjögren's Syndrome

Citation: Beckman, M.F.; Brennan, E.J.; Igba, C.K.; Brennan, M.T.; Mougeot, F.B.; Mougeot, J.-L.C. A Computational Text Mining-Guided Meta-Analysis Approach to Identify Potential Xerostomia Drug Targets. *J. Clin. Med.* **2022**, *11*, 1442. https://doi.org/10.3390/jcm11051442

Academic Editor: Margherita Sisto

Received: 3 February 2022
Accepted: 3 March 2022
Published: 5 March 2022

1. Introduction

1.1. Epidemiology and Symptomatology

Xerostomia, also known as the sensation or subjective complaint of dry mouth, is a common condition affecting the oral cavity, mainly due to functional and structural damage to the salivary glands [1]. Prevalence varies and is highly dependent on the population studied and methodologies implemented [2–4]. People most significantly impacted include women who are menopausal and individuals over 65 years of age [5,6]. However, younger individuals can also be affected, since approximately 20% of those who report this problem are between the ages of 18 to 34 [5]. Marcott et al. has recently suggested that the condition affects 10% to 46% of people amongst the US, Mexico, and several countries in Europe [7]. A study that analyzed population-based measures of the condition concluded that the prevalence of xerostomia ranges from 9.7 to 25.8% in men and 10.3 to 33.3% in women [8].

Symptoms of xerostomia vary physically and can result in general psychologic distress [9]. Symptoms often include the feeling of dryness and stickiness of the mouth, di ficulty swallowing, chewing or speaking, and having a dry tongue or grooved appearanc of the tongue [9]. Patients can also experience sore throat and an altered sense of taste [1(Because saliva acts to remove excess bacteria and plaque from the teeth, the lack of saliva i xerostomic patients can increase the risk of dental caries and infections [8]. In addition, th subjective perception of xerostomia is frequently, but not always, associated with reduce salivary flow [1,8,11].

1.2. Etiologies, Pathophysiology, and Treatment

Xerostomia etiologies include genetic predispositions (i.e., single-nucleotide polymo phisms associated with adverse drug reactions or salivary gland disorders), side effect from medications, radiation treatments to the head and neck, and certain chronic autoin mune diseases [3,5,12–14]. Most notably, dry mouth is commonly reported in patient suffering from Sjögren's Syndrome, rheumatoid arthritis (RA), chronic juvenile arthriti sarcoidosis, and systemic sclerosis [5].

Current treatments include products to stimulate saliva, mucosal comfort agent and/or saliva substitutes. These medications address the symptoms of xerostomia bu are unable to address the underlying biological mechanisms of the condition [5,15]. A recent study showed that 23.2% of patients in a xerostomia cohort used saliva substitute yet the effectiveness of such treatments remained unclear [7]. Vissink et al. found tha saliva substitutes can provide temporary relief of xerostomia symptoms [16]. However, Cochrane review did not find a significant difference in the effectiveness of oral lozenge sprays, gels, or other saliva substitutes when compared to a placebo [17]. The lack o targeted treatments available contributes to the diminished quality of life of those livin with this condition [7,8,15].

1.3. Data Mining and Objectives

A comprehensive knowledge-based resource detailing the pathways and biologica mechanisms of dry mouth pathophysiology could be beneficial to drug target discover in xerostomia therapeutic development. Advancements in biomedical research over th past decade have led to a significant increase in the number of publications and availabilit of open access research articles [18]. Data-mining and text-mining tools allow for th sorting and identification of information from a massive amount of research [19]. Man publications introduce individual approaches, yet fewer combine multiple methods t identify genes or expression pathways of interest [20].

Our objective was to utilize a combined data-mining approach to determine curate gene and protein interaction profiles of xerostomia and/or dry mouth to identify pc tential drugs that can target disease relevant molecular pathways. Our aims were t (i) perform literature mining for the identification of genetic and proteomic profiles asso ciated with xerostomia, (ii) establish the relationship of the concepts "xerostomia" anc "dry mouth" with genes, (iii) characterize xerostomia/dry mouth-related protein–protei interactions, and (iv) determine drug–gene interactions potentially useful for xerostomi therapeutic development.

2. Methods

2.1. Conventional Review of the Literature

The PubMed and PubMed Central biomedical databases were used to search fo articles in English relating to xerostomia and/or dry mouth [21]. We also sought to identif publications discussing the composition of saliva or providing information about wha constitutes low-, optimal-, and high-quality saliva. From this review, we selected keywords referred to as "search terms", thought to be linked to xerostomia and/or saliva to a variabl degree and risk of bias of each article was determined [22,23]. Search terms were used a input for the online tool pubmed2ensembl-biomartv0.7 (P2E) [24]. Results from P2E fo each search term were then combined with P2E results for "xerostomia" or "dry mouth" and duplicates were removed.

2.2. Protein–Protein Interaction and Visualization

The Search Tool for Recurring Instances of Neighboring Genes (STRINGv11.0) was used to analyze protein–protein interaction (PPI) networks of the gene sets for xerostomia and dry mouth separately using the maximum confidence level (CL) of 0.90 [25]. All genes without interactions were removed from further analysis.

STRING PPI networks of candidate genes with a CL > 0.90 for xerostomia and dry mouth target lists were imported into Cytoscapev3.8.2 via the stringAppv1.6.0 [26,27]. Using the imported PPI networks from STRINGv11.0, Cytoscape PPI networks were constructed with a confidence score (CS) of 0.98 for xerostomia and dry mouth gene sets separately to narrow results. These networks were then merged to create a PPI intersection network of xerostomia and dry mouth genes with matching name or Ensembl ID. Functional and enrichment data for these networks were retrieved using Cytoscapev3.8.2:stringAppv1.6.0 [27]. The filtered enrichment categories chosen were Kyoto Encyclopedia of Genes and Genomes (KEGG) pathways and Gene Ontology (GO) Biological Process [28,29]. Using the BiNGOv3.0.3 Cytoscapev3.8.1app, a network of overrepresented GO biological processes was created for the xerostomia/dry mouth intersection network using a hypergeometric test and false discovery rate ($p < 1.0 \times 10^{-4}$) [30]. AmiGO 2 was used to explore overrepresented GO biological processes [31]. Tissue expression of genes found in the intersection network of xerostomia/dry mouth was retrieved and plotted using histograms via Pythonv3.6.1:matplotlibv3.0.3 [32,33]. Cytoscapev3.8.2:stringAppv1.6.0 extracts information from TISSUESv2.0 database, using a confidence rating (CR) from zero to five on 20 tissue types, based on knowledge, experiments and text mining [34].

2.3. The Drug–Gene Interaction Database

The drug–gene interaction database (DGIdb) was used to identify drug interactions for genes found in the xerostomia/dry mouth intersection network [34]. Drugs and genes identified by DGIdb were then compared to drugs that have been or are currently being evaluated for treatment of xerostomia or dry mouth according to the ClinicalTrials.gov database [35,36].

3. Results

A flowchart showing the overall text- and data-mining methodology is presented in Figure 1.

3.1. Identification of Genetic and Proteomic Profiles Predominantly Associated with Xerostomia/Dry Mouth

From conventional searches for xerostomia and dry mouth using PubMed and PMC, 64 search terms were determined as related (Table 1). A table showing risk of bias for reviewed and selected articles is presented in Table S1. Search terms (n = 64) were split into six categories directly related to the etiology and/or pathobiology of xerostomia and/or dry mouth (Table 1). These categories are (i) autoimmune disorders (n = 12 terms), (ii) diet (n = 10 terms), (iii) genetics and physiology (n = 17 terms), (iv) medication (n = 14 terms), (v) radiation (n = 3 terms), and (vi) others (n = 8 terms). P2E analysis returned 1916 gene symbols and aliases (309 without duplicates) for "xerostomia" and 1134 (159 without duplicates) for "dry mouth. P2E result outputs are presented in Data File S1.

3.2. Xerostomia/Dry Mouth Protein–Protein Interactions

The STRINGv11.0 PPI network using a CL of 0.90 for the 'xerostomia' gene set (input = 309) returned a network of 229 genes (Figure 2a). PPI analysis using a CL of 0.90 for the 'dry mouth' gene set (input = 159) returned a network of 110 genes (Figure 2b).

Using STRINGv11.0 PPI networks imported into Cytoscapev3.8.2:stringAppv1.6.0, PPI networks of 128 genes from 229 genes and 55 genes from 110 genes for xerostomia and dry mouth, respectively, were returned as output with a CS of 0.98 (Figure S1). Using the "merge networks" feature in Cytoscapev3.8.2, an intersection network was created of the xerostomia/dry mouth networks (Figure S1a,b), and a total of 58 genes were returned at a CS of 0.98 (Figure 3).

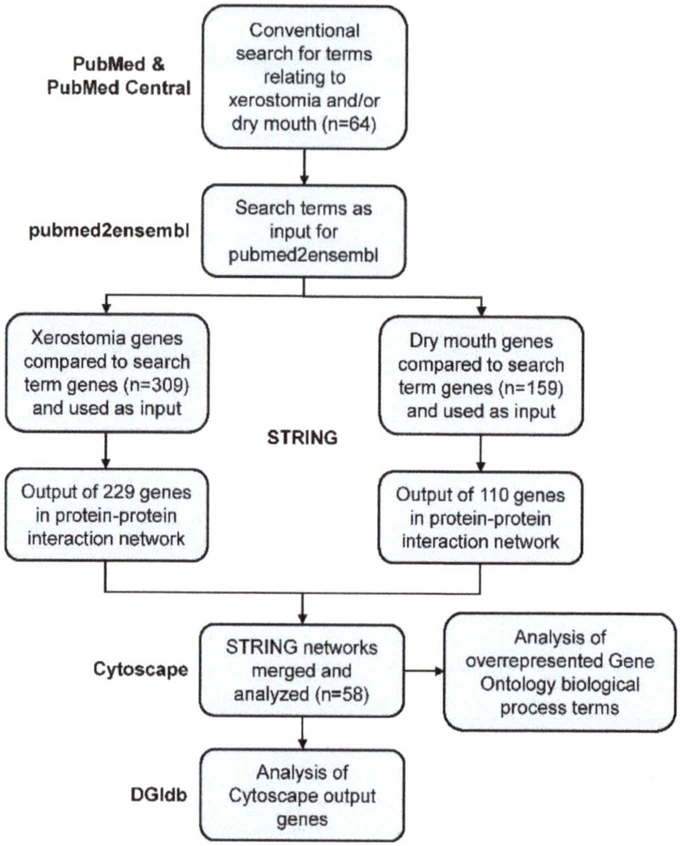

Figure 1. Overall Analytical Design. Search terms (n = 64) were determined to be related to xerostomia and/or dry mouth. Using search terms as input, pubmed2ensembl identified 1916 genes (309 without duplicates) and 1134 genes (159 without duplicates) to be related to xerostomia or dry mouth, respectively. Using STRINGv11.0, 229 genes were used as input for xerostomia and 110 genes were used as input for dry mouth with a confidence level of 0.90. STRINGv11.0 protein–protein interaction networks were used as input for Cytoscapev3.8.1 with a confidence score of 0.98. Network of 128 and 55 genes for xerostomia and dry mouth, respectively, were returned and merged, resulting in 58 genes with matching names or Ensembl IDs. The BiNGOv3.0.3 Cytoscapev3.8.1 app determined 360 gene ontology biological processes to be overrepresented in this intersection ($p < 1.0 \times 10^{-4}$). From 58 genes, 54 were found to have drug–gene interactions via the drug–gene interaction database (DGIdb). Using 54 total candidate gene targets, 27 drug trials consisting of 18 different drugs were identified using ClinicalTrials.gov that have been or are being evaluated for efficacy in treating xerostomia in general, head and neck cancer-related salivary gland dysfunction, or Sjögren's Syndrome.

Table 1. Xerostomia and/or Dry Mouth Search Terms. Search terms (n = 64) were determined using conventional methods. PubMed and PubMed Central were used to search for articles in English relating to xerostomia and/or dry mouth. Keywords or "search terms" thought to be linked to xerostomia and/or saliva were selected. Search terms were split into categories directly related to the etiology and/or pathobiology of xerostomia and/or dry mouth: [a] autoimmune conditions; [b] dietary and nutritional; [c] genetic and physical; [d] medication; [e] radiation therapy applied to head and neck cancer (HNC) patients; [f] other.

Category	Search Term (n = 64)
Autoimmune Disease [a]	Amyloid build up, chronic inflammatory autoimmune disorder, chronic juvenile arthritis, crest syndrome, dry mouth, hypohidrotic ectodermal dysplasia, juvenile rheumatoid arthritis, sarcoidosis, scleroderma, Sjögren's Syndrome; underactive thyroid gland, xerostomia (n = 12)
Diet [b]	Alcohol use, caffeine drink, food avoidance, food modification, morbidly obese, nutritional benefit, specialized metabolites, sugared beverages, tobacco use, unhealthy eating (n = 10)
Genetics and Physiology [c]	Burning mouth, difficulty swallowing, glycosylation, high flow salivary hypofunction, high-quality saliva, low-quality saliva, normal salivary composition, oncogenomics, optimal salivary function, poor saliva composition, saliva composition, salivary flow pH 5.5, salivary flow pH 7.8, salivary device, salivary flow between 0.4 mL and 0.5 mL, salivary hypofunction, sore throat (n = 17)
Medication [d]	Acetylcholine blocker, amphetamines, atropine, biotene, gustatory stimulants, histamine receptor inhibitor, lozenge, mucosal coating agent, opioid drug class, parasympathomimetic prescription, replacement saliva, saliva substitute, serotonin reuptake inhibition, valium (n = 14)
Radiation [e]	Radiation therapy, RTx, XRT (n = 3)
Other [f]	Feverishness, free water loss, impoverishment, multicultural populations, oral health care, oral thrush, thallium poisoning, vitamin A deficiency (n = 8)

Of the 95 FDR significant ($p < 1.0 \times 10^{-4}$) KEGG pathways, cytokine–cytokine receptor interaction (hsa04060; FDR = 1.06×10^{-49}), Hepatitis B (hsa05161; FDR = 1.89×10^{-25}), and pathways in cancer (hsa05200; FDR = 1.29×10^{-23}) were highly significant (Table S2). All significant KEGG pathways are presented in Data File S2. A total of 360 GO biological processes were determined as overrepresented, with the most significant being "immune system process" (GO:0002376; FDR = 2.61×10^{-29}) and "inflammatory response" (GO:0006954; FDR = 4.16×10^{-22}) (Data File S3). Although not significant, 31 GO biological processes were included in the overrepresented GO network due to being 'parents' of significant categories. A network of overrepresented GO biological processes is presented in Figure S2.

Of the 20 available tissue types from the TISSUESv2.0 database, our dataset had confidence ratings for 19 tissue types [34]. Albumin (ALB) and apolipoprotein A1 (APO1) had the highest confidence rating of 5.00 in heart. ALB also had the highest confidence rating in liver. The highest gene expression confidence among all genes was determined to be from blood, with an average expression confidence rating of 4.09. Saliva had an average tissue expression confidence rating of 1.94 among all genes. In saliva, myeloperoxidase (MPO) had the highest saliva expression confidence rating of 4.35, with the second highest being a confidence rating of 2.80 for epidermal growth factor receptor (EGFR). Histograms highlighting gene expression confidence ratings for the 19 tissue types are presented in Figure S3.

3.3. *The Drug–Gene Interaction Database*

Using an input of 58 genes from the Cytoscape xerostomia/dry mouth intersection network, 54 genes were determined to have drug–gene interactions via DGIdb (Table 2) [34]. The gene with the greatest number of drug–gene interactions was EGFR, with 178 drug interactions (Table S3). The second greatest number of drug interactions was nuclear factor kappa B subunit 1 (NFKB1) with 90 interactions (Table S3). For the 54 total gene targets, 27 associated clinical trials consisting of 18 different drugs have been evaluated for treatment of xerostomia, head and neck cancer-related salivary gland dysfunction, or

Sjögren's Syndrome per the ClinicalTrials.gov database (Table S3) [36]. No clinical trial were found to evaluate drugs with EGFR as a target and only one clinical trial has evaluate a drug with NFKB1 as a target for Sjögren's Syndrome (NCT00001599) [37]. Furthermor of the 18 drugs in trials, 13 were also identified by DGIdb [35]. Only two of these 13 drug identified by DGIdb had interaction scores greater than 10 [35]. These two drugs we belimumab (gene target tumor necrosis factor superfamily member 13b [TNFSF13B], wit an interaction score of 63.79) and tocilizumab (gene target interleukin 6 receptor [IL6R with an interaction score of 17.72) using the ratio of the average known gene partners fc all drugs to the known partners for a given drug depending on publications. The highes interaction score among all identified DGIdb genes was for the drug mogamulizuma which targets the gene C–C Motif Chemokine Receptor 4 (CCR4) [35]. DGIdb identifie 808 different drugs with gene interactions from our gene set that have not currently bee evaluated for treatment of dry mouth, xerostomia, or Sjögren's Syndrome [35]. Drug identified by DGIdb and their interaction scores are available in Data File S4 [35].

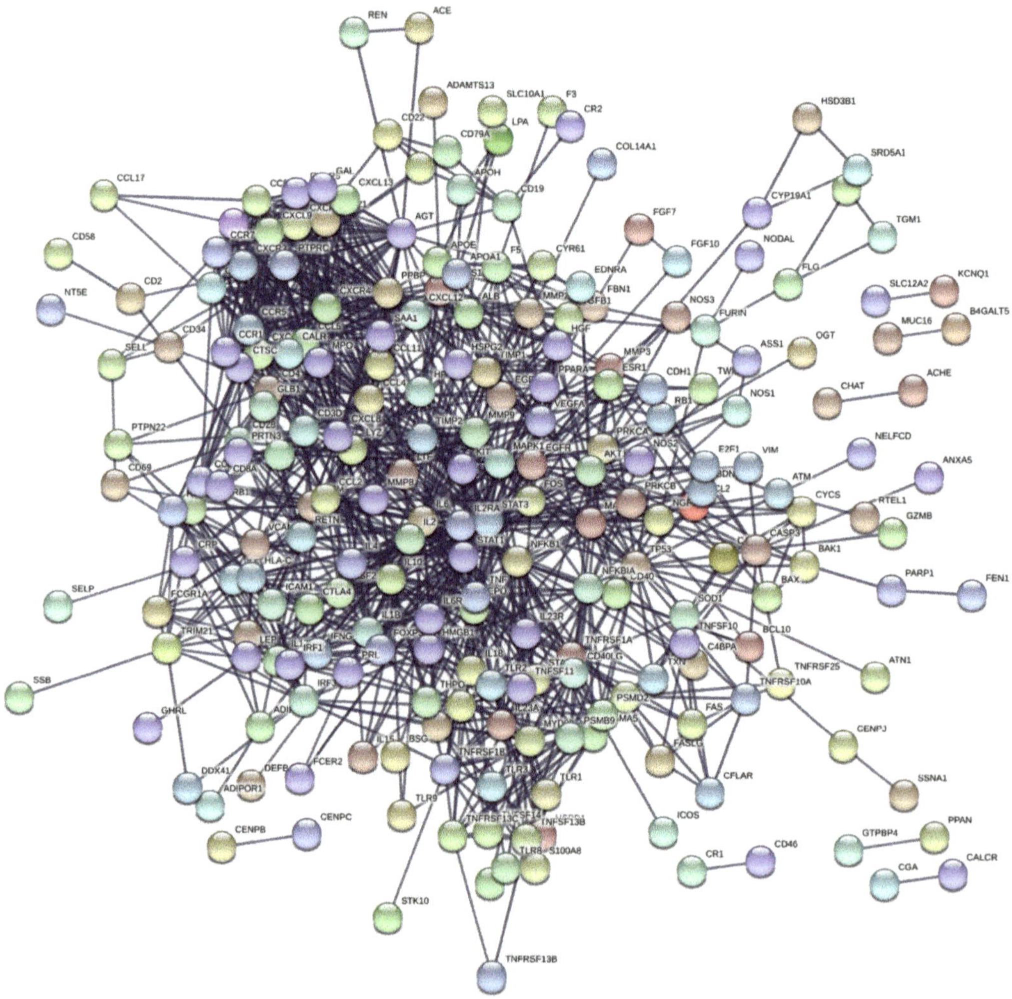

(a) Xerostomia

Figure 2. *Cont.*

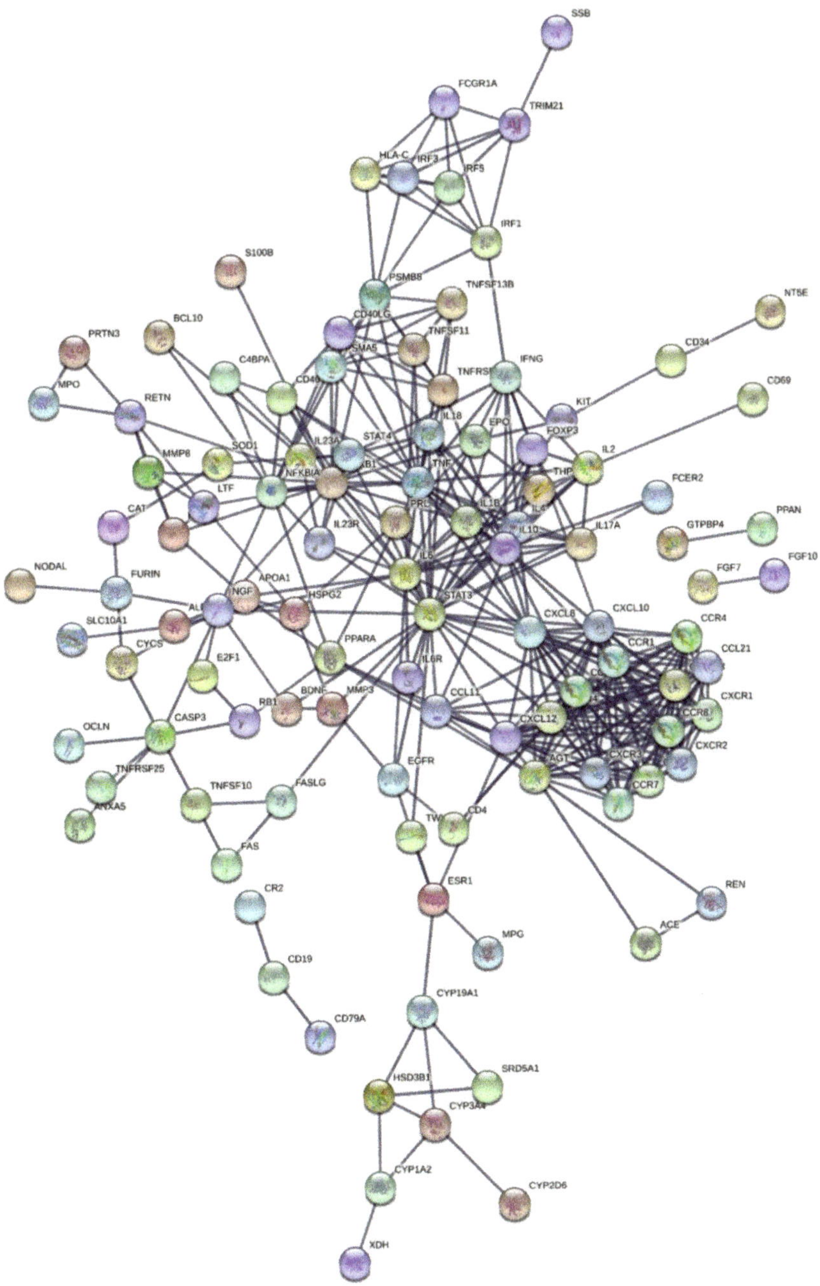

(b) Dry Mouth

Figure 2. STRING PPI Networks for Xerostomia and Dry Mouth. STRINGv11.0 protein–protein interaction networks for genes identified using search terms combined with (**a**) xerostomia (input = 309 genes; output = 229) and (**b**) dry mouth (input = 159 genes; output = 110) at a confidence level of 0.90.

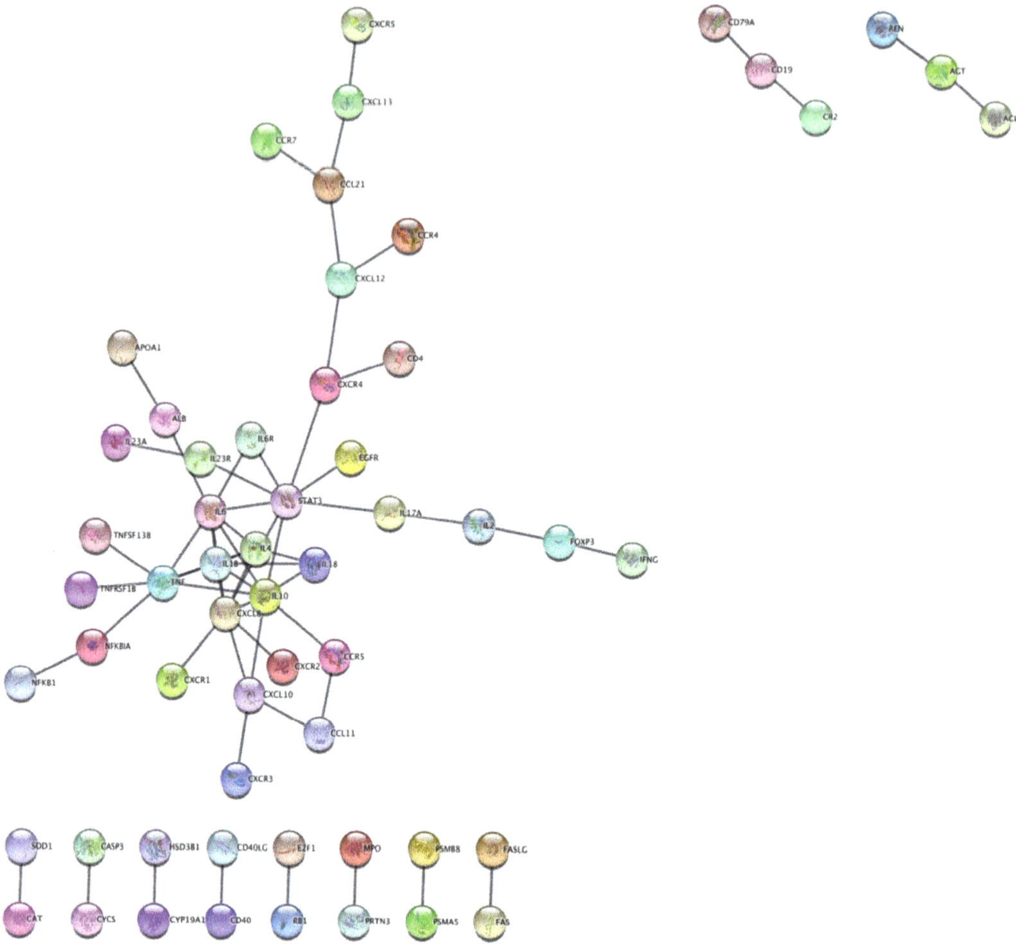

Figure 3. Cytoscape Protein–Protein Interaction Network of Xerostomia/Dry Mouth Network Intersection. Cytoscapev3.8.1:stringAppv1.6.0 protein–protein interaction network of xerostomia (input = 128 genes) and dry mouth (input = 55 genes) intersection (genes with matching name or Ensembl ID) with a 0.98 confidence score. The total number of returned genes in the network intersection is 58.

Table 2. Drugs Evaluated via ClinicalTrials.gov and the Drug–Gene Interaction Database Identified Drug–Gene Interactions. [a] Drug identified by Clinicaltrials.gov (https://ClinicalTrials.gov/) that has been/is being evaluated for diseases related to xerostomia/dry mouth. [b] Disease that the drug has been/is being evaluated for with an input search in ClinicalTrials.gov of "xerostomia" and "dry mouth". [c] ClinicalTrials.gov identifier. [d] Gene targets of drug identified using DrugBank (https://go.drugbank.com). Genes shown in bold are in common with the 54 genes identified with interactions using the Drug–Gene Interaction database (DGIdb) (https://www.dgidb.org/). [e] Genes identified by DGIdb (https://www.dgidb.org/) as having interactions with the drug. Note: HNC-OC is head and neck cancer oral complications; ND is not determined; SS is Sjögren's Syndrome.

Drug [a]	Disease [b]	Clinical Trial ID [c]	DrugBank Identified Drug Target [d]	DGIdb Gene [e]
Belimumab	SS	NCT02631538; NCT01160666	*TNFSF13B*	*TNFSF13B*
Cisplatin	HNC-OC; Xerostomia	NCT00057785; NCT04392622; NCT02990468	*DNA; MPG; A2M; TF; ATOX1;* ***MPO****; XDH; CYP4A11; PTGS2; NAT; CYP2C9; CYP2B6; BCHE; GSTT1; MT1A; MT2A;* ***SOD1****; GSTP1; NQO1; GSTM1;* ***ALB****; ABCC3; ABCC5; ABCC2; SLC22A2; SLC31A1; SLC31A2; ABCC6; ATP7B; ATP7A; ABCG2*	*E2F1; CXCR4; IL6; RB1; IFNG; EGFR; FAS*
Cyclosporine	SS	NCT00025818	*HRH1; HRH2; HRH3; S100A1; S100A2; S100B; S100A13; S100A2; CYP3A4; FMO1; FMO3;* ***ALB****; ABCB1*	*IL2; TNF; IL10*
Dexamethasone	SS; Xerostomia; HNC-OC	NCT01316770; NCT01748942; NCT00631358	*NR3C1; NR0B1; ANXA1; NOS2; NR1I2; HSD11B2; CYP3A4; HSD11B1; CYP3A5; CYP3A7; CYP17A1; CYP1A1; CYP2A6; CYP2B6; CYP2C19; CYP2C8; CYP2E1; CYP3A43; CYP4A11; CYP11B1;* ***ALB****; ABCB1; SLC22A8; ABCB11; ABCC2; ABCG2; SLCO1A2*	ND
Etanercept	SS	NCT00001954	***TNF****; FCGR1A; FCGR2A; FCGR2B; FCGR2C; FCGR3A; FCGR3B; LTA; C1Q PROTEIN GROUP*	*TNFRSF1B*
Fluorouracil	HNC-OC	NCT00057785	*TYMS; DNA; RNA; CYP2C9; CYP1A2; TYMP; DPYD; UPP1; UPP2; CYP2A6; CYP2C8; MTHFR; TYMS; UMPS; PPAT;* ***ALB****; SERPINA7; SLC22A7; SLC29A1; ABCG2; ABCC3; ABCC4; ABCC5*	*IL6R*
Hydroxychloroquine	SS	NCT01601028; NCT00431041; NCT00873496	*DNA; TLR7; TLR9; ACE2; CYP3A4; CYP2D6; CYP2C8;* ***ALB***	*TNF*
Levocarnitine	SS	NCT03953703	*SLC22A4; SLC22A5; CRAT; SLC24A29; SLC25A20; CROT; CPT2; CPT1A; XDH; CES1;* ***MPO****; SLC22A4; SLCO1B1; SLC22A5; SLC22A16; SLC22A8*	ND
Melatonin	HNC-OC	NCT02430298	*MTNR1A; MTNR1B; ESR1; RORB; CALM1;* ***MPO****; EPX; CALR; ASMT; NQO2; CYP1A1; CYP1A2; CYP1B1; CYP2C19; CYP2C9; ASMT; IDO1;* ***CYP19A1****; SLC22A8*	*IFNG*
Methotrexate	Autoimmune diseases	NCT03239600	*DHFR; TYMS; ATIC; DHFR; AOX1; MTHFR; PGD; FPGS; TYMS; ATIC; GGH; CYP3A4;* ***ALB****; ABCC3; ABCC4; ABCC1; SLC22A6; ABCC10; SLC22A8; ABCC2; ABCB1; SLC01A2; SLC16A1; ABCC11; SLCO1B3; SLC22A11; SLCO1C1; SLCO3A1; ABCG2; SLC22A7; SLC46A1; SLCO1B1; SLC04C1; SLC19A1; FOLR1; FOLR2; SLC15A1; SLC36A1*	*FOXP3; RB1; IL2; E2F1*
Mirabegron	SS	NCT04909255	*ADRB3; ADRB1; CYP3A4; CYP2D6; BCHE; UGT2B7; UGT1A3; UGT1A8;* ***ALB****; ORM1; ABCB1; SLCO1A2; SLC22A1; SLC22A2; SLC22A3*	ND
Oxybutynin	SS; Overactive bladder	NCT04909255; NCT00431041	*CHRM3; CHRM2; CHRM1; CYP3A4; CYP2C8; CYP2D6; CYP3A5; ORM1;* ***ALB***	ND

Table 2. *Cont.*

Drug [a]	Disease [b]	Clinical Trial ID [c]	DrugBank Identified Drug Target [d]	DGIdb Gene [e]
Paclitaxel	Xerostomia	NCT00095927	*TUBB1; BCL2; MAP4; MAP2; MAPT; NR1I2; CYP3A4; CYP3A5; CYP3A7;* ***CYP19A1****; CYP1B1; CYP2C8; ABCB11; ABCB1; ABCC1; ABCC10; SLCO1B3; ABCC2*	*E2F1; CYP19A1; CASP3; EGFR; CXCL8*
Prednisone	SS	NCT02370550	*NR3C1; CYP3A4; CYP2C19; CYP3A5; CYTOCHROME P450 3A SUBFAMILY GROUP; CYP2A6; CYP1B1; CYP2B6; CYP2CB; CYP2C9; HSD11B1;* ***ALB****; SERPINA6*	*CXCL12; IFNG*
Tacrolimus	SS; Dry eye	NCT03865888; NCT01850979	*FKBP1A; CYP3A5; CYP3A4;* ***ALB****; ORM1; ABCB1; ABCA5; SLCO1B1*	*IL18; FOXP3; IL10*
Thalidomide	SS; Xerostomia	NCT00001599	*CRBN;* ***TNF****;* ***NFKB1****; DNA; FGFR2; PTGS2; ALPHA1-ACID GLYCOPROTEIN GROUP*	*IL6R; NFKB1; TNF*
Tocilizumab	SS	NCT01782235	***IL6R****; CYP3A4*	*IL6R*
Tofacitinib	SS	NCT04496960	*JAK1; JAK2; JAK3; TYK2; CYP3A4; CYP2C19;* ***ALB***	ND

4. Discussion

This is the first study to apply a conventional review with bioinformatics tools to determine genetic and proteomic panels regarding the treatment of xerostomia (Figure 1). This approach has the potential to identify drug targets which could be used to create targeted treatments for xerostomic patients. We were able to identify search terms related to xerostomia and/or dry mouth (Table 1) and to combine P2E results for either xerostomia or dry mouth, thereby producing large networks of PPIs using $STRING_{v11\cdot0}$ at a high confidence (Figure 2). $STRING_{v11\cdot0}$ produced PPI networks of 229 xerostomia and 110 dry mouth genes using a CL of 0.90. Using a CS of 0.98, $Cytoscape_{v3\cdot8\cdot1}$ was able to narrow the $STRING_{v11\cdot0}$ results by returning networks of 128 genes from 229 xerostomia genes and 55 genes from 110 dry mouth genes (Figure S1). Using the 'intersection' option in $Cytoscape_{v3\cdot8\cdot1}$, we were able to focus our results to 58 genes from 128 xerostomia and 55 dry mouth genes with matching names or Ensembl IDs (Figure 3). Additionally, we were able to enrich our $Cytoscape_{v3\cdot8\cdot1}$ results with KEGG pathways as well as GO biological processes and to determine possible drug targets from our results.

When investigating the significant KEGG pathways identified by Cytoscape, we found that the 'cytokine–cytokine receptor interaction' pathway (hsa04060) is related to 'hypohidrotic ectodermal dysplasia' (KEGG DISEASE: H00651) and 'chronic mucocutaneous candidiasis' (KEGG DISEASE: H01109), both conditions causing symptoms related to xerostomia (Table S2 and Data File S2) [28]. Furthermore, the 'cytokine–cytokine receptor interaction' pathway was the most significant KEGG pathway (hsa04060; FDR = 1.06×10^{-49}) identified in the xerostomia/dry mouth intersection network. This pathway involves the gene *IL6R* which had the second-highest drug–gene interaction score of 17.72 (Table S2, Data File S2 and Data File S4) [35]. *IL6R* was also the target of a drug that we identified and has been evaluated in a clinical trial for its efficacy in primary Sjögren's Syndrome (pSS) patients (NCT01782235) (Table 2) [38]. The clinical trial was completed in July of 2018 and although results have not been posted, a publication of the trial determined that tocilizumab did not improve symptoms over a 24 week period compared to the placebo [39]. Indeed, *IL6R* has eight other drug–gene interactions according to DGIdb, which might explain this outcome (Table S3) [35]. Additionally, *IL6R* is a gene product of the 'inflammatory response' biological process (GO:0006954) which was found to be the second most overrepresented using BiNGO (Data File S3) [29–31].

IL6R was also identified in the third-most significant KEGG pathway, 'pathways in cancer' (hsa05200) (Table S2) [28]. We found that this pathway also involves the genes *NFKB1* and *EGFR*. *NFKB1* had 90 drug interactions according to the DGIdb database (Table S3) [34]. Our analysis revealed that only one clinical trial had evaluated the drug thalidomide targeting *NFKB1* for Sjögren's Syndrome (NCT00001599) (Table 2) [37]. This phase II trial was completed in June 2002, with no results posted. However, Pillemer et al. described that the administration of thalidomide was associated with unacceptable adverse effects when given at a dose of 50 or 100 mg [40]. All primary Sjögren's Syndrome patients (n = 4) had to discontinue the medication after the third week [40]. Furthermore, no clinical trials were identified that have evaluated *EGFR* as a drug target in xerostomia, dry mouth, or Sjögren's Syndrome. Indeed, *EGFR* had 178 drug–gene interactions in our gene set (the maximum), which could be exploited to partially restore the functionality of salivary glands by reducing inflammation (Table 2 and Table S3). We determined that *EGFR*, a gene belonging to the 'inflammatory response' biological process (GO:0006954), had the second-highest salivary expression confidence rating of 2.80 (Figure S3 and Data File S3) [29,31]. In addition, Lisi et al. determined that overexpression of nerve growth factor-beta, which is elevated in salivary gland epithelial cells in pSS, can be prevented with *EGFR* pathway inhibition [41]. Furthermore, Sisto et al. found that pro-inflammatory cytokine release can be reduced in salivary gland epithelial cells using an *EGFR* inhibitor combined with an *ADAM metallopeptidase domain 17* (*ADAM17*) inhibitor [42]. Further investigation into the involvement of these pathways and genes in xerostomia are warranted.

Other genes that may be of interest in the development and treatment of xerostomia are *MPO* and *TNFSF13B*, both of which are involved in the significantly overrepresented GO 'immune system process' (GO:002376) (Data File S3) [29,31]. Although *MPO* was not identified in a highly significant KEGG pathway, it had the highest expression confidence rating of 4.35 in saliva and had 21 drug–gene interactions via DGIdb (Figure S3 and Table S3) [35]. Moreover, *MPO* was a target of drugs in five clinical trials evaluating their effectiveness in the treatment of xerostomia, head and neck cancer oral complications, and Sjögren's Syndrome (NCT02430298, NCT00057785, NCT03953703, NCT04392622, and NCT02990468) (Table 2) [43–47]. One clinical trial determined that intensity modulated radiation therapy (IMRT) in patients with nasopharyngeal cancer combined with cisplatin and fluorouracil improved xerostomia scores significantly compared to previous radiation therapy oncology group trials [48]. Although some studies suggest that melatonin may have implications in the prevention and/or treatment of oral pathologies such as xerostomia, no clinical trials have reported its efficacy [49–51]. Clinical trials involving cisplatin, melatonin, and/or levocarnitine still hold the promise for better outcomes in the prevention and treatment of xerostomia. In addition, for disease conditions such as diabetes mellitus causing salivary gland dysfunction which results in salivary flow reduction and a change in saliva composition, significant mitigation of subjective xerostomia may be achieved through artificial saliva [52].

TNFSF13B is another gene of interest related to xerostomia, as, in our analysis, it had the greatest drug–gene interaction score of 63.79 among drugs that have been/are being evaluated in clinical trials (Data File S4). It is also the only identified target of the drug belimumab (Data File S4) [35,53]. Two clinical trials were found that evaluated this drug for efficacy and safety in pSS patients (NCT02631538 and NCT01160666) (Table 2) [54,55]. In clinical trial NCT02631538, of 24 patients receiving belimumab monotherapy, two patients had adverse effects and only one patient reached the stopping criteria for the study [54]. The other clinical trial (NCT01160666) found that lower blood cells and salivary natural killer cells were associated with a better response to belimumab [55,56]. This could be due to the high expression confidence of *TNFSF13B* in blood and saliva, 4.63 and 2.54, respectively (Figure S3). Furthermore, in patients with kidney renal clear cell carcinoma, it has been suggested that *TNFSF13B* may regulate the natural kill cell-mediated cytotoxicity pathway [57].

5. Limitations

For this study, several limitations related to our methodology and results must be recognized. There are few publications on xerostomia and limited human trials investigating the condition. Furthermore, xerostomia pathobiology is not well understood and there is much debate among investigators regarding the prevalence of xerostomia in different geographical locations and ethnic groups. The results reported in this study that may be relevant to xerostomia therapeutic development will require substantial validation in experimental preclinical models, since these were based on 'confidence' ranking of published research and scores provided by computational systems biology tools.

6. Conclusions

The *IL6R*, *EGFR*, *NFKB1*, *MPO*, and *TNFSF13B* genes might all have implications in the diagnosis and intervention of xerostomia. Our findings highlight the need for further investigation into these genes as candidate targets for treatment or treatment response follow-up in the future. However, the greatest challenge of such investigations resides in the difficulty to screen for relevant biomarkers, including those associated with genetic susceptibility, which would enable a better stratification of xerostomic patients at the molecular level.

Supplementary Materials: The following supporting information can be downloaded at: https://www.mdpi.com/article/10.3390/jcm11051442/s1, Table S1: Risk-of-Bias Assessment per PRISMA Guidelines. Risk-of-Bias assessment table using 'Cochran's Handbook for Systematic Reviews of Interventions' Risk-of-bias VISualization (robvis) tool for 40 publications manually curated using conventional searches of PubMed and PubMed Central for articles related to xerostomia, in English, between the years 2000 and 2020. Using Cochran's Risk-of-Bias 2 criteria, 19 publications were excluded. Of the total 40 publications, 21 publications were investigated to determine 'search terms' for xerostomia and dry mouth. Data File S1: P2E Results for Search Terms. Pubmed2ensembl results for 64 identified search terms. Figure S1: Cytoscape Xerostomia and Dry Mouth Protein–Protein Interaction Networks. $\text{Cytoscape}_{v3\cdot 8\cdot 1}$ protein–protein interaction networks using $\text{stringApp}_{v1\cdot 6\cdot 0}$ for (a) xerostomia (input = 229 genes; output = 128 genes) and (b) dry mouth (input = 110 genes; output = 55 genes) with a confidence score of 0.98 and a tissue expression filter for saliva set at 1.0. Data File S2: KEGG Pathways via STRING Enrichment from Cytosape for Xerostomia/Dry Mouth Intersection. Data File S3: GO Overrepresented Biological Processes from Cytoscape for Xerostomia/Dry Mouth Intersection. Table S2: Significant KEGG Pathways via STRING Enrichment in Cytoscape for Xerostomia/Dry Mouth Intersection. Table showing FDR significant ($p < 1.0 \times 10^{-4}$) KEGG pathways with more than 25 genes via $\text{Cytoscape}_{v3\cdot 8\cdot 1}$:$\text{stringApp}_{v1\cdot 6\cdot 0}$ STRING enrichment for xerostomia/dry mouth interaction network at a confidence score of 0.98. Genes in bold are in the gene xerostomia/dry mouth interaction gene set. Figure S2: BiNGO Overrepresentation of GO Terms for Xerostomia/Dry Mouth Intersection. Biological Networks Gene Ontology ($\text{BiNGO}_{v3\cdot 0\cdot 3}$) tool network of overrepresented Gene Ontology (GO) terms ($n = 360$) in the xerostomia/dry mouth intersection protein–protein interaction network for humans. Overrepresented GO terms shown are those at $p < 1 \times 10^{-4}$ using a hypergeometric test and false discovery rate correction. Figure S3: Gene Expression Confidences for 19 out of 20 Tissue Types. Histograms plotted using $\text{Python}_{v3\cdot 6\cdot 1}$:$\text{matplotlib}_{v3\cdot 0\cdot 3}$ package showing $\text{Cytoscape}_{v3\cdot 8\cdot 2}$ $\text{stringApp}_{v1\cdot 6\cdot 0}$ network gene expression for 19 out of 20 possible tissue types identified in the PPI network of xerostomia/dry mouth intersection with a confidence score of 0.98. Gene expression data from $\text{stringApp}_{v1\cdot 6\cdot 0}$ STRING enrichment feature that gathers information about expression of genes from $\text{TISSUES}_{v2\cdot 0}$ database (https://tissues.jensenlab.org/Search, accessed on 8 August 2021). $\text{TISSUES}_{v2\cdot 0}$ uses a "confidence" based rating from zero to five based on knowledge, experiments, and text mining. Table S3: The Drug–Gene Interaction Database Identified Drug–Gene Interaction Counts. [a] Gene identified in the xerostomia/dry mouth intersection network (54 of 58). [b] Number of drug–gene interactions identified using the Drug–gene Interaction database. Data File S4: The Drug–Gene Interaction Database Identified Interactions.

Author Contributions: J.-L.C.M. and F.B.M. conceived this study, contributed to the design of the analytical strategy, data interpretation and verification. M.F.B. designed the overall analytical strategy, conducted computational analyses, data interpretation, and curation of the data. E.J.B. and C.K.I. performed the initial analyses. All authors contributed to the writing/revision of the manuscript. All authors have read and agreed to the published version of the manuscript.

Funding: The research received no external funding.

Institutional Review Board Statement: Not applicable.

Informed Consent Statement: Not applicable.

Data Availability Statement: Publicly available data were used. All data used can be retrieved from the supplementary files or through our lab's GitHub repository (https://github.com/mbeckm01/Xerostomia.git, accessed on 12 January 2022).

Acknowledgments: This work was supported by the Atrium Health Foundation Research Fund (internal).

Conflicts of Interest: The authors declare no conflict of interest.

References

1. Thakkar, J.P.; Lane, C.J. Hyposalivation and Xerostomia and Burning Mouth Syndrome: Medical Management. *Oral Maxillofac. Surg. Clin. N. Am.* **2022**, *34*, 135–146. [CrossRef]
2. Sasportas, L.S.; Hosford, D.N.; Sodini, M.A.; Waters, D.J.; Zambricki, E.A.; Barral, J.K.; Graves, E.E.; Brinton, T.J.; Yock, P.G.; Le, Q.T.; et al. Cost-effectiveness landscape analysis of treatments addressing xerostomia in patients receiving head and neck radiation therapy. *Oral Surg. Oral Med. Oral Pathol. Oral Radiol.* **2013**, *116*, e37–e51. [CrossRef]

3. Field, E.A.; Fear, S.; Higham, S.M.; Ireland, R.S.; Rostron, J.; Willetts, R.M.; Longman, L.P. Age and medication are significant ris factors for xerostomia in an English population, attending general dental practice. *Gerodontology* **2001**, *18*, 21–24. [CrossRef]
4. Shinkai, R.S.; Hatch, J.P.; Schmidt, C.B.; Sartori, E.A. Exposure to the oral side effects of medication in a community-based samp *Spec. Care Dent.* **2006**, *26*, 116–120. [CrossRef]
5. Tanasiewicz, M.; Hildebrandt, T.; Obersztyn, I. Xerostomia of Various Etiologies: A Review of the Literature. *Adv. Clin. Exp. Me* **2016**, *25*, 199–206. [CrossRef]
6. Mirzaii-Dizgah, I.; Agha-Hosseini, F. Unstimulated whole saliva parathyroid hormone in postmenopausal women with xerost mia. *J. Contemp. Dent. Pract.* **2011**, *12*, 196–199. [CrossRef]
7. Marcott, S.; Dewan, K.; Kwan, M.; Baik, F.; Lee, Y.J.; Sirjani, D. Where Dysphagia Begins: Polypharmacy and Xerostomia. *Fe Pract.* **2020**, *37*, 234–241.
8. Hopcraft, M.S.; Tan, C. Xerostomia: An update for clinicians. *Aust. Dent. J.* **2010**, *55*, 238–244. [CrossRef]
9. Sivaramakrishnan, G.; Sridharan, K. Electrical nerve stimulation for xerostomia: A meta-analysis of randomised controlled trial *J. Tradit. Complement. Med.* **2017**, *7*, 409–413. [CrossRef]
10. American Dental Association. Available online: https://www.ada.org/en/member-center/oral-health-topics/xerostomi (accessed on 12 May 2020).
11. Glore, R.J.; Spiteri-Staines, K.; Paleri, V. A patient with dry mouth. *Clin. Otolaryngol.* **2009**, *34*, 358–363. [CrossRef]
12. Wu, L.S.; Huang, M.C.; Chen, C.K.; Shen, C.Y.; Fann, C.S.; Lin, C.Y.; Lin, C.C.; Cheng, A.T. Genome-Wide Association Study c Lithium-Induced Dry Mouth in Bipolar I Disorder. *J. Pers. Med.* **2021**, *11*, 1265. [CrossRef]
13. Thomson, W.M.; Chalmers, J.M.; Spencer, A.J.; Slade, G.D. Medication and dry mouth: Findings from a cohort study of olde people. *J. Public Health Dent.* **2000**, *60*, 12–20. [CrossRef]
14. Nederfors, T.; Isaksson, R.; Mörnstad, H.; Dahlöf, C. Prevalence of perceived symptoms of dry mouth in an adult Swedis population—Relation to age, sex and pharmacotherapy. *Community Dent. Oral Epidemiol.* **1997**, *25*, 211–216. [CrossRef] [PubMed
15. Assery, M.K.A. Efficacy of Artificial Salivary Substitutes in Treatment of Xerostomia: A Systematic Review. *J. Pharm. Bioallied Sc* **2019**, *11* (Suppl. S1), S1–S12. [CrossRef]
16. Vissink, A.; Mitchell, J.B.; Baum, B.J.; Limesand, K.H.; Jensen, S.B.; Fox, P.C.; Elting, L.S.; Langendijk, J.A.; Coppes, R.P.; Reylan M.E. Clinical management of salivary gland hypofunction and xerostomia in head-and-neck cancer patients: Successes an barriers. *Int. J. Radiat. Oncol. Biol. Phys.* **2010**, *78*, 983–991. [CrossRef]
17. Furness, S.; Worthington, H.V.; Bryan, G.; Birchenough, S.; McMillan, R. Interventions for the management of dry mouth: Topica therapies. *Cochrane Database Syst. Rev.* **2011**, *12*, CD008934. [CrossRef]
18. Singhal, A.; Leaman, R.; Catlett, N.; Lemberger, T.; McEntyre, J.; Polson, S.; Xenarios, I.; Arighi, C.; Lu, Z. Pressing needs o biomedical text mining in biocuration and beyond: Opportunities and challenges. *Database* **2016**, *2016*, baw161. [CrossRef]
19. Baxevanis, A.D. The importance of biological databases in biological discovery. *Curr. Protoc. Bioinform.* **2009**, *50*, 1. [CrossRef]
20. Jensen, L.J.; Saric, J.; Bork, P. Literature mining for the biologist: From information retrieval to biological discovery. *Nat. Re Genet.* **2006**, *7*, 119–129. [CrossRef]
21. NCBI Resource Coordinators. Database resources of the National Center for Biotechnology Information. *Nucleic Acids Res.* **201** *46*, D8–D13. [CrossRef]
22. Higgins, J.P.T.; Thomas, J.; Chandler, J.; Cumpston, M.; Li, T.; Page, M.J.; Welch, V.A. (Eds.) *Cochrane Handbook for Systemati Reviews of Interventions*, 2nd ed.; John Wiley & Sons: Chichester, UK, 2019.
23. McGuinness, L.A.; Higgins, J.P.T. Risk-of-bias VISualization (robvis): An R package and Shiny web app for visualizing risk-of-bia assessments. *Res. Syn. Methods* **2020**, *12*, 55–61. [CrossRef] [PubMed]
24. Baran, J.; Gerner, M.; Haeussler, M.; Nenadic, G.; Bergman, C.M. pubmed2ensembl: A resource for mining the biological literatur on genes. *PLoS ONE* **2011**, *6*, e24716. [CrossRef]
25. Szklarczyk, D.; Gable, A.L.; Lyon, D.; Junge, A.; Wyder, S.; Huerta-Cepas, J.; Simonovic, M.; Doncheva, N.T.; Morris, J.H Bork, P.; et al. STRING v11: Protein-protein association networks with increased coverage, supporting functional discovery i genome-wide experimental datasets. *Nucleic Acids Res.* **2019**, *47*, D607–D613. [CrossRef] [PubMed]
26. Shannon, P.; Markiel, A.; Ozier, O.; Baliga, N.S.; Wang, J.T.; Ramage, D.; Amin, N.; Schwikowski, B.; Ideker, T. Cytoscape: software environment for integrated models of biomolecular interaction networks. *Genome Res.* **2003**, *13*, 2498–2504. [CrossRef [PubMed]
27. Doncheva, N.T.; Morris, J.H.; Gorodkin, J.; Jensen, L.J. Cytoscape StringApp: Network Analysis and Visualization of Proteomic Data. *J. Proteome Res.* **2019**, *18*, 623–632. [CrossRef]
28. Kanehisa, M.; Goto, S. KEGG: Kyoto encyclopedia of genes and genomes. *Nucleic Acids Res.* **2000**, *28*, 27–30. [CrossRef]
29. Gene Ontology Consortium. Gene Ontology Consortium: Going forward. *Nucleic Acids Res.* **2015**, *43*, D1049–D1056. [CrossRef
30. Maere, S.; Heymans, K.; Kuiper, M. BiNGO: A Cytoscape plugin to assess overrepresentation of gene ontology categories i biological networks. *Bioinformatics* **2005**, *21*, 3448–3449. [CrossRef]
31. Carbon, S.; Ireland, A.; Mungall, C.J.; Shu, S.; Marshall, B.; Lewis, S.; AmiGO Hub; Web Presence Working Group. AmiGC Online access to ontology and annotation data. *Bioinformatics* **2009**, *25*, 288–289. [CrossRef]
32. Python Software Foundation. Python Laguage Reference. Version 3.6. Available online: http://www.python.org/ (accessed o 12 May 2021).
33. Hunter, J.D. Matplotlib: A 2D Graphics Environment. *Comput. Sci. Eng.* **2007**, *9*, 90–95. [CrossRef]

34. Palasca, O.; Santos, A.; Stolte, C.; Gorodkin, J.; Jensen, L.J. TISSUES 2.0: An integrative web resource on mammalian tissue expression. *Database* **2018**, *2018*, bay003. [CrossRef] [PubMed]
35. Freshour, S.L.; Kiwala, S.; Cotto, K.C.; Coffman, A.C.; McMichael, J.F.; Song, J.J.; Griffith, M.; Griffith, O.L.; Wagner, A.H. Integration of the Drug-Gene Interaction Database (DGIdb 4.0) with open crowdsource efforts. *Nucleic Acids Res.* **2021**, *49*, D1144–D1151. [CrossRef] [PubMed]
36. ClinicalTrials.gov. National Library of Medicine (US). Available online: http://clinicaltrials.gov/ (accessed on 10 August 2021).
37. ClinicalTrials.gov. National Library of Medicine (US). NCT00001599. Pilot Study of Thalidomide to Treat Sjögren's Syndrome. Available online: https://clinicaltrials.gov/ct2/show/NCT00001599 (accessed on 10 August 2021).
38. ClinicalTrials.gov. National Library of Medicine (US). NCT01782235. Efficacy of Tocilizumab in Primary Sjögren's Syndrome. Available online: https://clinicaltrials.gov/ct2/show/NCT01782235 (accessed on 10 August 2021).
39. Felten, R.; Devauchelle-Pensec, V.; Seror, R.; Duffau, P.; Saadoun, D.; Hachulla, E.; Pierre Yves, H.; Salliot, C.; Perdriger, A.; Morel, J.; et al. Interleukin 6 receptor inhibition in primary Sjögren syndrome: A multicentre double-blind randomised placebo-controlled trial. *Ann. Rheum. Dis.* **2020**, *80*, 329–338. [CrossRef]
40. Pillemer, S.R.; Leakan, R.A.; Sankar, V.; Manny, J.; Baum, B.J.; Smith, J.; Chaudhry, U.; Fox, P.C.; Radfar, L.; Ligier, S.; et al. Prominent adverse effects of thalidomide in primary Sjögren's syndrome. *Arthritis Rheum.* **2004**, *51*, 505–506. [CrossRef]
41. Lisi, S.; Sisto, M.; Ribatti, D.; D'Amore, M.; De Lucro, R.; Frassanito, M.A.; Lorusso, L.; Vacca, A.; Lofrumento, D.D. Chronic inflammation enhances NGF-β/TrkA system expression via EGFR/MEK/ERK pathway activation in Sjögren's syndrome. *J. Mol. Med.* **2014**, *92*, 523–537. [CrossRef] [PubMed]
42. Sisto, M.; Lisi, S.; D'Amore, M.; Lofrumento, D.D. The metalloproteinase ADAM17 and the epidermal growth factor receptor (EGFR) signaling drive the inflammatory epithelial response in Sjögren's syndrome. *Clin. Exp. Med.* **2015**, *15*, 215–225. [CrossRef]
43. ClinicalTrials.gov. National Library of Medicine (US). NCT02430298, Topical/Oral Melatonin for Preventing Concurrent Radiochemotherapy Induced Oral Mucositis/Xerostomia Cancer Patients. Available online: https://clinicaltrials.gov/ct2/show/NCT02430298 (accessed on 10 August 2021).
44. ClinicalTrials.gov. National Library of Medicine (US). NCT00057785. Radiation Therapy with or without Chemotherapy in Reducing Mouth Dryness in Patients with Nasopharyngeal Cancer. Available online: https://clinicaltrials.gov/ct2/show/NCT00057785 (accessed on 10 August 2021).
45. ClinicalTrials.gov. National Library of Medicine (US). NCT03953703. Levocarnitine for Dry Eye in Sjögren's Syndrome. Available online: https://clinicaltrials.gov/ct2/show/NCT03953703 (accessed on 10 August 2021).
46. ClinicalTrials.gov. National Library of Medicine (US). NCT04392622. d-Limonene +Radiation +Platinum Based Chemo for Xerostomia Prevention in Locally Advanced Head and Neck Squamous Cell Carcinoma. Available online: https://clinicaltrials.gov/ct2/show/NCT04392622 (accessed on 10 August 2021).
47. ClinicalTrials.gov. National Library of Medicine (US). NCT02990468. A Trial of Concurrent Radiation Therapy, Cisplatin, and BMX-001 in Locally Advanced Head and Neck Cancer (BMX-HN). Available online: https://clinicaltrials.gov/ct2/show/NCT02990468 (accessed on 10 August 2021).
48. Lee, N.; Harris, J.; Garden, A.S.; Straube, W.; Glisson, B.; Xia, P.; Bosch, W.; Morrison, W.H.; Quivey, J.; Thorstad, W.; et al. Intensity-modulated radiation therapy with or without chemotherapy for nasopharyngeal carcinoma: Radiation therapy oncology group phase II trial 0225. *J. Clin. Oncol.* **2009**, *27*, 3684–3690. [CrossRef] [PubMed]
49. Reiter, R.J.; Rosales-Corral, S.A.; Liu, X.Y.; Acuna-Castroviejo, D.; Escames, G.; Tan, D.X. Melatonin in the oral cavity: Physiological and pathological implications. *J. Periodontal. Res.* **2015**, *50*, 9–17. [CrossRef] [PubMed]
50. Mehta, A.; Kaur, G. Potential role of melatonin in prevention and treatment of oral carcinoma. *Indian J. Dent.* **2014**, *5*, 86–91. [CrossRef] [PubMed]
51. Gómez-Moreno, G.; Guardia, J.; Ferrera, M.J.; Cutando, A.; Reiter, R.J. Melatonin in diseases of the oral cavity. *Oral Dis.* **2010**, *16*, 242–247. [CrossRef] [PubMed]
52. Sinjari, B.; Feragalli, B.; Cornelli, U.; Belcaro, G.; Vitacolonna, E.; Santilli, M.; Rexhepi, I.; D'Addazio, G.; Zuccari, F.; Caputi, S. Artificial Saliva in Diabetic Xerostomia (ASDIX): Double Blind Trial of Aldiamed® Versus Placebo. *J. Clin. Med.* **2020**, *9*, 2196. [CrossRef] [PubMed]
53. Wishart, D.S.; Knox, C.; Guo, A.C.; Cheng, D.; Shrivastava, S.; Tzur, D.; Gautam, B.; Hassanali, M. DrugBank: A knowledgebase for drugs, drug actions and drug targets. *Nucleic Acids Res.* **2008**, *36*, D901–D906. [CrossRef] [PubMed]
54. ClinicalTrials.gov. National Library of Medicine (US). NCT02631538, Safety and Efficacy Study of Subcutaneous Belimumab and Intravenous Rituximab Co-administration in Subjects with Primary Sjögren's Syndrome. Available online: https://clinicaltrials.gov/ct2/show/NCT02631538 (accessed on 10 August 2021).
55. ClinicalTrials.gov. National Library of Medicine (US). NCT01160666. Efficacy and Safety of Belimumab in Subjects with Primary Sjögren's Syndrome (BELISS). Available online: https://clinicaltrials.gov/ct2/show/NCT01160666 (accessed on 10 August 2021).
56. Seror, R.; Nocturne, G.; Lazure, T.; Hendel-Chavez, H.; Desmoulins, F.; Belkhir, R.; Ravaud, P.; Benbijja, M.; Poirier-Colame, V.; Taoufik, Y.; et al. Low numbers of blood and salivary natural killer cells are associated with a better response to belimumab in primary Sjögren's syndrome: Results of the BELISS study. *Arthritis Res. Ther.* **2015**, *17*, 241. [CrossRef] [PubMed]
57. Li, S.; Hou, J.; Wang, Z.; Chang, J.; Xu, W. TNFSF13B correlated with poor prognosis and immune infiltrates in KIRC: A study based on TCGA data. *Int. J. Clin. Exp. Med.* **2019**, *12*, 12057–12067.

Journal of
Clinical Medicine

MDPI

eview

;jögren Syndrome: New Insights in the Pathogenesis and Role ›f Nuclear Medicine

ınzola Luz Kelly [1,2,3,*], Rivera Jose Nelson [4], Ramírez Sara [3] and Signore Alberto [5]

1 Nuclear Medicine Unit, Clinica Universitaria Colombia, Bogotá 111321, Colombia
2 Nuclear Medicine Unit, Clinica Reina Sofia, Bogotá 110121, Colombia
3 Fundacion Universitaria Sanitas, Bogotá 110111, Colombia
4 Internal Medicine Department Clinica Reina Sofia, Bogotá 110121, Colombia
5 Nuclear Medicine Unit, Department of Medical-Surgical Sciences and of Translational Medicine, Faculty of Medicine and Psychology, "Sapienza" University, 00185 Rome, Italy
* Correspondence: lkanzola@gmail.com; Tel.: +57-3112810545

Abstract: In the last years, new insights into the molecular basis of rheumatic conditions have been described, which have generated particular interest in understanding the pathophysiology of these diseases, in which lies the explanation of the diversity of clinical presentation and the difficulty in diagnostic and therapeutic approaches. In this review, we focus on the new pathophysiological findings for Sjögren syndrome and on the derived new SPECT and PET radiopharmaceuticals to detect inflammation of immunological origin, focusing on their role in diagnosis, prognosis, and the evaluation of therapeutic efficacy.

Keywords: Sjögren syndrome; nuclear medicine; radiopharmaceuticals; PET; SPECT

:**itation:** Kelly, A.L.; Nelson, R.J.; ara, R.; Alberto, S. Sjögren yndrome: New Insights in the 'athogenesis and Role of Nuclear Aedicine. *J. Clin. Med.* **2022**, *11*, 5227. ıttps://doi.org/10.3390/jcm11175227

\cademic Editor: Margherita Sisto

:eceived: 29 June 2022
\ccepted: 2 September 2022
'ublished: 4 September 2022

ublisher's Note: MDPI stays neutral vith regard to jurisdictional claims in ›ublished maps and institutional affil-ations.

1. Introduction

Sjögren syndrome (SS) belongs to the family of rheumatic autoimmune diseases characterized by systemic compromise with exocrine glands as target organs that are affected by chronic inflammation and immune-mediated destruction of the tissue, leading to severe dryness of the mouth and eyes. Extra-glandular symptoms are frequent and include fatigue, polyarthralgias, myositis, polyneuropathy, and gammaglobulinopathies, among others [1]. Since there is evidence of the presence of common pathophysiologic mechanisms shared by SS and thyroiditis, it is also common to find thyroid involvement in patients with SS as part of the peri-epithelial extra salivary manifestations of the disease [2]. Systemic complications regarding extra-glandular tissues are associated with vascular, respiratory, gastrointestinal, renal, and neurological systems, possibly affecting one-third of these patients [1].

SS may be present as a primary condition or accompanying other autoimmune diseases as secondary SS. In addition, SS has a predominant clinical presentation in females, with a female:male ratio of 9:1, higher than for all other autoimmune diseases [1]. The clinical phenotype of SS varies from benign conditions such as mild exocrinopathies to severe systemic manifestations such as B-cell non-Hodgkin's lymphoma (NHL) [3,4]. These lymphomas arise predominantly from memory B cells in the marginal zone of lymphoid tissue, with mucosa-associated lymphoid tissue (MALT) lymphomas being the most frequent type [5] and the parotid and minor salivary glands being the most frequent sites of involvement [6]. Patients at high risk of developing NHL are male and have clinical manifestations of severe systemic disease, such as vasculitis, splenomegaly, lymphadenopathy, glomerulonephritis, haematologic manifestations, high expression of autoantibodies, cryoglobulins and hypergammaglobulinemia, high biopsy focus scores, and presence of ectopic germinal centers, among others [7].

2. Pathogenesis

The pathogenesis of SS is complex, some fundamental concepts are in constructio and are still a matter of controversy; the lack of hard evidence has not been a barrier fc different authors to approach the subject through theoretical models, which have bee based on the results of observational studies in humans and in preclinical data.

a. Etiology

Several factors have been implicated in the etiology of SS, as follows:

- Genetic components: The importance of type I interferon has been recognized in th pathogenesis of SS. In pSS, labial salivary gland and peripheral blood gene expressio microarray studies, have demonstrated dysregulation of type I interferon-inducibl genes [8]. The Genome-Wide Association studies (GWS) reported a strong assoc ation in SS within the HLA region at 6p21 (OR = 3.5) and with IRF5 (transcriptio factor mediating type I interferon responses in monocytes, dendritic cells, and l cells that induces the transcription of interferon-alfa genes and the production c pro-inflammatory cytokines upon viral infection), STAT4, IL12A and TNIP1 loci [9 although genetic factors determine the baseline disease susceptibility and diseas phenotype, these factors contribute modestly to the clinical condition [10].
- Epigenetic mechanisms: Different epigenetic mechanisms, such as DNA methylatio histone modifications, and non-coding RNAs, are important factors for modulatin gene expression and generating an important link between the genome and phenotypi manifestations [11].
- Biological factors: several different types of infections can increase the risk of SS triggering a proinflammatory microenvironment that promotes autoimmunity. A it was mentioned above, the GWS reported a strong association with the presenc of IRF5 loci and the transcription of interferon-alfa genes, and the production o pro-inflammatory cytokines upon viral infection [9]. Both type I IFN and virus TLI ligands can stimulate the production of BAFF (B cell-activating factor of the tumo necrosis factor family) in cultured salivary glands epithelial cells, suggesting that vira infection could be responsible for the increase in BAFF production by ductal epithelia cells in pSS [12]. Different viruses have also been implicated in SS pathogenesis, such as Epstein–Barr virus (EBV), cytomegalovirus, hepatitis C, human T-lymphocyte viru type I, and hepatitis B [13]. Especially reactivation of latent EBV in genetically an hormonally susceptible individuals could play a role in the initiation and perpetua tion of the chronic inflammatory autoimmune response in the glands [14]. Curren evidence supports the fact that viral infections are factors that largely increase the risk of SS [10]. To this respect, it is important to clarify that epidemiologic studies only confirm association but do not prove causation.

Other biological factors that have been related to the pathogenesis of SS lack solic evidence, such as vaccination (information from case reports), vitamin D deficiency (fev studies with selection bias and confounding factors), stress, and hormones (few studies).

- Organic chemical factors: smoking, alcohol, solvents (prevalence studies with poo evidence) [15].
- Inorganic chemical factors: silicone breast implants and silica. In recent years, clini cians have become aware of the existence of autoimmune/inflammatory syndrom induced by adjuvants (ASIA) associated with previous agents such as vaccines anc silicone implants [16]; the authors described that such implants may lead to hetero geneous symptoms such as body aches, abnormal fatigue, depression, dry eyes, dry mouth, and chronic fatigue syndrome, among others. In a meta-analysis conducted to determine long-term health outcomes in women with silicone gel breast implants (Ox ford level of evidence III), the authors found an association between silicone implants and the risk of SS, but they highlighted the presence of information bias because the data were from studies on patients with the self-reported disease [17]. Thus, although the evidence is weak to date, the existence of an approach based on a theoretical mode

of Shoenfelds et al., which shows that silicone can enhance antigen-specific immune response, should be recognized. It is necessary to conduct validation studies in larger cohorts of patients as well as randomized trials.

b. **Immune response pathways**

SS pathophysiology includes concurrent dysregulation of an innate and adaptative immune pathway involving cell-mediated and humoral disease processes that are incompletely understood [18].

- Adaptative immunity: The involvement of this immunity in SS pathogenesis is evident through observations of autoreactive T and B cells, with pronounced B-cell hyperactivity, which appears to be the cornerstone of the disease process. Signs of this condition are well documented in the literature, as clinical findings in different tissues of the body and the observations in serological and histopathological markers (salivary glands, saliva, tears, serum, peripheral blood B cells, intrinsic B cell abnormalities, and the presence of germinal center-like structures, elevated levels of B cell-associated cytokines and chemokines, presence of anti-SSA/SSB autoantibodies, hypergammaglobulinemia, elevated levels of soluble CD27, amongst others) [19]. In spite of the recognized role of the B cells in the pathogenesis of SS, its exact contribution is partly understood, most data have been obtained from mouse models and some authors have shown the presence of a coordinated and integrated stimulation of B-cell receptor B, CD40 and Toll-like receptors (TLRs) with different cytokines during the process [20].
- Innate immunity: In most pSS, type I interferon (IFN) and type I IFN-induced genes and proteins are overexpressed, resulting in the so-called type I IFN signature of pSS; aberrancies have been described in the type I IFN system in salivary glands of pSS [21] as well as abnormalities in type I IFN-alfa in labial biopsies [22]; the effect of type I IFN is not only local on the salivary glands but is also systemic because of its up-regulation activity which could explain the main extraglandular manifestations of the disease [23].

Björk et al. have proposed a model to approach the possible pathogenic mechanisms associated with SS, which can be summarized as follows:

A trigger (e.g., viral infection) initiates disruption of the salivary gland epithelium, inducing the production of type I IFN, and auto-antigens released by the dying cells create an inflammatory microenvironment. Thereafter, antigen-presenting cells present viral and self-antigens, leading to the activation of autoreactive B and T cells with subsequent differentiation and activation of autoantibody-producing plasma cells. Tissue damage is induced by autoreactive T cells via the secretion of cytotoxic granules, disrupting the epithelium and amplifying exposure of the autoantigens. The autoantibodies and autoantigens form immune complexes that bind to receptors on plasmacytoid dendritic cells, enhancing the production of type I IFN, which promotes autoantibody production through the differentiation and activation of autoreactive B cells. Thus, a self-perpetuating cycle of autoimmunity is created (see Figure 1) [10].

c. **Ectopic Lymphoid-Like Structures (ELSs)**

Ectopic lymphoid-like structures (ELSs) play an important role in the pathogenesis of rheumatic autoimmune diseases. These structures belong to tertiary lymphoid organs, which are composed of clusters of mononuclear cells organized in target organs (non-lymphoid organs) at sites of chronic inflammation. It is known that ELSs can function as germinal centers, favoring B-cell selection and plasma cell differentiation and very often exhibiting an autoreactive phenotype to disease-specific autoantigens. A germinal center may be present within the structure, which in SS patients is associated with more severe systemic manifestations and a higher risk of B-cell lymphoma [24]. A schematic representation of an ELS is shown in Figure 2.

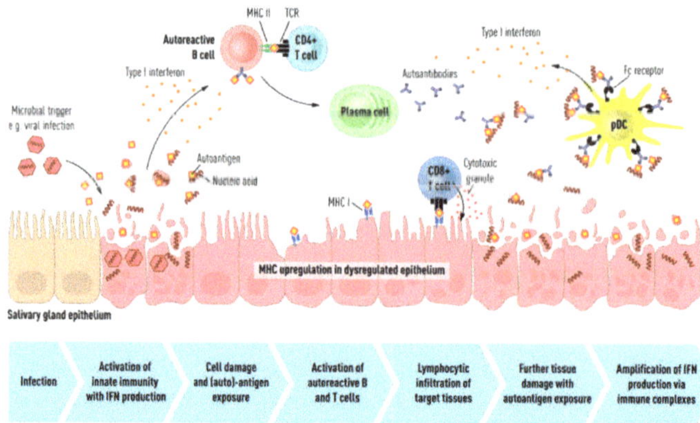

Figure 1. Schematic representation of the pathogenetic mechanisms at the basis of Sjogren syndrome **IFN**: interferon. **pDCs:** plasmacytoid dendritic cells. **MHC**: major histocompatibility complex. **TCR:** T cell receptor. Reprinted with permission from Environmental factors in the pathogenesis of primary Sjögren's syndrome, A. Björk, J. Mofors, M. Wahren-Herlenius., 2020, Journal of Internal Medicine, 287; 475–492.

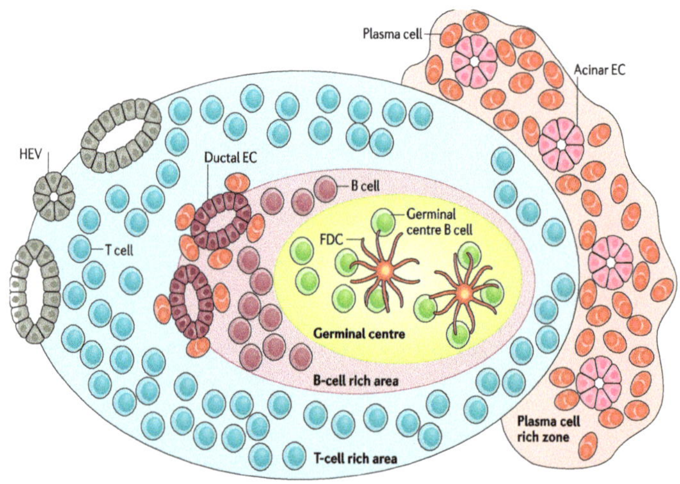

Figure 2. Schematic representation of an ectopic lymphoid-like structure (ELS), Segregation of T cells surrounding B cells. Development of high endothelial venules (HEVs) at the periphery of the ELS that enable lymphocytes expressing L-selectin to enter from the blood. Networks of follicular dendritic cells (FDCs) that support the germinal center response which expresses CD21 to facilitate the activation of B cells. Differentiation of hypermutated and class-switched plasma cells, which typically acquire a perifollicular localization with frequent infiltration of epithelial cells (ECs) from the ducts and acini. Reprinted by permission from Springer Nature Customer Service Centre GmbH: MDPI AG, Nature Reviews Rheumatology, Ectopic lymphoid neogenesis in rheumatic autoimmune diseases, Michele Bombardieri et al., COPYRIGHT, 2017.

The estimated prevalence of ELSs in SS is 30–40%, frequently around central duct structures, leading to the belief that ELSs may play an important role in antigen recognition and induction of an immune response against ductal epithelial cells [25]. The mechanisms responsible for ELS formation are grouped according to four different moments of the development of the ELS as follows:

a. Early activation of ELSs refers to the triggering process and depends on initiating factors.
b. Regulation and maintenance of ELSs depend on propagating factors that regulate progression towards organized ELSs as well as their maintenance.
c. Acquisition of the characteristics of a germinal center depends on functional factors.
d. Survival maintenance of germinal centers by other factors; in this setting, it is important to highlight the presence of IL-27, which has a negative regulatory role and acts as an inhibitor of ELS development [26].

The most important initiating factors are the chemokines CXCL13, IL-7, IL-22, CCL21, CCL19, and RANK ligand, the signal of which regulates the migration and survival of lymphoid tissue inducer cells [27]. Previous reports have documented high expression of these chemokines in ELSs, in salivary glands of patients with SS, and in the synovium of RA patients [28]. Other proinflammatory cytokines have also been described as initiating factors, such as IL-23 and IL-17 [29]. The above concept supports the fact that cells of the adaptative immune system become capable of releasing key mediators that are crucial for the progression and maintenance of ELSs. Some chemokines and their cellular sources involved in ELS activation and organizational processes are summarized in Table 1 [24].

Table 1. Cellular sources of the chemokines regulating ectopic lymphoid organogenesis.

Pathway	ELS-Positive Target Tissues in Rheumatic Autoimmune Diseases
CXCL13	$CD4^+$ T Cells, $CD14^+$ monocytes, $CD68^+$ macrophages or DC, Endothelial cells, epithelial cells, fibroblast-like synoviocytes, and Follicular DCs.
CCL19	Myofibroblast-like stroma
CCL21	Myofibroblast-like stroma, Lymphatic endothelial cells, DCs.
RANKL	B cells, Fibroblast-like synoviocytes
IL-7	Fibroblast-like synoviocytes, Siblining synovial macrophages
IL-22	$CD4^+$ T cells, NKp44 NK cells.

Abbreviations: CCL, CC: chemokine ligand; DCs: dendritic cells, NK: natural killer.

Factors considered mediators of ELS function are secreted by specialized T helper cell subsets that migrate into B-cell follicles, where the development of functional germinal centers requires a strong interaction between T and B cells [30]. Moreover, several factors, such as cytokines and membrane-bound ligands, are required to activate the function of these germinal centers; as a result of the strong interaction between T follicular helper cells ($_{\text{TFHs}}$) and B cells, IL-21 is released. This cytokine is a potent cofactor for B-cell survival and proliferation and plasma cell differentiation [31] that has been implicated in the development of ELSs in rheumatic disease, particularly in SS and RA [32,33]. Indeed, in the salivary glands of SS patients, the interaction between $CD4^+$ cells and activated epithelial cells promotes T_{FH} cell differentiation and IL-21 production [34]. Regarding facilitating factors, the role of IL-17 as a down-regulator of ELS development deserves mention, and it has attracted scientific interest as a potential factor for the treatment of rheumatic diseases via gene therapy [35].

The ectopic germinal centers of ELSs are associated with the local production of autoantibodies and have been associated with the maintenance of autoimmunity within a target organ. In SS patients with ELSs, the prevalence of circulating anti-Ro/SSA and anti-La/SSB antibodies is 20% higher than that in patients without ELSs [36]. ELSs promote affinity maturation and differentiation of plasma cells reactive against disease-specific autoantigens; these autoantigens are exposed as a result of the chronic inflammatory process and are presented to B cells and T cells by antigen-presenting cells.

Although the processes involved in the formation of ELSs in the synovium and in the salivary glands in AR and SS patients share common pathways, the antigen-driven autoimmune response appears to be disease-specific.

Under the pathological condition of rheumatic autoimmune disease, the autoreactiv plasma cells generated in the ELSs are retained within the target tissue by the action c CXCL12, IL-6, and APRIL [37,38].

There is evidence that in SS patients, the presence of ELSs is associated with diseas progression, high levels of circulating autoantibodies, and systemic manifestations, such a lymphadenopathy and peripheral neuropathy [36]. Indeed, there are reports of a stron relationship between the presence of ELSs in salivary gland biopsy and a higher risk c developing lymphoma [39].

Thus far, we have reviewed how the study of ELSs has allowed the investigators t build a theoretical model that undoubtedly will serve as a fundament for future invest gations. Overall, a better understanding of the physiopathology and histopathologica heterogeneity of target tissue in rheumatic conditions might lead to the identification c different molecules and markers to be used for diagnostic and therapeutic purposes, thoug clinical evidence from research with larger cohorts of patients and randomized studie is necessary.

The two most difficult situations in SS are as follows:

- the difficulty of early and accurate diagnosis, which is crucial to avoid major complication
- a means of evaluating the efficacy of therapy.

To facilitate diagnostic and prognostic approaches for SS, several tools have bee validated, such as the following:

- for diagnostic purposes: ACR-EULAR criteria [40],
- for calculating systemic disease activity: ESSDAI (Eular Sjögren Syndrome Diseas Activity Index) [41],
- for patient-reported symptoms: ESSPRI (EULAR Sjogren Patient-Reported Symp toms) [41] and
- for evaluating response to different therapies: CRESS (Composite of Relevant End points for Sjögren's Syndrome) [42].

Despite these available tools, SS diagnosis remains underrecognized, with misdiagno sis occurring in some cases, impacting prognosis and the possibility of implementing th appropriate treatment.

The discouraging results in this field emphasize the heterogeneous characteristic of this systemic autoimmune disease and the urgent need to find better biomarkers tha could elucidate the disease process for faster diagnosis (glandular function and the sicc symptoms are not always coupled) to provide better bases for further therapies.

3. Role of New Molecular Image Strategies in Sjogren's Syndrome

The goal of SS is to be able to stratify pSS through the integration of clinical, laborator histopathology, and imaging data; thus, it could be possible to identify which patient have clinical manifestations related to inflammatory activity or sequelae; the possibilit to identify which patients are on the risk of lymphoma development it is also importan Because new treatment strategies are emerging, there is also evident the need for nev probes for a more reliable treatment response evaluation [43].

The potential for diagnosis and classification of pSS of the salivary glands ultrasoun (SGUS) has been pointed out previously by different authors [44]; nowadays this techniqu is emerging as a complementary tool for biopsy purposes. In a recent study the author reported that by adding SGUS as a minor item to ACR/EULAR criteria, the sensitivit could rise to 95.6% [45]. Other authors have reported that a combined positivity of SGU and anti-SSA antibodies provides a high predictive value for the diagnosis of pSS [46 The main limitation of SGUS is the lack of a standardized scoring system, however, a an initiative to overcome this issue, the Outcome Measures in Rheumatology Clinica Trials (OMERACT) proposed a four-grade semiquantitative score with good intra an interobserver agreement results [47]. Last generation ultra-high resolution ultrasoun (UHFUS) transducers, which produce frequencies up to 70 MHz with resolution up t

30 um, offer new possibilities to visualize labial salivary glands and to guide diagnostic biopsy procedures [48]. Recently, Baldini et al. demonstrated that the mean labial glandular surface area obtained by the high-resolution ultrasound-guided procedure was significantly higher than the area obtained by the traditional biopsy procedure. This procedure could facilitate the assessment of the focus score [49].

Promising innovations are ultrasound elastography (with algorithms to evaluate quantitatively the tissue stiffness of the salivary gland tissue [50], the application of artificial intelligence to automatically score for biopsy purposes [51], and the ultrasound-guided core needle biopsy of major salivary glands which could represent an alternative to surgical biopsy [52].

MRI does not belong to the common standard tools used for the diagnostic approach of pSS. Because of its high spatial resolution the major impact in such patients is for local staging of pSS associated with salivary glands lymphomas [53].

Salivary gland scintigraphy is a nuclear medicine technique that through the administration intravenously of ^{99m}Tc-04 allows for to evaluate of the function of major salivary glands (perfusion, concentration, and elimination characteristics) [54]. Sialoscintigraphy is no longer part of the recent classification criteria for pSS [40]; the reported diagnostic approach shows a sensitivity of up to 90% with specificity of around 50%, making this tool not able to distinguish the functional compromise of SS and other salivary glands pathologies. It is possible that this technique could have some potential indication in the future as part of the tools available for the follow-up of patients [54].

Molecular nuclear medicine imaging has emerged with several biomarkers with potential clinical impact for its contribution to diagnosing, assessing the inflammatory status, and assessing disease progression. These images allow in vivo the characterization of cells and the phenomena involved in inflammatory diseases. For this purpose, by using radiolabeled molecules (administered in nanomolar amounts), that participate in the biochemical and pathophysiological process of chronic inflammation, it is possible to make a qualitative and quantitative assessment of the inflammatory burden in vivo. Recent advances in the development of target-specific imaging agents, allow us to perform a non-invasive evaluation of various molecular events such as angiogenesis, apoptosis, and cell trafficking in living organisms. Cellular and molecular changes occur a long time before structural changes, therefore, non-invasive visualization and quantification of molecular processes facilitate the early detection of the disease, establish a prognosis, and could potentially estimate the potential impact of biologic therapies.

In this review, we focus on radiopharmaceuticals that provide in vivo pathophysiological information about the disease not only in the salivary glands but also in other tissues that may be affected as part of the spectrum of the SS, such as the joints and thyroid gland.

a. Somatostatin Receptor Imaging

Radiolabelled peptides are highly specific and are used to reveal the presence of target molecules in inflammatory disease through molecular imaging. The peptides used in nuclear medicine images are easily synthesized, stabilized, and modified with good pharmacokinetic parameters; they also show high receptor binding affinity and are internalized into cells [55]. One of the most commonly used radiolabelled peptides for the inflammatory disease clinical approach is somatostatin, which has been used for inflammatory diseases for more than two decades, particularly in rheumatoid arthritis, SS, and autoimmune thyroid disease [56,57]. This is supported by the well-known presence of active and over-expressed somatostatin receptors in inflammatory and immunological cells from different tissues [58]. The diagnostic accuracy is also high because of the strong binding affinity of somatostatin to its five receptors. Different radiopharmaceuticals for somatostatin receptor scintigraphy are available, such as ^{68}Ga-DOTA-TATE, ^{68}Ga-DOTA-TOC, ^{68}Ga-DOTA-NOC, and ^{99m}Tc-EDDA/HYNIC-TOC [59], offering the possibility of detecting active inflammation in tissues affected by SS. Some of the evidence that supports the use of these radiopharmaceuticals in SS has been provided by Anzola et al., who reported the normal biodistribution of ^{68}-Ga-DOTA-NOC and reference values for salivary glands, thyroid glands, and major joints, constituting the starting point for PET studies for further analysis in patients affected by rheumatic inflammatory disorders [60]. Using a cohort of 62 patients with confirmed SS by AECG criteria, the same group [61] reported the ability of ^{99m}Tc-HYNIC-TOC scintigraphy to identify active inflammatory processes not only in salivary glands but also in many joints. This work highlighted the capability of the molecule to evaluate inflammatory compromise in sites different from the salivary glands, to evaluate the inflammation status of the salivary glands, and to hypothesize the usefulness of the probe to assess response to treatment. In a pilot study in 18 patients with rheumatoid arthritis and secondary SS who received infliximab as treatment, the authors [62] showed uptake of ^{99m}Tc HYNIC-TOC in all affected joints and in the salivary glands in 12 of 18 patients. They also demonstrated a significant reduction in uptake by joints but not salivary glands after treatment with infliximab, enhancing the potential of the molecule to assess disease activity in rheumatoid arthritis and to detect secondary SS (Figures 3 and 4). It is important to highlight that because the synovia of patients with SS and rheumatoid arthritis highly express somatostatin receptors [63], radiolabelled somatostatin can identify sites of active inflammation in joints accompanying salivary gland compromise in primary or secondary SS.

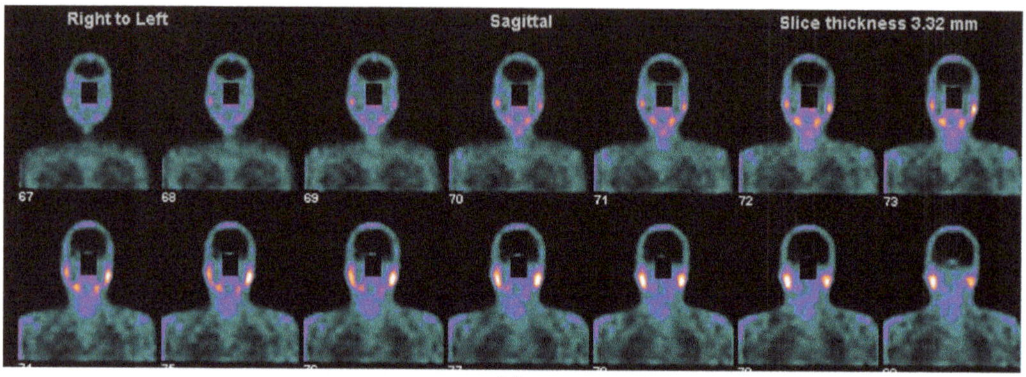

(a)

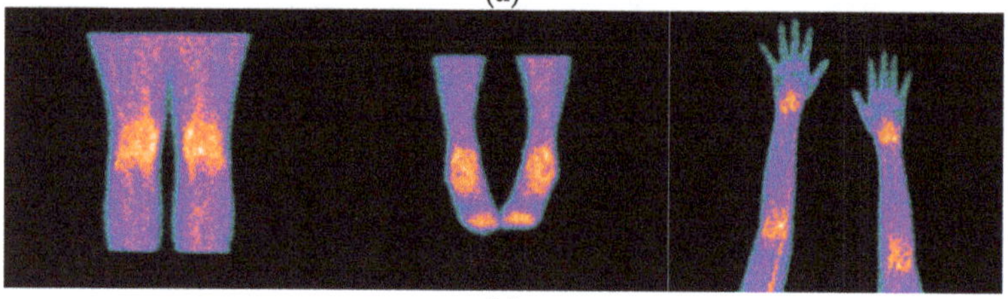

(b)

Figure 3. Images acquired after ^{99m}Tc-HYNIC-TOC administration i.v in a patient with SS, sicca symptoms, and painful joints. In (**a**) high abnormal uptake in parotids and submandibular salivary glands. In (**b**) shows high abnormal uptake in knees, ankles, elbows, and carpal joints.

One systematic review [56] reported promising results of radiolabelled somatostatin analogs as diagnostic tools for localizing and identifying sites of active inflammation in joints as well as extra-articular involvement, such as the salivary glands, in patients with chronic inflammatory diseases (Figures 3a,b and 4a,b).

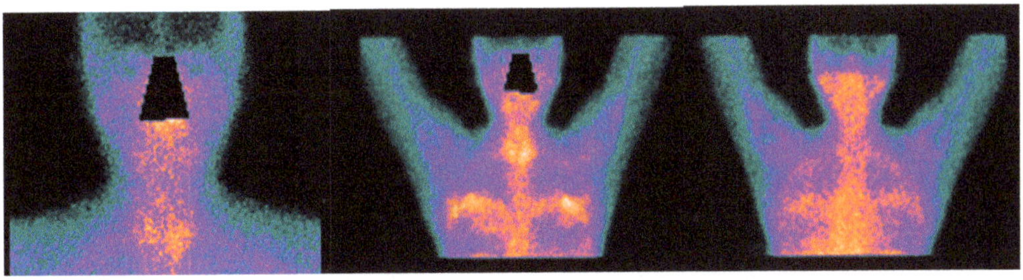

(a)

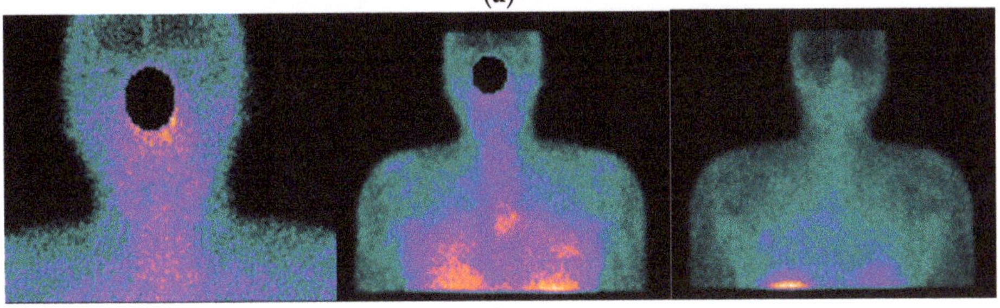

(b)

Figure 4. 42-year-old female patient with the previous history of bilateral mammoplasty; four years later she complained of dryness (VAS 5/10), fatigue (VAS 10/10), pain (VAS:8/10) ESSPRI: 23, and thyroiditis. She was diagnosed with SS under ACR-EULAR criteria and she started treatment with DMARDS for two years without relieving symptoms. She asked her surgeon to remove the implants and six months after the removal of the implants there was an improvement in her clinical condition, dryness (VAS: 2/10), fatigue (VAS:6/10), pain (VAS: 5/10) post-surgery ESSPRI: 13. In (**a**) ^{99m}Tc HYNIC-TOC images show high abnormal uptake of the radiotracer in the thyroid gland, submandibular glands, with a high abnormal bilateral mammary periprosthetic distribution of the radiotracer. SS was diagnosed under ACR-EULAR criteria. In (**b**) ^{99m}Tc HYNIC-TOC images 6 months post removal of prosthesis show a significant decrease in uptake of the radiotracer in submandibular glands and thyroid gland. There was a concern that silicone could be associated with SS.

b. B-lymphocyte Imaging in SS

Currently, the importance of the role of B lymphocytes in the pathogenesis of rheumatic inflammatory diseases through the production of auto-antibodies, T-cell activation, and pro-inflammatory cytokines is well recognized [64]. We previously reviewed how these cells are found in pathological infiltrates of affected tissues and are implicated in disease progression, with B-cell hyperactivity being fundamental to the disease. The maturation of B cells from stem cells suggests several steps, with changes in cell surface markers. Indeed, these surface markers have gained attention for use in B-cell-depleting therapies through the use of different monoclonal antibodies against them, acting directly (CD19, CD20, CD22) or indirectly via blockade of cytokine pathways (TNF-alpha, interleukin-6, B lymphocyte stimulator (BLyS) and proliferation-inducing ligand APRIL) [65,66]. Although some molecules are commonly used, scarce evidence is available, and the results of trials are inconclusive. No biologic drug has yet been approved for the treatment of pSS, though three biologics, i.e., rituximab, belimumab, and abatacept, have shown effectiveness in open studies for extra-glandular symptoms but not for dryness [67]. Anti-tumor necrosis factor-alpha (TNF-alpha) drug trials in pSS have failed to show promising results; although a potential protective role for TNF-alfa against lymphoproliferation has been hypothesized, it has been demonstrated that depletion of TNF-alpha may increase BAFF (B-cell activating factor) levels in humans, discouraging its use for pSS in clinical practice [68]. Rituximab i a chimeric monoclonal antibody directed against CD20, which is expressed on membrane cells. Expert opinion [69–71] supports its use as a therapeutic option in pSS with system compromise and as second-line therapy for hematological manifestations. In additio a radiolabelled anti-CD20 mAb probe for in vivo imaging of CD20-positive lymphocyt infiltration in inflammatory diseases has been described, offering the possibility of a bette approach to disease staging [72].

In vivo imaging of lymphocyte B through the use of anti-CD20 radiotracer has pote tial applicability for SS patients. Malviya et al. [73] used radiolabelled anti-CD20 (rituxima and showed B Lymphocyte infiltration in affected tissues of patients with different chron inflammatory autoimmune diseases and who were candidates for rituximab treatment. Th authors reported the in vivo localization pattern of the B-lymphocytes mediating the i flammatory process, with variable uptake by salivary glands and lacrimal glands in two S patients. Despite the small sample size, this work provides the basis for further studies a sessing whether an antibody accumulates in inflamed tissue before using the same antibod for therapeutic purposes, thereby improving the selection of patients who might benef from the therapy, which is called immune scintigraphy for therapeutic decision-making.

c. T-lymphocyte Imaging in SS

Because activated T lymphocytes are involved in chronic inflammatory diseases an IL2 is mainly secreted by these cells to play a regulatory role during inflammation, som authors have developed a means of detecting these cells in vivo through the synthesis o different radiopharmaceuticals for SPECT and PET systems [74]. Reports to date hav demonstrated its usefulness in different clinical inflammatory scenarios, such as in insuliti in type 1 diabetes [75], Crohn's disease [76], and Hashimoto thyroiditis, among others, fo diagnostic and prognostic purposes and for therapy follow-up.

In a recently published study [77], in a cohort of 48pSS, the authors reported the utilit of ^{99m}Tc-IL2 for evaluating in vivo the extent and severity of lympho-mononuclear ce infiltration in the salivary glands. When they compared the results with a control grou they found a statistically significant difference ($p < 0.0001$) in the radiotracer uptake i salivary glands between the two groups; they also observed that the uptake in patients wit a longer history of the disease was lower compared with the recently diagnosed patient They highlighted the capacity of the molecule to detect active inflammation mediated b IL2 and the possibility to treat those patients with immune-modulatory drugs and usin the probe for evaluating the efficacy of the treatment (Figure 5).

New radiotracers, such as ^{18}F-fluorbenzoyl interleukin-2, have also been develope for PET systems, allowing detection of activated T lymphocytes for the same purposes. In preclinical study, Di Gialleonardo et al. [78] identified activated T lymphocytes in inflame tissues, highlighting the potential of the probe for detecting activated T lymphocytes i autoimmune diseases such as SS. Because T lymphocytes are also mainly implicated in th pathogenesis of SS, molecular images for detecting T lymphocyte activity would play a important role in diagnostic approaches [44].

d. Other PET Radiopharmaceuticals Used in SS

Recently, in an age- and sex-matched study with SS patients and healthy voluntee using MRI, ^{11}C-MET-PET, and ^{18}F-FDG-PET, Jimenez-Royo et al. [79] reported how molec ular imaging findings correlate with disease characteristics, providing information abou the inflammatory and functional status of the salivary glands. ^{11}C-MET PET (a protei synthesis marker incorporated into cellular proteins) information [80] was used to evaluat residual salivary gland function, and ^{18}F-FDG PET information was used to evaluate th inflammatory condition through glucose utilization by the inflamed cell [81]. Their mai findings were significantly lower ^{11}C-MET uptake in the parotid and submandibular gland in SS patients than in volunteers and higher uptake of ^{18}F-FDG in the salivary glands o SS patients, indicating the presence of inflammation. Furthermore, a negative correlatio between ^{11}C-MET and ^{18}F-FDG uptake (loss of function with highly inflamed tissues was reported. Regarding histological analysis, the most relevant finding was related to a moderate positive correlation between ^{18}F-FDG uptake in the parotid gland and CD20+ B-cell infiltration in the minor salivary gland of patients, suggesting that ^{18}F-FDG uptake shows B-cell tissue infiltration By using ^{18}F-FDG PET in SS patients, Cohen et al. [82] found evidence of the added value of the tool, demonstrating systemic compromise in SS. These authors observed that although the most frequent site of uptake was the salivary glands, the lymph nodes and lungs were equally affected. They also described a PETC/CT inflammation score that correlated with ESSDAI and gammaglobulin levels, suggesting that ^{18}F-FDG PET may help in assessing disease activity and represent an inflammation biomarker for SS.

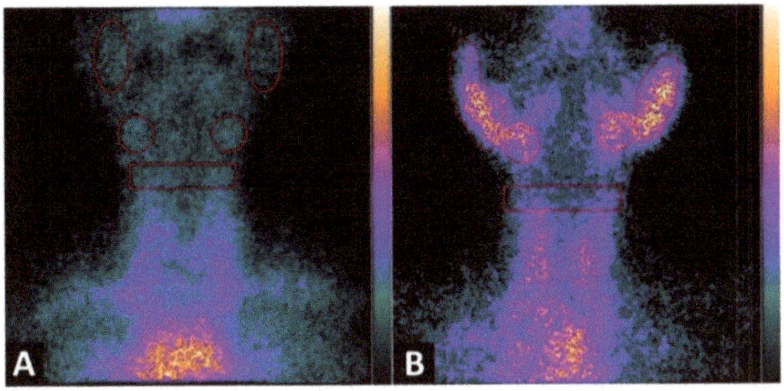

Figure 5. Planar image of the neck was obtained 1h after ^{99m}Tc-IL2 injection in a control subject (**A**) and in a patient with Sjögren syndrome at the time of diagnosis (**B**). In (**A**) the scan shows no ^{99m}Tc-IL2 uptake by the salivary glands. In (**B**) an evident accumulation of ^{99m}Tc-IL2 can be observed in both parotids and submandibular glands, indicating the presence of activated lymphocytes. The calculated parotid to background (P/B) ratios are 1.35 and 1.30 in right and left glands, respectively, and the submandibular gland to background (S/B) ratios are 1.57 and 1.64 in right and left glands, respectively. Reprinted with permission from Imaging Activated-T-Lymphocytes in the Salivary Glands of Patients with Sjögren's Syndrome by 99mTc-Interleukin-2: Diagnostic and Therapeutic Implications Campagna, G.; Anzola, L. K.; Varani, M.; Lauri, C.; Gentiloni Silveri, G.; Chiurchioni, L.; et al. *J. Clin. Med.* **2022**, *11* (15), 4368. [77].

Although interesting characteristics of ^{18}F-FDG PET have been described as inflammation markers in SS, it is important to take into consideration that new probes would make possible more specific detection of inflammation by targeting specific molecules and cells expressed in compromised tissues, providing good characteristics not only for diagnostic purposes but also for therapy decision-making and follow-up [83].

Because primary SS may be associated with lymphoma with a risk of 5–7% [84] and this diagnosis might be difficult because of the common clinical findings with SS, the usefulness of ^{18}F-FDG in the case of lymphoma for initial staging, biopsy guidance, evaluation of response to therapy and detection of relapse is well recognized [85]. Keraen et al. [86] compared ^{18}F-FDG patterns in patients with active primary SS with lymphoma and those without lymphoma. They observed that salivary gland enlargement, particularly the parotid glands, was more frequent in lymphoma patients ($p = 0.003$) and that the presence of focal compromise in the lungs was highly suggestive of lymphoma ($p = 0.01$); they observed the highest SUVmax (maximum standardized uptake value) on whole scans in patients with lymphoma ($p = 0.02$); in ROC curve analysis, they reported a parotid gland cut-off > 4.7 on SUV max has a sensitivity and specificity of 73.3% and 86.7%, respectively, for the presence of lymphoma.

Other radiopharmaceuticals with the potential to detect inflammation in SS patients include ^{68}Ga-pentixafor, a radioligand of the chemokine receptor CXCR4 that plays an important role in the trafficking of progenitor and inflammatory cells [87]. Cytawa et al. [88] demonstrated in a case report bilateral intense radiotracer uptake in the parotid and submandibular salivary glands, consistent with inflammatory cell infiltration in a patient with SS.

4. Conclusions

The more we investigate the pathogenesis of diseases, the more we understand how to prevent and treat them. However, we also define new important molecular targets for diagnostic purposes by tailoring new radiopharmaceuticals. This strategy certainly applies to rheumatic diseases and to SS in particular, and understanding the role of several molecules, receptors, and immune cells in SS has allowed the application of specific radiopharmaceuticals for targeting these molecules and cells in vivo. Furthermore, the availability of SPECT and PET studies has offered the possibility to show in vivo the presence, homing, and trafficking of different immune cells involved in the pathogenesis of SS, providing further understanding of the pathogenetic role of these cells. Current evidence supports conducting robust studies to determine the appropriate place for molecular imaging in the diagnostic flowchart of SS and for therapy decision-making and follow-up of therapy efficacy.

Author Contributions: Review design: all authors. Manuscript drafting/manuscript revision for important intellectual content: A.L.K., S.A. Literature research: A.L.K., R.J.N., R.S. All authors have read and agreed to the published version of the manuscript.

Funding: No additional funding was received for this work.

Institutional Review Board Statement: Not applicable.

Informed Consent Statement: Not applicable.

Data Availability Statement: Not applicable.

Conflicts of Interest: The authors declare no conflict of interest.

References

1. Mariette, X.; Criswell, L.A. Primary Sjögren's Syndrome. *N. Engl. J. Med.* **2018**, *378*, 931–939. [CrossRef] [PubMed]
2. Anaya, J.-M.; Restrepo-Jiménez, P.; Rodríguez, Y.; Rodríguez-Jiménez, M.; Acosta-Ampudia, Y.; Monsalve, D.M.; Pacheco, Y.; Ramírez-Santana, C.; Molano-González, N.; Mantilla, R.D. Sjögren's Syndrome and Autoimmune Thyroid Disease: Two Sides of the Same Coin. *Clin. Rev. Allergy Immunol.* **2019**, *56*, 362–374. [CrossRef] [PubMed]
3. Brito-Zerón, P.; Kostov, B.; Solans, R.; Fraile, G.; Suárez-Cuervo, C.; Casanovas, A.; Rascón, F.J.; Qanneta, R.; Pérez-Alvarez, R.; Ripoll, M.; et al. Systemic Activity and Mortality in Primary Sjögren Syndrome: Predicting Survival Using the EULAR-SS Disease Activity Index (ESSDAI) in 1045 Patients. *Ann. Rheum. Dis.* **2016**, *75*, 348–355. [CrossRef]
4. Kassan, S.S. Increased Risk of Lymphoma in Sicca Syndrome. *Ann. Intern. Med.* **1978**, *89*, 888. [CrossRef] [PubMed]
5. Ioannidis, J.P.A.; Vassiliou, V.A.; Moutsopoulos, H.M. Long-Term Risk of Mortality and Lymphoproliferative Disease and Predictive Classification of Primary Sjögren's Syndrome: Classification of Sjögren's Syndrome. *Arthritis Rheum.* **2002**, *46*, 741–747. [CrossRef]
6. Kapsogeorgou, E.K.; Voulgarelis, M.; Tzioufas, A.G. Predictive Markers of Lymphomagenesis in Sjögren's Syndrome: From Clinical Data to Molecular Stratification. *J. Autoimmun.* **2019**, *104*, 102316. [CrossRef] [PubMed]
7. Goules, A.V.; Tzioufas, A.G. Lymphomagenesis in Sjögren's Syndrome: Predictive Biomarkers towards Precision Medicine. *Autoimmun. Rev.* **2019**, *18*, 137–143. [CrossRef] [PubMed]
8. Hjelmervik, T.O.R.; Petersen, K.; Jonassen, I.; Jonsson, R.; Bolstad, A.I. Gene Expression Profiling of Minor Salivary Glands Clearly Distinguishes Primary Sjögren's Syndrome Patients from Healthy Control Subjects. *Arthritis Rheum.* **2005**, *52*, 1534–1544. [CrossRef]
9. Lessard, C.J.; Registry, F.U.P.S.S.; Li, H.; Adrianto, I.; Ice, J.A.; Rasmussen, A.; Grundahl, K.M.; Kelly, J.; Dozmorov, M.; Miceli-Richard, C.; et al. Variants at Multiple Loci Implicated in Both Innate and Adaptive Immune Responses Are Associated with Sjögren's Syndrome. *Nat. Genet.* **2013**, *45*, 1284–1292. [CrossRef]
10. Björk, A.; Mofors, J.; Wahren-Herlenius, M. Environmental Factors in the Pathogenesis of Primary Sjögren's Syndrome. *J. Intern. Med.* **2020**, *287*, 475–492. [CrossRef]
11. Imgenberg-Kreuz, J.; Rasmussen, A.; Sivils, K.; Nordmark, G. Genetics and Epigenetics in Primary Sjögren's Syndrome. *Rheumatology* **2021**, *60*, 2085–2098. [CrossRef] [PubMed]

2. Ittah, M.; Miceli-Richard, C.; Eric Gottenberg, J.-; Lavie, F.; Lazure, T.; Ba, N.; Sellam, J.; Lepajolec, C.; Mariette, X. B Cell-Activating Factor of the Tumor Necrosis Factor Family (BAFF) Is Expressed under Stimulation by Interferon in Salivary Gland Epithelial Cells in Primary Sjögren's Syndrome. *Arthritis Res. Ther.* **2006**, *8*, R51. [CrossRef] [PubMed]
3. Bartoloni, E.; Alunno, A.; Gerli, R. The Dark Side of Sjögren's Syndrome: The Possible Pathogenic Role of Infections. *Curr. Opin. Rheumatol.* **2019**, *31*, 505–511. [CrossRef] [PubMed]
4. Inoue, H.; Mishima, K.; Yamamoto-Yoshida, S.; Ushikoshi-Nakayama, R.; Nakagawa, Y.; Yamamoto, K.; Ryo, K.; Ide, F.; Saito, I. Aryl Hydrocarbon Receptor-Mediated Induction of EBV Reactivation as a Risk Factor for Sjögren's Syndrome. *J. Immunol. Baltim.* **2012**, *188*, 4654–4662. [CrossRef]
5. Olsson, P.; Turesson, C.; Mandl, T.; Jacobsson, L.; Theander, E. Cigarette Smoking and the Risk of Primary Sjögren's Syndrome: A Nested Case Control Study. *Arthritis Res. Ther.* **2017**, *19*, 50. [CrossRef]
6. Watad, A.; Quaresma, M.; Brown, S.; Cohen Tervaert, J.W.; Rodríguez-Pint, I.; Cervera, R.; Perricone, C.; Shoenfeld, Y. Autoimmune/Inflammatory Syndrome Induced by Adjuvants (Shoenfeld's Syndrome)—An Update. *Lupus* **2017**, *26*, 675–681. [CrossRef]
7. Balk, E.M.; Earley, A.; Avendano, E.A.; Raman, G. Long-Term Health Outcomes in Women With Silicone Gel Breast Implants: A Systematic Review. *Ann. Intern. Med.* **2016**, *164*, 164–175. [CrossRef]
8. Cobb, B.L.; Lessard, C.J.; Harley, J.B.; Moser, K.L. Genes and Sjögren's Syndrome. *Rheum. Dis. Clin. N. Am.* **2008**, *34*, 847–868. [CrossRef]
9. Kroese, F.G.M.; Abdulahad, W.H.; Haacke, E.; Bos, N.A.; Vissink, A.; Bootsma, H. B-Cell Hyperactivity in Primary Sjögren's Syndrome. *Expert Rev. Clin. Immunol.* **2014**, *10*, 483–499. [CrossRef]
0. Rawlings, D.J.; Schwartz, M.A.; Jackson, S.W.; Meyer-Bahlburg, A. Integration of B Cell Responses through Toll-like Receptors and Antigen Receptors. *Nat. Rev. Immunol.* **2012**, *12*, 282–294. [CrossRef]
1. Wildenberg, M.E.; van Helden-Meeuwsen, C.G.; van de Merwe, J.P.; Drexhage, H.A.; Versnel, M.A. Systemic Increase in Type I Interferon Activity in Sjögren's Syndrome: A Putative Role for Plasmacytoid Dendritic Cells. *Eur. J. Immunol.* **2008**, *38*, 2024–2033. [CrossRef] [PubMed]
2. Båve, U.; Nordmark, G.; Lövgren, T.; Rönnelid, J.; Cajander, S.; Eloranta, M.-L.; Alm, G.V.; Rönnblom, L. Activation of the Type I Interferon System in Primary Sjögren's Syndrome: A Possible Etiopathogenic Mechanism. *Arthritis Rheum.* **2005**, *52*, 1185–1195. [CrossRef] [PubMed]
3. Bodewes, I.L.A.; Al-Ali, S.; van Helden-Meeuwsen, C.G.; Maria, N.I.; Tarn, J.; Lendrem, D.W.; Schreurs, M.W.J.; Steenwijk, E.C.; van Daele, P.L.A.; Both, T.; et al. Systemic Interferon Type I and Type II Signatures in Primary Sjögren's Syndrome Reveal Differences in Biological Disease Activity. *Rheumatol. Oxf. Engl.* **2018**, *57*, 921–930. [CrossRef] [PubMed]
4. Bombardieri, M.; Lewis, M.; Pitzalis, C. Ectopic Lymphoid Neogenesis in Rheumatic Autoimmune Diseases. *Nat. Rev. Rheumatol.* **2017**, *13*, 141–154. [CrossRef] [PubMed]
5. Barone, F.; Bombardieri, M.; Manzo, A.; Blades, M.C.; Morgan, P.R.; Challacombe, S.J.; Valesini, G.; Pitzalis, C. Association of CXCL13 and CCL21 Expression with the Progressive Organization of Lymphoid-like Structures in Sjögren's Syndrome. *Arthritis Rheum.* **2005**, *52*, 1773–1784. [CrossRef] [PubMed]
6. Jones, G.W.; Bombardieri, M.; Greenhill, C.J.; McLeod, L.; Nerviani, A.; Rocher-Ros, V.; Cardus, A.; Williams, A.S.; Pitzalis, C.; Jenkins, B.J.; et al. Interleukin-27 Inhibits Ectopic Lymphoid-like Structure Development in Early Inflammatory Arthritis. *J. Exp. Med.* **2015**, *212*, 1793–1802. [CrossRef]
7. Mebius, R.E. Organogenesis of Lymphoid Tissues. *Nat. Rev. Immunol.* **2003**, *3*, 292–303. [CrossRef]
8. Salomonsson, S.; Jonsson, M.V.; Skarstein, K.; Brokstad, K.A.; Hjelmström, P.; Wahren-Herlenius, M.; Jonsson, R. Cellular Basis of Ectopic Germinal Center Formation and Autoantibody Production in the Target Organ of Patients with Sjögren's Syndrome: Ectopic Germinal Center Formation in Sjögren's Syndrome. *Arthritis Rheum.* **2003**, *48*, 3187–3201. [CrossRef]
9. Xanthou, G.; Polihronis, M.; Tzioufas, A.G.; Paikos, S.; Sideras, P.; Moutsopoulos, H.M. "Lymphoid" Chemokine Messenger RNA Expression by Epithelial Cells in the Chronic Inflammatory Lesion of the Salivary Glands of Sjögren's Syndrome Patients: Possible Participation in Lymphoid Structure Formation. *Arthritis Rheum.* **2001**, *44*, 408–418. [CrossRef]
0. Shulman, Z.; Gitlin, A.D.; Weinstein, J.S.; Lainez, B.; Esplugues, E.; Flavell, R.A.; Craft, J.E.; Nussenzweig, M.C. Dynamic Signaling by T Follicular Helper Cells during Germinal Center B Cell Selection. *Science* **2014**, *345*, 1058–1062. [CrossRef]
1. Karnell, J.L.; Ettinger, R. The Interplay of IL-21 and BAFF in the Formation and Maintenance of Human B Cell Memory. *Front. Immunol.* **2012**, *3*, 2. [CrossRef] [PubMed]
2. Kwok, S.-K.; Cho, M.-L.; Park, M.-K.; Oh, H.-J.; Park, J.-S.; Her, Y.-M.; Lee, S.-Y.; Youn, J.; Ju, J.H.; Park, K.S.; et al. Interleukin-21 Promotes Osteoclastogenesis in Humans with Rheumatoid Arthritis and in Mice with Collagen-Induced Arthritis. *Arthritis Rheum.* **2012**, *64*, 740–751. [CrossRef] [PubMed]
3. Liu, H.; Liu, G.; Gong, L.; Zhang, Y.; Jiang, G. Local Suppression of IL-21 in Submandibular Glands Retards the Development of Sjögren's Syndrome in Non-Obese Diabetic Mice. *J. Oral Pathol. Med.* **2012**, *41*, 728–735. [CrossRef] [PubMed]
4. Gong, Y.-Z.; Nititham, J.; Taylor, K.; Miceli-Richard, C.; Sordet, C.; Wachsmann, D.; Bahram, S.; Georgel, P.; Criswell, L.A.; Sibilia, J.; et al. Differentiation of Follicular Helper T Cells by Salivary Gland Epithelial Cells in Primary Sjögren's Syndrome. *J. Autoimmun.* **2014**, *51*, 57–66. [CrossRef]
5. Pitzalis, C.; Jones, G.W.; Bombardieri, M.; Jones, S.A. Ectopic Lymphoid-like Structures in Infection, Cancer and Autoimmunity. *Nat. Rev. Immunol.* **2014**, *14*, 447–462. [CrossRef]

36. Risselada, A.P.; Looije, M.F.; Kruize, A.A.; Bijlsma, J.W.J.; van Roon, J.A.G. The Role of Ectopic Germinal Centers in th Immunopathology of Primary Sjögren's Syndrome: A Systematic Review. *Semin. Arthritis Rheum.* **2013**, *42*, 368–376. [CrossRe
37. Nutt, S.L.; Hodgkin, P.D.; Tarlinton, D.M.; Corcoran, L.M. The Generation of Antibody-Secreting Plasma Cells. *Nat. Rev. Immunc* **2015**, *15*, 160–171. [CrossRef]
38. Szyszko, E.A.; Brokstad, K.A.; Oijordsbakken, G.; Jonsson, M.V.; Jonsson, R.; Skarstein, K. Salivary Glands of Primary Sjögren' Syndrome Patients Express Factors Vital for Plasma Cell Survival. *Arthritis Res. Ther.* **2011**, *13*, R2. [CrossRef]
39. Theander, E.; Vasaitis, L.; Baecklund, E.; Nordmark, G.; Warfvinge, G.; Liedholm, R.; Brokstad, K.; Jonsson, R.; Jonsson, M. Lymphoid Organisation in Labial Salivary Gland Biopsies Is a Possible Predictor for the Development of Malignant Lymphom in Primary Sjögren's Syndrome. *Ann. Rheum. Dis.* **2011**, *70*, 1363–1368. [CrossRef]
40. Shiboski, C.H.; Shiboski, S.C.; Seror, R.; Criswell, L.A.; Labetoulle, M.; Lietman, T.M.; Rasmussen, A.; Scofield, H.; Vitali, C Bowman, S.J.; et al. 2016 ACR-EULAR Classification Criteria for Primary Sjögren's Syndrome: A Consensus and Data-Drive Methodology Involving Three International Patient Cohorts. *Arthritis Rheumatol* **2017**, *69*, 35–45. [CrossRef]
41. Seror, R.; Bootsma, H.; Saraux, A.; Bowman, S.J.; Theander, E.; Brun, J.G.; Baron, G.; Le Guern, V.; Devauchelle-Pensec, V Ramos-Casals, M.; et al. Defining Disease Activity States and Clinically Meaningful Improvement in Primary Sjögren's Syndrom with EULAR Primary Sjögren's Syndrome Disease Activity (ESSDAI) and Patient-Reported Indexes (ESSPRI). *Ann. Rheum. Di* **2016**, *75*, 382–389. [CrossRef] [PubMed]
42. Arends, S.; de Wolff, L.; van Nimwegen, J.F.; Verstappen, G.M.P.J.; Vehof, J.; Bombardieri, M.; Bowman, S.J.; Pontarini, E Baer, A.N.; Nys, M.; et al. Composite of Relevant Endpoints for Sjögren's Syndrome (CRESS): Development and Validation of Novel Outcome Measure. *Lancet Rheumatol.* **2021**, *3*, e553–e562. [CrossRef]
43. Zandonella Callegher, S.; Giovannini, I.; Zenz, S.; Manfrè, V.; Stradner, M.H.; Hocevar, A.; Gutierrez, M.; Quartuccio, L.; De Vita, S Zabotti, A. Sjögren Syndrome: Looking Forward to the Future. *Ther. Adv. Musculoskelet. Dis.* **2022**, *14*, 1759720X22110029. [CrossRef]
44. Van Ginkel, M.S.; Glaudemans, A.W.J.M.; van der Vegt, B.; Mossel, E.; Kroese, F.G.M.; Bootsma, H.; Vissink, A. Imaging i Primary Sjögren's Syndrome. *J. Clin. Med.* **2020**, *9*, 2492. [CrossRef] [PubMed]
45. Jousse-Joulin, S.; Gatineau, F.; Baldini, C.; Baer, A.; Barone, F.; Bootsma, H.; Bowman, S.; Brito-Zerón, P.; Cornec, D Dorner, T.; et al. Weight of Salivary Gland Ultrasonography Compared to Other Items of the 2016 ACR/EULAR Classificatio Criteria for Primary Sjögren's Syndrome. *J. Intern. Med.* **2020**, *287*, 180–188. [CrossRef]
46. Kroese, F.G.M.; Haacke, E.A.; Bombardieri, M. The Role of Salivary Gland Histopathology in Primary Sjögren's Syndrom Promises and Pitfalls. *Clin. Exp. Rheumatol.* **2018**, *36* (Suppl. 112), 222–233.
47. Zabotti, A.; Callegher, S.Z.; Tullio, A.; Vukicevic, A.; Hocevar, A.; Milic, V.; Cafaro, G.; Carotti, M.; Delli, K.; De Lucia, O.; et a Salivary Gland Ultrasonography in Sjögren's Syndrome: A European Multicenter Reliability Exercise for the HarmonicSS Projec *Front. Med.* **2020**, *7*, 581248. [CrossRef]
48. Manfrè, V.; Cafaro, G.; Riccucci, I.; Zabotti, A.; Perricone, C.; Bootsma, H.; De Vita, S.; Bartoloni, E. One Year in Review 202 Comorbidities, Diagnosis and Treatment of Primary Sjögren's Syndrome. *Clin. Exp. Rheumatol.* **2020**, *38* (Suppl. 126), 10–22.
49. Baldini, C.; Ferro, F.; Izzetti, R.; Vitali, S.; Fonzetti, S.; Governato, G.; Aringhieri, G.; Elefante, E.; Mosca, M.; Donati, V.; et a Fri0153 Ultra High-Resolution Ultrasound (Uhfus) of Labial Salivary Glands: Potential Applications in Primary Sjögren' Syndrome. *Ann. Rheum. Dis.* **2020**, *79* (Suppl. 1), 660–661. [CrossRef]
50. Cindil, E.; Oktar, S.O.; Akkan, K.; Sendur, H.N.; Mercan, R.; Tufan, A.; Ozturk, M.A. Ultrasound Elastography in Assessment c Salivary Glands Involvement in Primary Sjögren's Syndrome. *Clin. Imaging* **2018**, *50*, 229–234. [CrossRef]
51. Radovic, M.; Vukicevic, A.; Zabotti, A.; Milic, V.; De Vita, S.; Filipovic. Deep Learning Based Approach for Assessment of Primar Sjögren's Syndrome from Salivary Gland Ultrasonography Images. Available online: https://www.springerprofessional.de/en deep-learning-based-approach-for-assessment-of-primary-sjoegren-/17790232 (accessed on 23 August 2022).
52. Lorenzon, M.; Di Franco, F.T.; Zabotti, A.; Pegolo, E.; Giovannini, I.; Manfrè, V.; Mansutti, E.; De Vita, S.; Zuiani, C.; Girometti, I Sonographic Features of Lymphoma of the Major Salivary Glands Diagnosed with Ultrasound-Guided Core Needle Biopsy i Sjögren's Syndrome. *Clin. Exp. Rheumatol.* **2021**, *39* (Suppl. 133), 175–183. [CrossRef]
53. Grevers, G.; Ihrler, S.; Vogl, T.J.; Weiss, M. A Comparison of Clinical, Pathological and Radiological Findings with Magneti Resonance Imaging Studies of Lymphomas in Patients with Sjögren's Syndrome. *Eur. Arch. Otorhinolaryngol.* **1994**, *251*, 214–21 [CrossRef] [PubMed]
54. Baldini, C.; Zabotti, A.; Filipovic, N.; Vukicevic, A.; Luciano, N.; Ferro, F.; Lorenzon, M.; De Vita, S. Imaging in Primary Sjögren' Syndrome: The "Obsolete and the New". *Clin. Exp. Rheumatol.* **2018**, *36* (Suppl. 112), 215–221. [PubMed]
55. Sosabowsky, J.; Melendez-Alafort, L.; Mather, S. Radiolabelling of Peptides for Diagnosis and Therapy of Non-Oncologica Diseases. *Q. J. Nucl. Med.* **2003**, *47*, 223–237.
56. Anzola, L.K.; Glaudemans, A.W.J.M.; Dierckx, R.A.J.O.; Martinez, F.A.; Moreno, S.; Signore, A. Somatostatin Receptor Imaging b SPECT and PET in Patients with Chronic Inflammatory Disorders: A Systematic Review. *Eur. J. Nucl. Med. Mol. Imaging* **2019**, *4* 2496–2513. [CrossRef]
57. Signore, A.; Anzola, K.L.; Auletta, S.; Varani, M.; Petitti, A.; Pacilio, M.; Galli, F.; Lauri, C. Current Status of Molecular Imaging i Inflammatory and Autoimmune Disorders. *Curr. Pharm. Des.* **2018**, *24*, 743–753. [CrossRef]
58. Duet, M.; Lioté, F. Somatostatin and Somatostatin Analog Scintigraphy: Any Benefits for Rheumatology Patients? *Joint Bone Spin* **2004**, *71*, 530–535. [CrossRef]

59. Cascini, G.L.; Cuccurullo, V.; Tamburrini, O.; Rotondo, A.; Mansi, L. Peptide Imaging with Somatostatin Analogues: More than Cancer Probes. *Curr. Radiopharm.* **2013**, *6*, 36–40. [CrossRef] [PubMed]
60. Anzola, L.; Lauri, C.; Granados, C.; Lagana, B.; Signore, A. Uptake Pattern of [68Ga]Ga-DOTA-NOC in Tissues: Implications for Inflammatory Diseases. *Q. J. Nucl. Med. Mol. Imaging* **2019**, *66*, 156–161. [CrossRef]
61. Anzola, L.K.; Rivera, J.N.; Dierckx, R.A.; Lauri, C.; Valabrega, S.; Galli, F.; Lopez, S.M.; Glaudemans, A.W.J.M.; Signore, A. Value of Somatostatin Receptor Scintigraphy with 99mTc-HYNIC-TOC in Patients with Primary Sjögren Syndrome. *J. Clin. Med.* **2019**, *8*, 763. [CrossRef]
62. Anzola-Fuentes, L.K.; Chianelli, M.; Galli, F.; Glaudemans, A.W.J.M.; Martin, L.M.; Todino, V.; Migliore, A.; Signore, A. Somatostatin Receptor Scintigraphy in Patients with Rheumatoid Arthritis and Secondary Sjögren's Syndrome Treated with Infliximab: A Pilot Study. *EJNMMI Res.* **2016**, *6*, 49. [CrossRef] [PubMed]
63. Reubi, J.C.; Waser, B.; Markusse, H.M.; Krenning, E.P.; VanHagen, M.; Laissue, J.A. Vascular Somatostatin Receptors in Synovium from Patients with Rheumatoid Arthritis. *Eur. J. Pharmacol.* **1994**, *271*, 371–378. [CrossRef]
64. Tedder, T.F.; Boyd, A.W.; Freedman, A.S.; Nadler, L.M.; Schlossman, S.F. The B Cell Surface Molecule B1 Is Functionally Linked with B Cell Activation and Differentiation. *J. Immunol. Baltim. Md* **1985**, *135*, 973–979.
65. Malviya, G.; Galli, F.; Sonni, I.; Pacilio, M.; Signore, A. Targeting T and B Lymphocytes with Radiolabelled Antibodies for Diagnostic and Therapeutic Applications. *Q. J. Nucl. Med. Mol. Imaging* **2010**, *54*, 654–676. [PubMed]
66. Dörner, T.; Kinnman, N.; Tak, P.P. Targeting B Cells in Immune-Mediated Inflammatory Disease: A Comprehensive Review of Mechanisms of Action and Identification of Biomarkers. *Pharmacol. Ther.* **2010**, *125*, 464–475. [CrossRef]
67. Gandolfo, S.; De Vita, S. Emerging Drugs for Primary Sjögren's Syndrome. *Expert Opin. Emerg. Drugs* **2019**, *24*, 121–132. [CrossRef]
68. Mavragani, C.P.; Niewold, T.B.; Moutsopoulos, N.M.; Pillemer, S.R.; Wahl, S.M.; Crow, M.K. Augmented Interferon-Alpha Pathway Activation in Patients with Sjögren's Syndrome Treated with Etanercept. *Arthritis Rheum.* **2007**, *56*, 3995–4004. [CrossRef]
69. Giacomelli, R.; Afeltra, A.; Alunno, A.; Baldini, C.; Bartoloni-Bocci, E.; Berardicurti, O.; Carubbi, F.; Cauli, A.; Cervera, R.; Ciccia, F.; et al. International Consensus: What Else Can We Do to Improve Diagnosis and Therapeutic Strategies in Patients Affected by Autoimmune Rheumatic Diseases (Rheumatoid Arthritis, Spondyloarthritides, Systemic Sclerosis, Systemic Lupus Erythematosus, Antiphospholipid Syndrome and Sjogren's Syndrome)?: The Unmet Needs and the Clinical Grey Zone in Autoimmune Disease Management. *Autoimmun. Rev.* **2017**, *16*, 911–924. [CrossRef]
70. Gottenberg, J.-E.; Cinquetti, G.; Larroche, C.; Combe, B.; Hachulla, E.; Meyer, O.; Pertuiset, E.; Kaplanski, G.; Chiche, L.; Berthelot, J.-M.; et al. Efficacy of Rituximab in Systemic Manifestations of Primary Sjogren's Syndrome: Results in 78 Patients of the AutoImmune and Rituximab Registry. *Ann. Rheum. Dis.* **2013**, *72*, 1026–1031. [CrossRef]
71. Carubbi, F.; Cipriani, P.; Marrelli, A.; Benedetto, P.D.; Ruscitti, P.; Berardicurti, O.; Pantano, I.; Liakouli, V.; Alvaro, S.; Alunno, A.; et al. Efficacy and Safety of Rituximab Treatment in Early Primary Sjögren's Syndrome: A Prospective, Multi-Center, Follow-up Study. *Arthritis Res. Ther.* **2013**, *15*, R172. [CrossRef]
72. Malviya, G.; Conti, F.; Chianelli, M.; Scopinaro, F.; Dierckx, R.A.; Signore, A. Molecular Imaging of Rheumatoid Arthritis by Radiolabelled Monoclonal Antibodies: New Imaging Strategies to Guide Molecular Therapies. *Eur. J. Nucl. Med. Mol. Imaging* **2010**, *37*, 386–398. [CrossRef] [PubMed]
73. Malviya, G.; Anzola, K.L.; Podestà, E.; Laganà, B.; Del Mastro, C.; Dierckx, R.A. (99m)Tc-Labeled Rituximab for Imaging B Lymphocyte Infiltration in Inflammatory Autoimmune Disease Patients. *Mol. Imaging Biol.* **2012**, *14*, 637–646. [CrossRef] [PubMed]
74. Signore, A.; Picarelli, A.; Annovazzi, A.; Britton, K.E.; Grossman, A.B.; Bonanno, E.; Maras, B.; Barra, D.; Pozzilli, P. 123I-Interleukin-2: Biochemical Characterization and in Vivo Use for Imaging Autoimmune Diseases. *Nucl. Med. Commun.* **2003**, *24*, 305–316. [CrossRef] [PubMed]
75. Signore, A.; Parman, A.; Pozzilli, P.; Andreani, D.; Beverley, P.C. Detection of Activated Lymphocytes in Endocrine Pancreas of BB/W Rats by Injection of 123I-Interleukin-2: An Early Sign of Type 1 Diabetes. *Lancet Lond. Engl.* **1987**, *2*, 537–540. [CrossRef]
76. Signore, A.; Chianelli, M.; Alessio, A.; Bonanno, E.; Spagnoli, L.G.; Pozzilli, P.; Pallone, F.; Biancone, L. 123I-Interleukin-2 Scintigraphy for in Vivo Assessment of Intestinal Mononuclear Cell Infiltration in Crohn's Disease. *J. Nucl. Med. Off. Publ. Soc. Nucl. Med.* **2000**, *41*, 242–249.
77. Campagna, G.; Anzola, L.K.; Varani, M.; Lauri, C.; Silveri, G.G.; Chiurchioni, L.; Spinelli, F.R.; Priori, R.; Conti, F.; Signore, A. Imaging Activated-T-Lymphocytes in the Salivary Glands of Patients with Sjögren's Syndrome by 99mTc-Interleukin-2: Diagnostic and Therapeutic Implications. *J. Clin. Med.* **2022**, *11*, 4368. [CrossRef]
78. Di Gialleonardo, V.; Signore, A.; Glaudemans, A.W.J.M.; Dierckx, R.A.J.O.; De Vries, E.F.J. *N* -(4- ^{18} F-Fluorobenzoyl)Interleukin-2 for PET of Human-Activated T Lymphocytes. *J. Nucl. Med.* **2012**, *53*, 679–686. [CrossRef]
79. Jimenez-Royo, P.; Bombardieri, M.; Ciurtin, C.; Kostapanos, M.; Tappuni, A.R.; Jordan, N.; Saleem, A.; Fuller, T.; Port, K.; Pontarini, E.; et al. Advanced Imaging for Quantification of Abnormalities in the Salivary Glands of Patients with Primary Sjögren's Syndrome. *Rheumatology* **2021**, *60*, 2396–2408. [CrossRef]
80. Glaudemans, A.W.J.M.; Enting, R.H.; Heesters, M.A.A.M.; Dierckx, R.A.J.O.; Van Rheenen, R.W.J.; Walenkamp, A.M.E.; Slart, R.H.J.A. Value of 11C-Methionine PET in Imaging Brain Tumours and Metastases. *Eur. J. Nucl. Med. Mol. Imaging* **2013**, *40*, 615–635. [CrossRef]
81. Ziakas, P.D.; Poulou, L.S.; Thanos, L. Towards Integrating Positron Emission Tomography for Work-up of Patients with Sjögren's Syndrome and Associated Lymphomas. *Autoimmun. Rev.* **2014**, *13*, 327–329. [CrossRef]

82. Cohen, C.; Mekinian, A.; Uzunhan, Y.; Fauchais, A.-L.; Dhote, R.; Pop, G.; Eder, V.; Nunes, H.; Brillet, P.-Y.; Valeyre, D.; et al. 18F-Fluorodeoxyglucose Positron Emission Tomography/Computer Tomography as an Objective Tool for Assessing Disease Activity in Sjögren's Syndrome. *Autoimmun. Rev.* **2013**, *12*, 1109–1114. [CrossRef] [PubMed]
83. Signore, A.; Lauri, C.; Auletta, S.; Anzola, K.; Galli, F.; Casali, M.; Versari, A.; Glaudemans, A.W. mmuno-Imaging to Predict Treatment Response in Infection, Inflammation and Oncology. *J. Clin. Med.* **2019**, *8*, 681. [CrossRef] [PubMed]
84. Zintzaras, E. The Risk of Lymphoma Development in Autoimmune Diseases: A Meta-Analysis. *Arch. Intern. Med.* **2005**, *165*, 2337. [CrossRef] [PubMed]
85. Weiler-Sagie, M.; Bushelev, O.; Epelbaum, R.; Dann, E.J.; Haim, N.; Avivi, I.; Ben-Barak, A.; Ben-Arie, Y.; Bar-Shalom, R.; Israel, O. ^{18}F-FDG Avidity in Lymphoma Readdressed: A Study of 766 Patients. *J. Nucl. Med.* **2010**, *51*, 25–30. [CrossRef]
86. Keraen, J.; Blanc, E.; Besson, F.L.; Leguern, V.; Meyer, C.; Henry, J.; Belkhir, R.; Nocturne, G.; Mariette, X.; Seror, R. Usefulness of ^{18}F-Labeled Fluorodeoxyglucose–Positron Emission Tomography for the Diagnosis of Lymphoma in Primary Sjögren's Syndrome. *Arthritis Rheumatol.* **2019**, *71*, 1147–1157. [CrossRef]
87. Döring, Y.; Pawig, L.; Weber, C.; Noels, H. The CXCL12/CXCR4 Chemokine Ligand/Receptor Axis in Cardiovascular Disease. *Front. Physiol.* **2014**, *5*, 212. [CrossRef]
88. Cytawa, W.; Kircher, S.; Schirbel, A.; Shirai, T.; Fukushima, K.; Buck, A.K.; Wester, H.-J.; Lapa, C. Chemokine Receptor 4 Expression in Primary Sjögren's Syndrome. *Clin. Nucl. Med.* **2018**, *43*, 835–836. [CrossRef]

Journal of
Clinical Medicine

MDPI

'eview

?leomorphic Adenoma of the Salivary Glands and :pithelial–Mesenchymal Transition

'uka Matsumiya-Matsumoto, Yoshihiro Morita * and Narikazu Uzawa

Department of Oral and Maxillofacial Surgery II, Graduate School of Dentistry, Osaka University, 1-8 Yamadaoka, Suita-shi 565-0871, Osaka, Japan; matsumiya.yuka.dent@osaka-u.ac.jp (Y.M.-M.); uzawa.narikazu.dent@osaka-u.ac.jp (N.U.)

* Correspondence: morita.yoshihiro.dent@osaka-u.ac.jp

Abstract: Pleomorphic adenoma (PA) is a localized tumor that presents pleomorphic or mixed characteristics of epithelial origin and is interwoven with mucoid tissue, myxoid tissue, and chondroid masses. The literature reported that PA most often occurs in adults aged 30–60 years and is a female predilection; the exact etiology remains unclear. Epithelial–mesenchymal transition (EMT) is the transdifferentiation of stationary epithelial cells primarily activated by a core set of transcription factors (EMT-TFs) involved in DNA repair and offers advantages under various stress conditions. Data have suggested that EMTs represent the basic principle of tissue heterogeneity in PAs, demonstrating the potential of adult epithelial cells to transdifferentiate into mesenchymal cells. It has also been reported that multiple TFs, such as TWIST and SLUG, are involved in EMT in PA and that SLUG could play an essential role in the transition from myoepithelial to mesenchymal cells. Given this background, this review aims to summarize and clarify the involvement of EMT in the development of PA, chondrocyte differentiation, and malignant transformation to contribute to the fundamental elucidation of the mechanisms underlying EMT.

Keywords: pleomorphic adenoma; epithelial–mesenchymal transition; carcinoma ex-pleomorphic adenoma

:itation: Matsumiya-Matsumoto, Y.; Aorita, Y.; Uzawa, N. Pleomorphic adenoma of the Salivary Glands and pithelial–Mesenchymal Transition. *J. 'lin. Med.* **2022**, *11*, 4210. https:// oi.org/10.3390/jcm11144210

Academic Editor: Margherita Sisto

Received: 28 May 2022
Accepted: 18 July 2022
Published: 20 July 2022

1. What Is Pleomorphic Adenoma (PA)?

PA is the most common salivary gland tumor, representing up to two-thirds of all salivary gland neoplasms [1]. First termed as PA by Willis [1], it has also been referred to as branchioma, enclavoma, enchondroma, endothelioma, and mixed tumor, among others [2]. It most frequently occurs in the parotid glands (85%), followed by the minor salivary (10%) and submandibular glands (5%) [3]. The World Health Organization defines PA as a localized tumor that presents pleomorphic or mixed characteristics of epithelial origin and is interwoven with mucoid tissue, myxoid tissue, and chondroid masses.

Although PA most commonly appears in the parotid glands, it can also be located in the hard and soft palate and saliva glands of the upper lip, cheek, tongue, and floor of the mouth [4]. The morphological complexity of PA, which presents with pathognomic histopathologic features across glands and individuals, is the basis of the term. PA is a single cell that differentiates into epithelial or myoepithelial cells as opposed to multiplying carcinogenic epithelium and myoepithelium cells concurrently [5]. The recognition of PA is conceptualized by identifying three components: epithelial, myoepithelial, and mesenchymal. Histologically, PA presents as a variable epithelium pattern in a loose fibrous myxoid-, chondroid-, or mucoid-type stroma. Myoepithelial cells have a polygonal shape with pale eosinophilic cytoplasm.

Microscopic identification is needed for a definitive diagnosis of PA [6]. It is known that the incidence of PA increases from 15 to 20 years after radiation exposure. However, the exact etiology is unknown, and the cause of PA remains unclear. A few previous studies have reported an association between PA and simian virus 40 (SV40). Furthermore, cytogenetics and molecular studies have suggested an association with chromosoma aberrations involving 8q12 and 12q [7]. Moreover, the use of tobacco, exposure to chemical and genetic predisposition are suggested to play a role in the etiology of the disease [8 PA typically appears as an irregular nodular lesion with a firm consistency. If the PA i superficial and does not show any fixation, areas of cystic degeneration can be palpate PA in the minor salivary glands most frequently occurs in the palate, upper lips, and bucca mucosa [1,9] and is typically asymptomatic, painless, and does not involve the facial nerv If no interventions are implemented in the early stages, PA can grow to massive proportion and may become malignant. In tissue sections, PA appears as an irregular ovoid mass wit well-defined borders and may remain unencapsulated or be covered by an incomplet fibrous capsule. PA can have a rubbery, fleshy, or mucoid consistency interspersed wit areas of hemorrhage and infarction [10].

Although computed tomography (CT) and magnetic resonance imaging (MRI) can b used to confirm the presence of the tumor, MRI is preferred. MRI allows a better delineatio of the tumor margins and their location concerning surrounding tissues. However, t differentiate malignant and benign lesions, fine-needle aspiration is used. Although P is encapsulated, it is still excised with adequate margins involving surrounding health tissue; this is because pseudopodic cells exhibit microscopic extensions into the surroundin tissues due to dehiscences in the false capsule. Therefore, to prevent the spillage of tumo cells, incisional biopsy is avoided [11]. Surgical excision is the most common treatmen Superficial parotidectomy with facial nerve preservation is frequently performed for th PA at the superficial lobe of the parotid gland. If the tumor involves the deep lobe, tota parotidectomy is carried out. Wide local excision involving the periosteum or bone is use to treat PA in the minor salivary glands, as enucleation is associated with an increase risk of local recurrence [5]. The prognosis of PA is good, with a 95% overall cure rat Radiotherapy is not indicated because the tumor is radio-resistant [5,12].

Clinically, PA can be diagnosed as a palatal abscess, odontogenic or nonodont genic cyst, or soft tissue tumors such as fibroma, lipoma, neurofibroma, neurilemmoma lymphoma, or other salivary gland tumors. A palatal abscess can be differentiated b identifying its source, such as a nonvital tooth in the immediate surroundings. Neithe odontogenic nor nonodontogenic cysts show a cystic nature during an exploration int the mass [5]. Due to its varied histopathological presentation, PA can be confused wit myoepithelioma, mucoepidermoid carcinoma, adenoid cystic carcinoma (ACC), basal ce adenoma, or epithelial–myoepithelial carcinoma [6,13]. Myoepitheliomas are relatively rar benign salivary gland tumors consisting of neoplastic myoepithelial cells. The ductal stru ture is lacking or only slightly noticeable. It tends to occur in adults, and there seem to b no gender differences. It occurs most often in the parotid glands in the large salivary gland and in the palatine glands in the minor salivary glands. Clinically, it is a slow-growin mass with bulging elastic toughness. Macroscopically, it is a well-defined solid tumor wit a capsule around it. Histologically, it is classified into spindle cell type, epithelioid cell typ epithelioid cell type, clear cell type, and mixed type in which these are mixed. Howeve myoepithelioma does not exhibit typical features such as glanduloductal differentiation o the absence of chondromyxoid or chondroid foci [6,13]. Intermediary cells are a commo feature in both mucoepidermoid carcinoma and PA. Mucoepidermoid carcinoma consist of mucus-producing cells, epithelioid cells, and intermediate cells, which are smaller in siz and morphologically do not belong to either of these cells. It originates from the salivar glands, the exocrine glands in the area covered by the respiratory tract hair epithelium and the cervix. It is one of the most common malignant salivary gland tumors. The 5-yea survival rate is as good as 80%, and it has a relatively good prognosis. However, some hav a poor prognosis and a low degree of differentiation. Mostly in the parotid glands, 40% i the minor salivary glands occur in the palate. It is common among women in their 30 s and 40 s. It is rare in children under 10 years of age, but it is common among malignan tumors in children. The capsule is indistinct, and infiltration into surrounding tissues i conspicuous in poorly differentiated ones. There is no pain at the beginning, but when i grows larger, it causes pain and neuropathy, and it is usually noticed within one year. It may occur in the jawbone. Histopathologically, cystically dilated ducts and irregular ducts show bright cytoplasmic cells with clear mucus production. In the surrounding area, the proliferation of flat epithelial-like cells showing the paving stone-like arrangement and intermediate type cells forming solid follicles is observed. Squamous cell-like cells show no keratinization, the stroma is fibrotic tissue, and the tumor capsule is unclear. However, in mucoepidermoid carcinoma, they produce extracellular material and cannot create myxochondroid stroma [5,6,13]. ACC is produced from exocrine glands such as lacrimal glands, salivary glands, and mammary glands, which have a structure called myoepithelial cells and have a function of actively squeezing secretions. In extremely rare cases, it may occur in organs that would not normally have myoepithelial cells, such as the uterus, and is thought to be derived from metaplastic cells or pluripotent epithelial stem cells. In salivary gland tumors, the frequency is high, the cell atypia is not high, but the infiltration tendency is strong, and the metastasis rate is high. Relapses may repeatedly occur, eventually resulting in a poor prognosis. The sieving structure is characteristic, but there are many other cases in which solidity or ductal structure is predominant. ACC has a tendency to directly invade the adjacent nerve sheaths close to the primary tumor and spread along the nerve [14]. Furthermore, it often causes neurological symptoms and may be accompanied by facial nerve paralysis. Hematogenous metastases to the lungs, bones, and skin have also been reported. It usually occurs in women around the age of 50. The recurrence rate is high, and the growth is relatively slow, but the prognosis is poor, especially in the submandibular and sublingual glands. Since there is infiltration around the nerve, it is necessary to secure a sufficient safety margin when excising. The identification of ACC is made based on its tendency for perineural invasion and infiltrative growth patterns [6,13]. Basal cell adenoma is a benign tumor that develops in the salivary gland and is a localized tumor with a clear capsule consisting of uniform proliferation of basal cell-like cells. It is relatively rare among salivary gland tumors. In particular, it is extremely rare to occur in the submandibular gland [6,13]. Basal cell adenocarcinoma is a malignant type of basal cell adenoma, but it lacks atypia and polyphasic cells and is difficult to distinguish by cytopathology alone. Histologically, the presence or absence of infiltration and proliferation to the surroundings is essential for differentiation. However, in the case of pleomorphic adenoma, there may be cases in which basal cell-like cells are the main constituents, but even in such cases, a certain number of myoepithelial cells showing other types of morphology are usually mixed, which is a clue for differentiation [6,13]. Epithelial–myoepithelial carcinoma is a tumor consisting of a follicle of myoepithelial cells in the form of clear cells and a bilayer duct, and clear cells are usually arranged in the outer layer of the duct. However, in recent years, cases with prominent basal cell-like traits and cases with peculiar images that can be called histological modifications such as apocrine-like characteristics and differentiation into sebaceous glands have been reported. In general, since it shows a monotonous image mainly composed of clear cells, it is unlikely that pleomorphic adenoma is mistaken for this tumor, but this tumor is clinically low malignant and histologically atypical is conspicuous. However, the boundaries may be relatively clear, and it is possible that this tumor may be mistaken for pleomorphic adenoma. It lacks myxomatous stroma and osteochondral, and the presence or absence of plasma cell-like cells appears to be a major indicator of differentiation [6,13,15].

In PA, malignancy occurs in three forms: mostly as carcinoma ex-pleomorphic adenoma (Ca ex PA), and rarely as carcinosarcoma and metastasizing pleomorphic adenoma (MPA) [16,17]. A systematic review of 81 cases of MPA by Knight et al. [18] found that bone, lung, and cervical lymph nodes were the most common sites for MPA, with occurrences of 36.6% (28 cases), 33.8% (26 cases), and 20.1% (17 cases), respectively; other sites included the kidneys (8.6%), cutaneous (8.6%), hepatic (4.9%), and brain (3.7%). The risk of recurrence of PA is typically associated with a poor surgical procedure, resulting in spillage of the tumor or tumor capsule. Furthermore, the recurrence of PA occurs as multiple, separate nodules. The associated surgical risks are pseudopodia, capsular penetration, and tumor rupture [19].

2. Epithelial–Mesenchymal Transition (EMT) in Tumor Progression

Epithelial–mesenchymal transition (EMT), first observed in early development, is a term used to describe the transdifferentiation of quiescent epithelial cells to mesenchymal and motile phenotypes [20]. EMT is known to contribute to embryonal processes such as gastrulation, heart development, and neural crest formation [21,22] and physiological processes such as wound healing [23] and tissue homeostasis [24]. In addition, pathological reactivation of EMT is known to play a fundamental role in diseases such as organ fibrosis and the progression of cancer to metastasis. Cancer is a very complex and diverse disease that varies not only between entities but also within the same entity, between different subtypes, and even within subtypes. In particular, within the same individual, tumors exhibit not only spatial heterogeneity but also temporal heterogeneity. This can be triggered by continuous mutations and clonal evolution [25]. However, the EMT process mediates the plasticity of cancer cells, allowing for continuous and reversible adaptation to constantly changing conditions. Furthermore, it is not genetically fixed because it depends on the mutations that accumulate. It is epigenetically tuned by signals from the microenvironment, making the entire program reversible (i.e., by activating mesenchymal–epithelial transformation) and highly dynamic [26].

EMT is mainly activated by a core set of transcription factors (EMT-TFs), including *SNAIL* (also *SNAI1*) and *SLUG* (also *SNAI2*), the basic helix–loop–helix factors *TWIST1* (*TWIST*) and *TWIST2*, and the zinc finger E-box binding homeobox factors *ZEB1* and *ZEB2* All of these factors can repress epithelial genes such as the E-cadherin-encoding gene *CDH1* via binding to E-box motifs in cognate promoter regions [21], as shown regarding *SNAIL* [27,28], *TWIST* [29], *ZEB1* [30], and *ZEB2* [31]. In parallel, EMT-TF directly or indirectly activates genes associated with mesenchymal phenotypes such as *VIM* (vimentin), *FN1* (fibronectin), and *CDH2* (N-cadherin) [21,32]. However, many functions are performed by separate, unshared EMT-TFs due to differences in expression patterns and protein sizes and structures [33]. Beyond the "classical" EMT properties, EMT-TF is widely important in cancer biology, as demonstrated by its additional pleiotropic function [34]. EMT-TF helps maintain stem cell properties, enhances tumorigenicity, and links to cancer stem cells. In addition, EMT-TF provides a survival-promoting phenotype that is involved in DNA repair, antigenic escape, treatment resistance, aging, and escape from apoptosis and provides benefits under a variety of stress conditions. Altogether, the combination of classical EMT functions and the highly diverse, context-dependent, nonredundant, and nonclassical functions of EMT-TFs, which is also dynamically regulated by the tumor microenvironment, enables cancer cells to adapt permanently to changing conditions [35]. As a result, therapeutic interventions, including EMT/plasticity, are thought to help combat many aspects of tumor progression with a single blow.

We have been studying lymph node metastasis using human oral cancer cell lines. Human oral cancer cells were inoculated into the tongue of nude mice, metastasized to the submandibular lymph nodes, and oral cancer cells were isolated and cultured from the metastatic lesions to establish a highly metastatic strain. It was found that this highly metastatic cell line to the lymph node promoted EMT induction as compared with the parental line. Furthermore, it was reported that the mesenchymal marker Fibronectin induces the expression of *VEGF-C* and promotes lymphangiogenesis. This indicates that EMT of cancer cells indirectly induces lymph node metastasis of malignant tumors [36]. Further in vivo studies on the relationship between EMT of cancer cells and the tumor microenvironment are desired.

2.1. EMT Marker

The following is a brief description of typical EMT markers.

2.1.1. Major Epithelial Markers

E-Cadherin

E-cadherin is an essential molecule in maintaining epithelial integrity and is involved in the regulatory mechanisms of epithelial cell proliferation, differentiation, and survival. It has also been suggested that E-cadherin may also be interested in tumorigenesis.

Cytokeratin

Cytokeratin is a family of intermediate filaments that provide mechanical support in epithelial cells. Cytokeratin expression is organ/tissue-specific and differentiation-dependent. Cytokeratin is used as a diagnostic tumor marker because epithelial malignancies maintain specific cytokeratin patterns associated with a cellular origin.

2.1.2. Major Mesenchymal Markers

N-Cadherin

N-cadherin (nerve cadherin) is a 130-kDa transmembrane glycoprotein, also known as CDH2 (cadherin 2), and is one of the classic members of the cadherin superfamily. The expression of N-cadherin has been reported in various cells, including neurons, endothelial cells, and cardiomyocytes.

Vimentin

Vimentin is an intermediate filament unique to mesenchymal cells. Vimentin is a major cytoskeletal protein distributed in various cells such as fibroblasts, vascular endothelial cells, smooth muscle cells, collateral muscle cells, bone/cartilage cells, and nerve sheath cells that make up the connective tissue.

Fibronectin

Fibronectin is a glycoprotein that forms an extracellular matrix, and a polypeptide with a molecular weight of about 250 kDa forms a dimer. It mainly promotes the adhesion of fibroblasts, hepatocytes, nerve cells, etc. Integrin, a specific receptor on the surface of cell membranes, is involved in cell adhesion, cell migration, phagocytosis, etc. It works in the field of tissue damage.

3. EMT in PAs

Frequently, PA involves areas in which myoepithelial cells lose adhesion and disperse in copious chondroid/myxoid stroma; this has been recognized as EMT [37,38]. As a feature of PA, Masson favored mesenchymatous transformation, which may have been influenced by his investigations on Wilms tumor, where similar transformations occur [38–40]. In this process, which was subsequently described as mesenchymalization or stromalization, attributable to the activation of dormant mesenchymal genes in tumor epithelial cells [41], formerly polarized tumor epithelial cells lose cell adhesion molecules (E-cadherin) and secrete matrix [42,43] before separating and dispersing in the copious myxoid stroma, where they have been observed to simulate primitive mesenchyme or "swarming bees" and to express α5-integrin, Fibroblastic and chondrocyte collagens (types I–III) [44,45].

Mesenchymalization/romanization, as described above, falls within the range of EMT [46]. Immunohistochemistry has revealed that in PA, much of the tumor parenchyma shows transitional, epithelial, and mesenchymal phenotypes [37]. The aggrecan (chondroitin sulfate proteoglycan 1) and *CK14* mRNAs are localized in luminal and non-luminal cells of the epithelial and mesenchymal phenotypes, respectively, by in situ hybridization [37,47]. The variable immunohistochemical localization of transforming growth factor (TGF)-β isoforms in luminal and non-luminal tumor cells is further supported by EMT in PA [48] because TGF-β affects EMT [49]. EMT can also account for the hyalinization/collagenous structures, elastosis and cartilaginous, osseous, myoid (smooth muscular and adipocytic [50,51] phenotypes of PA, which in turn, explains its complex microstructur Therefore, assessing the expression of Snail1 (a protein that influences EMT through th transcriptional repression of E-cadherin) in PA is of interest. As a feature of PA, EMT i most undoubtedly appealing, but the argument that PA does not originate in the exocrin pancreas, where myoepithelial cells are absent, anchors and reinforces the notion of ne plastic or modified myoepithelial [52]. Langman et al. [53] reported that Wilms tumo 1 protein (WT1) is co-expressed by calponin (+) and p63 (+) in non-luminal cells in PA suggesting the usefulness of WT1 as a myoepithelial marker. Interestingly, they did no report any WT1 immunoreactivity in normal salivary myoepithelial cells [53]. A mor recent study confirmed the absence of WT1 immunoreactivity and suggested that WT (+) cells undergo EMT in PA [54], which would be consistent with the role played by th WT1 gene in affecting epithelial or mesenchymal status [55]. Caution is needed befor interpreting the immunoreactivities of purported pathological analogs as markers whe particular macromolecules are not expressed in normal cells. The trend of discoverin novel myoepithelial features continues, with podoplanin being a recent example [56].

EMT and neoplastic or modified myoepithelial may not be mutually exclusive. In tumor cell undergoing myoid EMT, a loss of intercellular cohesion and the cytoplasmi accumulation of myofibrils would be expected, thereby qualifying the entity as a neoplasti myoepithelial or modified myoepithelial cell [54]. However, EMT allows a broader pe spective and explains non-myoid cell phenotypes separating from the intervening phas of modified myoepithelium [38]. Although outside the scope of the present article, "my oepitheliomas" are considered members of the PA family [57], as it is likely that the are PAs that feature widespread myoid EMT, eventually resulting in the "depletion" o luminal structures [38]. PAs of the parotid gland were analyzed by Aigner et al. [37] a a model that shows morphological features of epithelial and mesenchymal tissue type They demonstrated areas with unequivocal epithelial and mesenchymal differentiatio by using matrix gene expression profiles as an additional criterion to identify cellula phenotypes. Many regions showed a transitional phenotype, with cells demonstratin epithelial and mesenchymal features. These data suggested that EMTs represent the basi principle of tissue heterogeneity in PAs and concluded that PAs illustrate the potential o adult (neoplastic) epithelial cells to transdifferentiate into mesenchymal cells in vivo.

4. EMT-Activating Transcription Factors (EMT-TFs) in PAs

4.1. TWIST and SLUG Are Expressed as EMT-TFs in PAs

Histologic diversity due to myoepithelial cells with morphologic plasticity, which can be attributed to EMT, is the hallmark of PAs. The occurrence of EMT within PA ha been demonstrated by immunohistochemical and ultrastructural analyses [48,58,59], bu no specific TFs have been identified. To our knowledge, only four studies have investigate the expression of EMT-TFs in PAs through the examination of *TWIST* or *SLUG* expressio by immunohistochemical or reverse transcription-quantitative polymerase chain reactio (RT–qPCR) analysis [60–63].

Pardis et al. [60] reported observing TWIST expression in 12 cases of PA, predominantl with a cytoplasmic pattern and moderate intensity, evaluated immunohistochemicall Furthermore, Yuen et al. [64] reported that the cytoplasmic expression of TWIST wa associated with neoplastic transformation in prostate tissues. In Pardis et al.'s study, th overexpression of *TWIST* also seemed to be related to neoplasm formation in the salivar glands. In agreement with Pardis et al., Shen et al. [62] identified the overexpression o *TWIST* in 30% of PAs, which had only previously been demonstrated in some benign an malignant tumors. TWIST had been observed in the parenchymal cells of benign tumors o the prostate, parathyroid, and lung and precancerous lesions of the oral cavity [60,64–67]

4.2. TWIST1 Inhibits Chondrocyte Differentiation in PAs

We have previously provided conclusive but indirect evidence that epithelial cells differentiate into chondrocytes during salivary gland PA tumorigenesis [61]. Our study found that epithelial cells express Sox9 and Sox6 and produce aggrecan and type II collagen, which are substances in the extracellular matrix peculiar to cartilage. Sox9, Sox6, and Sox5 make up a trio of TFs essential for chondrocyte differentiation. Sox9 functions in concert with Sox6 or Sox5 as a master regulator of chondrocyte differentiation [37]. The TF of this trio induces chondrocyte differentiation in both chondrogenic and non-chondrogenic mesenchymal cells already involved in other lineages, such as epithelial cells from the cervix, liver, and kidneys [68]. Both human and mouse salivary gland cells have been shown to express Sox9 [59], as well as ductal and acinar cells. These cells are similar to PA epithelial cells because they express Sox6. However, it differs from PA because it does not produce genes that are not transcribed in the salivary glands, such as aggrecan and type II collagen. The most crucial step in controlling gene expression is RNA transcription, which depends on the balance of positive and negative TFs. Negative TF suppresses positive TF when cartilage-specific genes such as *δEF1*, *AP-2α*, *SNAIL*, *SLUG*, *Twist1*, and *C/EBPβ* [48,69–72] are not expressed. Among these genes, *δEF1*, *AP-2α*, and *Twist1* are expressed by chondrocyte progenitor cells and can remain undifferentiated [58,69,71,72]. Therefore, their expression in salivary glands was compared to that in PA. The mRNAs of *δEF1* and *AP-2α* were detected in both salivary glands and PA. *Twist1* mRNA was found in the salivary glands but not in three of the four PAs. Based on the results of RT-qPCR analysis, significantly less *Twist1* mRNA was found in the remaining tumors than in the salivary glands. Based on immunohistochemistry results, the Twist1 and Sox9 proteins were localized to the same salivary gland cells. These results suggest that Twist1 expression can suppress the potential transactivation of the Sox protein in salivary gland cells. In addition, the depletion of Twist1 that occurs during the neoplastic transformation of salivary gland cells allows the Sox protein to transcribe the aggrecan and type II collagen genes. *Twist1*, a member of the TF's basic helix-loop-helix family, is essential for the development of tissues of mesoderm origin, emphasizing its function in EMT and metastasis [73]. *Twist1* has also been identified as a downstream mediator of standard Wnt signaling, known to suppress cartilage cell differentiation in cartilage [72]. Furthermore, ectopic expression of *Twist1* suppressed the expression of chondrocyte marker genes such as type II collagen and aggrecan in mouse chondrocyte progenitor cells. In contrast, *Twist1* depletion enhanced the expression of these genes [72]. *Twist1* can directly or indirectly regulate the expression of the target gene. During chondrocyte differentiation, it acts indirectly by binding to Sox9 and blocking its transactivation potential [58]. It also binds to MyoD and Runx2, the master transcriptional regulators of myogenesis and bone formation, respectively, and inhibits the differentiation of mesenchymal precursor cells into these lines [73]. Therefore, we hypothesized that Twist1 interferes with the differentiation of salivary gland cells into chondrocytes. To test this hypothesis, we conducted in vitro gain-of-function and loss-of-function experiments with Twist1 to examine the expression of aggrecan and type II collagen in human submandibular gland (HSG) cells [74]. Although HSG cells are neoplastic when inoculated into immunodeficient mice, they have been found to retain many of the characteristics of PA-generating salivary duct cells [74]. We also found that HSG cells contained the elements of salivary duct cells. They expressed Sox9, Sox6, and Twist1, but not aggrecan or type II collagen. The knockdown of Twist1 by small interfering RNA resulted in upregulation of both aggrecan and type II collagen gene expression. In contrast, overexpression of Twist1 led to the downregulation of these two genes. These results supported our hypothesis [61].

4.3. SLUG Is an Important EMT-TF for EMT Induction of Myoepithelial Cells in PA

The localization of *TWIST1* expression has also varied (i.e., nuclear vs. cytoplasmic) between studies. To improve the sensitivity and specificity for detecting the expression of EMT-TFs, including *SNAIL*, *SLUG*, *ZEB1*, and *TWIST1*, Kim et al. used RNA in situ hybridization (ISH) as opposed to immunohistochemistry in a series of PAs [63]. They also investigated the association between *PLAG1* and *SLUG* expression and the functional roles of *SLUG* in EMT using primary cultured PA cells and the expression of four significant EMT-TFs. As a result, they found that *SLUG* was upregulated in PAs and restricted its expression to neoplastic myoepithelial and stromal cells. Furthermore, using primary cultured PA cells reported that *SLUG* was involved in tumor growth and the regulation of EMT marker expression, revealing that *SLUG* was a significant TF in EMT in PAs.

In contrast to negligible *SNAIL*, *ZEB1*, and *TWIST1* expression, they found low but significant levels of *SLUG* expression in normal salivary glands according to RT–qPCR analysis. Using a mixed approach by combining RNA ISH for *SLUG* and multiplex immunohistochemistry for *CK19* and *P63* allowed them to observe the co-localization of *SLUG* and *P63*, confirming that myoepithelial cells in the salivary glands express *SLUG* commonly. Their findings suggested that *SLUG* is a critical TF that confers mesenchymal features such as contractile function and elongated morphology to myoepithelial cells, which are present in Bartholin's glands and the mammary, sweat, lacrimal, and mucous glands of the aerodigestive tract [68]. Furthermore, these findings concluded that the expression of *SLUG* in the myoepithelium of other organs should be examined. Indeed, Guo et al. [75] found that the Slug protein is specifically expressed in basal cell nuclei in murine mammary epithelium and that Slug and Sox9 act cooperatively to determine the mammary stem cell state. Kim et al. [63] reported that myoepithelial cells start to separate and disperse into the myxoid stroma at the periphery of tumor glands in PAs, in contrast to cohesive luminal structures. They did not observe SLUG expression in luminal epithelial cells. Only SLUG-positive myoepithelial cells were observed to exhibit changes in EMT markers, i.e., the downregulation of E-cadherin and the upregulation of N-cadherin and vimentin. In addition, no histological evidence has been found to suggest a direct transition from luminal epithelial to stromal cells in PAs. Therefore, EMT in PAs can technically be described as a transition from myoepithelial to mesenchymal cells. However, luminal epithelial cells may have the potential to transform into mesenchymal cells. It remains unclear whether a change between luminal epithelial and myoepithelial cells can occur under certain circumstances in PAs.

These findings suggest that multiple TFs, including *TWIST* and *SLUG*, are involved in EMT in PA. That *SLUG* may play an essential role in the transition from myoepithelial to mesenchymal cells. Furthermore, there seems to be a complicated mechanism in which *TWIST* expression is reduced to induce the differentiation into chondrocytes (Figure 1).

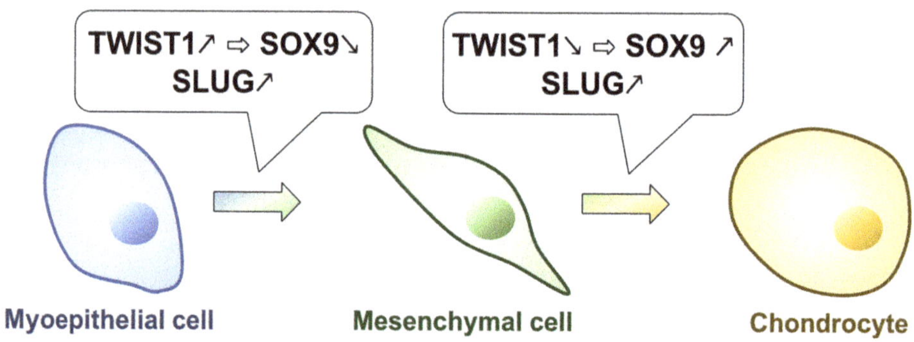

Figure 1. EMT induction and chondrocyte differentiation by changes of TFs expression in PAs.

5. Carcinoma Ex-Pleomorphic Adenoma (Ca ex PA) and EMT

A characteristic of EMT, mediated by the signaling molecule TGF-β1 [76], is the loss of E-cadherin expression. In general, changes in gene expression are achieved primarily by genetic and epigenetic methods. Genetic changes broadly alter the structure or number of specific genes, whereas epigenetic changes occur at the transcriptional level [77]. The standard epigenetic method for modifying gene expression is methylation of CpG islands in the promoter region. CpG methylation is primarily associated with various types of cancer, including squamous cell carcinoma of the esophagus (SCC) [78,79], oral SCC [80], salivary Ca ex PA [81], and ACC [82]. It regulates tumor progression through the inactivation of tumor suppressor genes such as *p16*, *MGMT*, *DAPK*, and *RASSF1A*. Changes in the methylation status of the *CDH1* promoter have been reported to be essential contributors to E-cadherin silence in many tumors [77,83,84], and *CDH1* silence is the stage and attack of advanced tumors. It is directly related to the typical expression type [83].

Xia et al. [85] first investigated the methylation status of the *CDH1* promoter in salivary Ca ex PA. They found a link between the methylation of the *CDH1* promoter and the expression of E-cadherin in 35.14% (13/37) of cases of Ca ex PA in terms of the absence of expression of E-cadherin. Similar to the findings reported by Zhang et al. [86], a negative E-cadherin detection rate of 38.33% was observed in 60 cases of CAC. Nevertheless, they also found negative E-cadherin expression in 68.42% (26/38) of eyelid SCCs and 87.26% (18/23) of oral SCC cases. In another study [83], a 42.33% (58/137) rate of decreased E-cadherin expression was found in breast cancer. Therefore, decreased E-cadherin expression appears to occur at varying frequencies in different tumor types and relatively infrequently, especially in salivary gland tumors. In the same study, methylation of the *CDH1* promoter was also detected using bisulfite sequencing PCR. It can detect methylation at each CpG site individually and is considered the "gold standard" for determining DNA methylation. They found a *CDH1* methylation rate of 67.57% (25/37) in Ca ex PA, similar to many other tumors such as primary lung cancer (88%) [87], breast carcinoma (65–95%) [83,88–90], and colorectal carcinoma (52%) [91]. They also reported that DNA methylation occurred preferentially in the first four compared to other CpG islands. Furthermore, they investigated the link between the methylation state of *CDH1* and the expression of E-cadherin in patients with Ca ex PA. Methylation of *CDH1* was significantly associated with decreased expression of E-cadherin in clinical samples ($p < 0.001$). In addition, they evaluated *CDH1* mRNA and protein levels corresponding to *CDH1* methylation status in two Ca ex PA cell lines, SM-AP1 and SM-AP4. According to the above results, they found that cells with higher levels of *CDH1* methylation had a weaker E-cadherin expression. In addition, TGF-β1 treatment of SM-AP1 cells led to the downregulation of E-cadherin and the upregulation of vimentin in vitro experiments, suggesting that EMT might play a character in the repression of E-cadherin in salivary Ca ex PA.

In spite of these results, no association was found between the methylation of the *CDH1* promoter and the downward regulation of e-cadherin expression levels. Many studies have shown that *CDH1* expression may be suppressed by mechanisms other than the methylation of the promoter. These include chromatin structural changes, loss of heterozygosity at 16q22.1, inactivated genetic mutations, specific transcription factors, and translational and posttranslational regulation [92–94]. Xia et al. concluded that E-cadherin expression levels are regulated primarily by DNA methylation of Ca ex PA, both in vivo and in vitro. They also stated that tumors with methylation of the *CDH1* promoter showed the following histopathological tendencies: Lumen differentiation ($p = 0.004$), high tumor grade ($p = 0.005$), high T stage ($p = 0.024$), and high TNM stage ($p = 0.038$). In other words, it was suggested that the malignancy of Ca ex PA increases due to the decreased expression of E-cadherin. Still, they are not the only other regulators that affect *CDH1* in Ca ex PA. It suggests that the mechanism needs to be investigated in future studies.

6. Conclusions

Pleomorphic adenoma is the most frequently occurring tumor of the salivary gland. This tumor is benign but can have a relapse after an incomplete excision and can turn into a malignant tumor.

Pleomorphic adenoma is an encapsulated tumor, but the capsule may be incomplete or show infiltration by a tumor. CT and MRI are used for diagnostic imaging, and puncture aspiration biopsy is preferred. PA is confirmed by histopathological examination. It is characterized by a mixed appearance of epithelial, myoepithelial, and mesenchyma components. The mesenchymal component may include mucoid tissue, myxoid tissu and infrequently chondroid tissue. From several ultrastructural and immunohistochemica studies, it was suggested that the mesenchymal component is epithelial in origin.

Although EMT is highly likely to be involved in developing PA, chondrocyte differe tiation, and malignant transformation, many points remain unclear, and further researc seems to be required. A more detailed study of EMT in PA would be expected to contribut to the fundamental elucidation of the mechanisms underlying EMT.

Funding: This work was supported by JSPS KAKENHI Grant Nos. JP21K16945.

Institutional Review Board Statement: Not applicable.

Informed Consent Statement: Not applicable.

Data Availability Statement: No new data were created or analyzed in this study. Data sharing i not applicable to this article.

Conflicts of Interest: The authors declare no conflict of interest.

References

1. Rajendran, R. *Shafer's Textbook of Oral Pathology*; Elsevier: Amsterdam, The Netherlands, 2009.
2. Regezi, J.A.; Batsakis, J.G. Histogenesis of Salivary Gland Neoplasms. *Otolaryngol. Clin. N. Am.* **1977**, *10*, 297–307. [CrossRef]
3. Luna, M.A. Head and neck surgical pathology. In *Salivary Glands*; Pilch, B.Z., Ed.; Lippincott Williams & Wilkins: Philadelphi PA, USA, 2001; pp. 284–349.
4. Pons Vicente, O.; Almendros Marqués, N.; Berini Aytés, L.; Gay Escoda, C. Tumors of Minor Salivary Glands. *Med. Oral Pato Oral Cir. Bucal* **2008**, *13*, 582–590.
5. Almeslet, A.S. Pleomorphic Adenoma: A Systematic Review. *Int. J. Clin. Pediatric Dent.* **2020**, *13*, 284–287. [CrossRef] [PubMed
6. Zarbo, R.J. Salivary Gland Neoplasia: A Review for the Practicing Pathologist. *Mod. Pathol.* **2002**, *15*, 298–323. [CrossRef]
7. Mittal, D.G.; Aggrawal, D.A.; Garg, D.R.; Rathi, D.A.; Ganguly, D.A. Pleomorphic Adenoma: A Case Report. *Int. J. Appl. Den Sci.* **2017**, *3*, 154–155.
8. Martinelli, M.; Martini, F.; Rinaldi, E.; Caramanico, L.; Magri, E.; Grandi, E.; Carinci, F.; Pastore, A.; Tognon, M. Simian Virus 4 Sequences and Expression of the Viral Large T Antigen Oncoprotein in Human Pleomorphic Adenomas of Parotid Glands. *Am. Pathol.* **2002**, *161*, 1127. [CrossRef]
9. Friedrich, R.E.; Li, L.; Knop, J.; Giese, M.; Schmelzl, R. Pleomorphic Adenoma of the Salivary Glands: Analysis of 94 Patient *Anticancer Res.* **2005**, *25*, 1703–1705.
10. Nagaraj, H.; Raikar, R.; Rajalakshmi, T.A.; Asha, M.; Mutgi, A. The World's Biggest Benign Parotid Tumour "Pleomorphi Adenoma": A Rare Case Report. *IOSR J. Dent. Med. Sci.* **2014**, *13*, 8–12. [CrossRef]
11. Sergi, B.; Limongelli, A.; Scarano, E.; Fetoni, A.R.; Paludetti, G. Giant Deep Lobe Parotid Gland Pleomorphic Adenom Involving the Parapharyngeal Space. Report of Three Cases and Review of the Diagnostic and Therapeutic Approaches. *Act Otorhinolaryngol. Ital.* **2008**, *28*, 261.
12. Auclair, P.L.; Ellis, G.L. Atypical Features in Salivary Gland Mixed Tumors: Their Relationship to Malignant Transformation. *Mo Pathol.* **1996**, *9*, 652–657.
13. Harada, H.; Kawahara, A. *Salivary Gland Tumors: Practical Learning with Consultation Cases*, 1st ed.; Medical View Co., Ltd.: Toky Japan, 2018; ISBN 978-4-7583-0397-2.
14. Liu, X.; Yang, X.; Zhan, C.; Zhang, Y.; Hou, J.; Yin, X. Perineural Invasion in Adenoid Cystic Carcinoma of the Salivary Gland Where We Are and Where We Need to Go. *Front. Oncol.* **2020**, *10*, 1493. [CrossRef]
15. Morita, Y.; Kashima, K.; Suzuki, M.; Kinosada, H.; Teramoto, A.; Matsumiya, Y.; Uzawa, N. Differential Diagnosis between Ora Metastasis of Renal Cell Carcinoma and Salivary Gland Cancer. *Diagnostics* **2021**, *11*, 506. [CrossRef]
16. Auclair, P.L.; Langloss, J.M.; Weiss, S.W.; Corio, R.L. Sarcomas and Sarcomatoid Neoplasms of the Major Salivary Gland Region A Clinicopathologic and Immunohistochemical Study of 67 Cases and Review of the Literature. *Cancer* **1986**, *58*, 1305–131 [CrossRef]
17. Ghosh, A.; Arundhati; Asthana, A.K. Pleomorphic Adenoma of the Parotid Gland Metastasizing to the Scapular Region: A Cas Report. *Acta Cytol.* **2008**, *52*, 733–735. [CrossRef]
18. Knight, J.; Ratnasingham, K. Metastasising Pleomorphic Adenoma: Systematic Review. *Int. J. Surg.* **2015**, *19*, 137–145. [CrossRef
19. Bradley, P.J. Recurrent Salivary Gland Pleomorphic Adenoma: Etiology, Management, and Results. *Curr. Opin. Otolaryngol. Hea Neck Surg.* **2001**, *9*, 100–108. [CrossRef]
20. Hay, E.D. An Overview of Epithelio-Mesenchymal Transformation. *Acta Anat.* **1995**, *154*, 8–20. [CrossRef]
21. Nieto, M.A.; Huang, R.Y.Y.J.; Jackson, R.A.A.; Thiery, J.P.P. EMT: 2016. *Cell* **2016**, *166*, 21–45. [CrossRef] [PubMed]

22. Thiery, J.P.; Acloque, H.; Huang, R.Y.J.; Nieto, M.A. Epithelial-Mesenchymal Transitions in Development and Disease. *Cell* **2009**, *139*, 871–890. [CrossRef]
23. Arnoux, V.; Nassour, M.; L'Helgoualc'h, A.; Hipskind, R.A.; Savagner, P. Erk5 Controls Slug Expression and Keratinocyte Activation during Wound Healing. *Mol. Biol. Cell* **2008**, *19*, 4738–4749. [CrossRef]
24. Ahmed, N.; Maines-Bandiera, S.; Quinn, M.A.; Unger, W.G.; Dedhar, S.; Auersperg, N. Molecular Pathways Regulating EGF-Induced Epithelio-Mesenchymal Transition in Human Ovarian Surface Epithelium. *Am. J. Physiol. Cell Physiol.* **2006**, *290*, C1532–C1542. [CrossRef] [PubMed]
25. McGranahan, N.; Swanton, C. Clonal Heterogeneity and Tumor Evolution: Past, Present, and the Future. *Cell* **2017**, *168*, 613–628. [CrossRef] [PubMed]
26. Brabletz, S.; Schuhwerk, H.; Brabletz, T.; Stemmler, M.P. Dynamic EMT: A Multi-Tool for Tumor Progression. *EMBO J.* **2021**, *40*, e108647. [CrossRef] [PubMed]
27. Batlle, E.; Sancho, E.; Francí, C.; Domínguez, D.; Monfar, M.; Baulida, J.; García De Herreros, A. The Transcription Factor Snail Is a Repressor of E-Cadherin Gene Expression in Epithelial Tumour Cells. *Nat. Cell Biol.* **2000**, *2*, 84–89. [CrossRef]
28. Cano, A.; Pérez-Moreno, M.A.; Rodrigo, I.; Locascio, A.; Blanco, M.J.; del Barrio, M.G.; Portillo, F.; Nieto, M.A. The Transcription Factor Snail Controls Epithelial-Mesenchymal Transitions by Repressing E-Cadherin Expression. *Nat. Cell Biol.* **2000**, *2*, 76–83. [CrossRef]
29. Yang, J.; Mani, S.A.; Donaher, J.L.; Ramaswamy, S.; Itzykson, R.A.; Come, C.; Savagner, P.; Gitelman, I.; Richardson, A.; Weinberg, R.A. Twist, a Master Regulator of Morphogenesis, Plays an Essential Role in Tumor Metastasis. *Cell* **2004**, *117*, 927–939. [CrossRef]
30. Eger, A.; Aigner, K.; Sonderegger, S.; Dampier, B.; Oehler, S.; Schreiber, M.; Berx, G.; Cano, A.; Beug, H.; Foisner, R. DeltaEF1 Is a Transcriptional Repressor of E-Cadherin and Regulates Epithelial Plasticity in Breast Cancer Cells. *Oncogene* **2005**, *24*, 2375–2385. [CrossRef]
31. Comijn, J.; Berx, G.; Vermassen, P.; Verschueren, K.; van Grunsven, L.; Bruyneel, E.; Mareel, M.; Huylebroeck, D.; van Roy, F. The Two-Handed E Box Binding Zinc Finger Protein SIP1 Downregulates E-Cadherin and Induces Invasion. *Mol. Cell* **2001**, *7*, 1267–1278. [CrossRef]
32. Dongre, A.; Weinberg, R.A. New Insights into the Mechanisms of Epithelial-Mesenchymal Transition and Implications for Cancer. *Nat. Rev. Mol. Cell Biol.* **2019**, *20*, 69–84. [CrossRef]
33. Stemmler, M.P.; Eccles, R.L.; Brabletz, S.; Brabletz, T. Non-Redundant Functions of EMT Transcription Factors. *Nat. Cell Biol.* **2019**, *21*, 102–112. [CrossRef]
34. Brabletz, T.; Kalluri, R.; Nieto, M.A.; Weinberg, R.A. EMT in Cancer. *Nat. Rev. Cancer* **2018**, *18*, 128–134. [CrossRef]
35. Puisieux, A.; Brabletz, T.; Caramel, J. Oncogenic Roles of EMT-Inducing Transcription Factors. *Nat. Cell Biol.* **2014**, *16*, 488–494. [CrossRef]
36. Morita, Y.; Hata, K.; Nakanishi, M.; Omata, T.; Morita, N.; Yura, Y.; Nishimura, R.; Yoneda, T. Cellular Fibronectin 1 Promotes VEGF-C Expression, Lymphangiogenesis and Lymph Node Metastasis Associated with Human Oral Squamous Cell Carcinoma. *Clin. Exp. Metastasis* **2015**, *32*, 739–753. [CrossRef]
37. Aigner, T.; Neureiter, D.; Völker, U.; Belke, J.; Kirchner, T. Epithelial–Mesenchymal Transdifferentiation and Extracellular Matrix Gene Expression in Pleomorphic Adenomas of the Parotid Salivary Gland. *J. Pathol.* **1998**, *186*, 178–185. [CrossRef]
38. Triantafyllou, A.; Thompson, L.D.R.; Devaney, K.O.; Bell, D.; Hunt, J.L.; Rinaldo, A.; Vander Poorten, V.; Ferlito, A. Functional Histology of Salivary Gland Pleomorphic Adenoma: An Appraisal. *Head Neck Pathol.* **2015**, *9*, 387–404. [CrossRef]
39. Masson, P. *Human Tumors: Histology Diagnosis and Technique*, 2nd ed.; Wayne State University Press: Detroit, MI, USA, 1970; 1103p.
40. Masson, P. The Rôle of the Neural Crests in the Embryonal Adenosarcomas of the Kidney1. *Am. J. Cancer* **1938**, *33*, 1–32. [CrossRef]
41. Harrison, J.D.; Auger, D.W. Mucosubstance Histochemistry of Pleomorphic Adenoma of Parotid and Submandibular Salivary Glands of Man: Light and Electron Microscopy. *Histochem. J.* **1991**, *23*, 293–302. [CrossRef]
42. Zhao, M.; Takata, T.; Kudo, Y.; Sato, S.; Ogawa, I.; Wakida, K.; Uchida, T.; Nikai, H. Biosynthesis of Glycosaminoglycans and Aggrecan by Tumor Cells in Salivary Pleomorphic Adenoma: Ultrastructural Evidence. *J. Oral Pathol. Med.* **1999**, *28*, 442–450. [CrossRef]
43. Economopoulou, P.; Hanby, A.; Odell, E.W. Expression of E-Cadherin, Cellular Differentiation and Polarity in Epithelial Salivary Neoplasms. *Oral Oncol.* **2000**, *36*, 515–518. [CrossRef]
44. Franchi, A.; Santoro, R.; Paglierani, M.; Bondi, R. Immunolocalization of Alpha 2, Alpha 5, and Alpha 6 Integrin Subunits in Salivary Tissue and Adenomas of the Parotid Gland. *J. Oral Pathol. Med.* **1994**, *23*, 457–460. [CrossRef]
45. Neureiter, D.; Böhmer, J.; Kirchner, T.; Aigner, T. Pleomorphic Adenomas of the Parotid Express Different Mesenchymal Phenotypes: Demonstration of Matrix Gene Expression Products Characteristic of the Fibroblastic and Chondrocytic Cell Lineages. *Histopathology* **1999**, *35*, 373–379. [CrossRef] [PubMed]
46. Thiery, J.P. Epithelial-Mesenchymal Transitions in Development and Pathologies. *Curr. Opin. Cell Biol.* **2003**, *15*, 740–746. [CrossRef] [PubMed]
47. Su, L.; Morgan, P.R.; Harrison, D.L.; Waseem, A.; Lane, E.B. Expression of Keratin MRNAs and Proteins in Normal Salivary Epithelia and Pleomorphic Adenomas. *J. Pathol.* **1993**, *171*, 173–181. [CrossRef] [PubMed]
48. Kusafuka, K.; Yamaguchi, A.; Kayano, T.; Takemura, T. Immunohistochemical Localization of Members of the Transforming Growth Factor (TGF)-Beta Superfamily in Normal Human Salivary Glands and Pleomorphic Adenomas. *J. Oral Pathol. Med.* **2001**, *30*, 413–420. [CrossRef]

49. Nawshad, A.; Lagamba, D.; Polad, A.; Hay, E.D. Transforming Growth Factor-Beta Signaling during Epithelial-Mesenchymal Transformation: Implications for Embryogenesis and Tumor Metastasis. *Cells Tissues Organs* **2005**, *179*, 11–23. [CrossRef]
50. Seifert, G.; Donath, K.; Schäfer, R. Lipomatous Pleomorphic Adenoma of the Parotid Gland. Classification of Lipomatous Tissue in Salivary Glands. *Pathol. Res. Pract.* **1999**, *195*, 247–252. [CrossRef]
51. Haskell, H.D.; Butt, K.M.; Woo, S.-B. Pleomorphic Adenoma with Extensive Lipometaplasia: Report of Three Cases. *Am. J. Surg Pathol.* **2005**, *29*, 1389–1393. [CrossRef]
52. Garrett, J.R.; Lenninger, S.; Ohlin, P. Concerning Possible Contractile Mechanisms in the Pancreas–Myoepithelial Cells. *Experientia* **1970**, *26*, 741. [CrossRef]
53. Langman, G.; Andrews, C.L.; Weissferdt, A. WT1 Expression in Salivary Gland Pleomorphic Adenomas: A Reliable Marker of the Neoplastic Myoepithelium. *Mod. Pathol.* **2011**, *24*, 168–174. [CrossRef]
54. Leader, R.; Deol-Poonia, R.K.; Sheard, J.; Triantafyllou, A. Immunohistochemical Localization of WT1 in Epithelial Salivary Tumors. *Pathol. Res. Pract.* **2014**, *210*, 726–732. [CrossRef]
55. Hohenstein, P.; Hastie, N.D. The Many Facets of the Wilms' Tumour Gene, WT1. *Hum. Mol. Genet.* **2006**, *15*, R196–R201 [CrossRef]
56. Tsuneki, M.; Maruyama, S.; Yamazaki, M.; Essa, A.; Abé, T.; Babkair, H.A.; Ahsan, M.S.; Cheng, J.; Saku, T. Podoplanin Is a Novel Myoepithelial Cell Marker in Pleomorphic Adenoma and Other Salivary Gland Tumors with Myoepithelial Differentiation *Virchows Arch.* **2013**, *462*, 297–305. [CrossRef]
57. Cheuk, W.; Chan, J.K. Salivary Gland Tumors. In *Diagnostic Histopathology of Tumors;* Churchill Livingstone Elsevier: Philadelphia, PA, USA, 2007; pp. 239–325.
58. Enescu, A.; Enescu, A.Ş.; Florou, C.; Petrescu, F. E-Cadherin and α-SMA Expression in the Epithelial-Mesenchymal Transition of Salivary Glands Pleomorphic Adenomas. *Rom. J. Morphol. Embryol.* **2014**, *55*, 1383–1387.
59. Devi, A.; Yadav, A.B.; Kamboj, M.; Narwal, A.; Kumar, V.; Singh, V. Potential Immmunohistochemical Markers to Characterize Epithelial-Mesenchymal Transition in Pleomorphic Adenoma. *J. Exp. Ther. Oncol.* **2019**, *13*, 1–7.
60. Pardis, S.; Zare, R.; Jaafari-Ashkavandi, Z.; Ashraf, M.J.; Khademi, B. Twist Expression in Pleomorphic Adenoma, Adenoid Cystic Carcinoma and Mucoepidermoid Carcinoma of Salivary Glands. *Turk. Patoloji. Derg.* **2016**, *32*, 15–21. [CrossRef]
61. Matsumoto, Y.; Sato, S.; Maeda, T.; Kishino, M.; Toyosawa, S.; Usami, Y.; Iwai, S.; Nakazawa, M.; Yura, Y.; Ogawa, Y. Transcription Factors Related to Chondrogenesis in Pleomorphic Adenoma of the Salivary Gland: A Mechanism of Mesenchymal Tissue Formation. *Lab. Investig.* **2016**, *96*, 16–24. [CrossRef]
62. Shen, M.; Wen, Y.; Hua, C.; Xiao, J. The Expression of Twist in Salivary Adenoid Cystic Carcinoma and Its Clinicopathological Significance. *Chin. Ger. J. Clin. Oncol.* **2010**, *9*, 187–192. [CrossRef]
63. Kim, H.; Lee, S.B.; Myung, J.K.; Park, J.H.; Park, E.; Kim, D.I.; Lee, C.; Kim, Y.; Park, C.-M.; Kim, M.B.; et al. SLUG Is a Key Regulator of Epithelial-Mesenchymal Transition in Pleomorphic Adenoma. *Lab. Investig.* **2022**, *102*, 631–640. [CrossRef]
64. Yuen, H.-F.; Chua, C.-W.; Chan, Y.-P.; Wong, Y.-C.; Wang, X.; Chan, K.-W. Significance of TWIST and E-Cadherin Expression in the Metastatic Progression of Prostatic Cancer. *Histopathology* **2007**, *50*, 648–658. [CrossRef]
65. Fendrich, V.; Waldmann, J.; Feldmann, G.; Schlosser, K.; König, A.; Ramaswamy, A.; Bartsch, D.K.; Karakas, E. Unique Expression Pattern of the EMT Markers Snail, Twist and E-Cadherin in Benign and Malignant Parathyroid Neoplasia. *Eur. J. Endocrinol.* **2009**, *160*, 695–703. [CrossRef]
66. Merikallio, H.; Pääkkö, P.; Salmenkivi, K.; Kinnula, V.; Harju, T.; Soini, Y. Expression of Snail, Twist, and Zeb1 in Malignant Mesothelioma. *APMIS* **2013**, *121*, 1–10. [CrossRef]
67. De Freitas Silva, B.-S.; Yamamoto, F.-P.; Corrêa Pontes, F.-S.; Cury, S.-E.; Fonseca, F.-P.; Rebelo-Pontes, H.; Pinto-Júnior, D.S. TWIST and P-Akt Immunoexpression in Normal Oral Epithelium Oral Dysplasia and in Oral Squamous Cell Carcinoma. *Med. Oral Patol. Oral Cir. Bucal.* **2012**, *17*, e29–e34. [CrossRef]
68. Savera, A.T.; Zarbo, R.J. Defining the Role of Myoepithelium in Salivary Gland Neoplasia. *Adv. Anat. Pathol.* **2004**, *11*, 69–85. [CrossRef]
69. Jang, B.G.; Kim, H.S.; Chang, W.Y.; Bae, J.M.; Kim, W.H.; Kang, G.H. Expression Profile of LGR5 and Its Prognostic Significance in Colorectal Cancer Progression. *Am. J. Pathol.* **2018**, *188*, 2236–2250. [CrossRef]
70. Maruyama, S.; Cheng, J.; Shingaki, S.; Tamura, T.; Asakawa, S.; Minoshima, S.; Shimizu, Y.; Shimizu, N.; Saku, T. Establishment and Characterization of Pleomorphic Adenoma Cell Systems: An in-Vitro Demonstration of Carcinomas Arising Secondarily from Adenomas in the Salivary Gland. *BMC Cancer* **2009**, *9*, 247. [CrossRef]
71. Kim, Y.; Kang, K.; Lee, S.B.; Seo, D.; Yoon, S.; Kim, S.J.; Jang, K.; Jung, Y.K.; Lee, K.G.; Factor, V.M.; et al. Small Molecule-Mediated Reprogramming of Human Hepatocytes into Bipotent Progenitor Cells. *J. Hepatol.* **2019**, *70*, 97–107. [CrossRef]
72. Park, J.-H.; Kim, Y.-H.; Shim, S.; Kim, A.; Jang, H.; Lee, S.-J.; Park, S.; Seo, S.; Jang, W.I.; Lee, S.B.; et al. Radiation-Activated PI3K/AKT Pathway Promotes the Induction of Cancer Stem-Like Cells via the Upregulation of SOX2 in Colorectal Cancer. *Cells* **2021**, *10*, 135. [CrossRef]
73. De Brito, B.S.; Giovanelli, N.; Egal, E.S.; Sánchez-Romero, C.; do Nascimento, J.D.S.; Martins, A.S.; Tincani, Á.J.; Negro, A.D.; Gondak, R.D.O.; Almeida, O.P.D.; et al. Loss of Expression of Plag1 in Malignant Transformation from Pleomorphic Adenoma to Carcinoma Ex Pleomorphic Adenoma. *Hum. Pathol.* **2016**, *57*, 152–159. [CrossRef]
74. Voz, M.L.; Mathys, J.; Hensen, K.; Pendeville, H.; Van Valckenborgh, I.; Van Huffel, C.; Chavez, M.; Van Damme, B.; De Moor, B.; Moreau, Y.; et al. Microarray Screening for Target Genes of the Proto-Oncogene PLAG1. *Oncogene* **2004**, *23*, 179–191. [CrossRef]

5. Guo, W.; Keckesova, Z.; Donaher, J.L.; Shibue, T.; Tischler, V.; Reinhardt, F.; Itzkovitz, S.; Noske, A.; Zürrer-Härdi, U.; Bell, G.; et al. Slug and Sox9 Cooperatively Determine the Mammary Stem Cell State. *Cell* **2012**, *148*, 1015–1028. [CrossRef] [PubMed]
6. Dong, C.; Wu, Y.; Yao, J.; Wang, Y.; Yu, Y.; Rychahou, P.G.; Evers, B.M.; Zhou, B.P. G9a Interacts with Snail and Is Critical for Snail-Mediated E-Cadherin Repression in Human Breast Cancer. *J. Clin. Investig.* **2012**, *122*, 1469–1486. [CrossRef] [PubMed]
7. Wang, Y.-Q.; Yuan, Y.; Jiang, S.; Jiang, H. Promoter Methylation and Expression of CDH1 and Susceptibility and Prognosis of Eyelid Squamous Cell Carcinoma. *Tumour Biol.* **2016**, *37*, 9521–9526. [CrossRef] [PubMed]
8. Guo, W.; Cui, L.; Wang, C.; Guo, Y.; Shen, S.; Kuang, G.; Dong, Z. Decreased Expression of RASSF1A and Up-Regulation of RASSF1C Is Associated with Esophageal Squamous Cell Carcinoma. *Clin. Exp. Metastasis* **2014**, *31*, 521–533. [CrossRef]
9. Bai, J.; Zhang, X.; Hu, K.; Liu, B.; Wang, H.; Li, A.; Lin, F.; Zhang, L.; Sun, X.; Du, Z.; et al. Silencing DNA Methyltransferase 1 (DNMT1) Inhibits Proliferation, Metastasis and Invasion in ESCC by Suppressing Methylation of RASSF1A and DAPK. *Oncotarget* **2016**, *7*, 44129–44141. [CrossRef]
0. Contaldo, M.; Domenico, M.D.; Caraglia, M.; Giordano, A.; Tombolini, V.; Giovane, A.; Papagerakis, S.; Rubini, C.; Rosa, A.D.; Serpico, R.; et al. The Role of E-Cadherin Down-Regulation in Oral Cancer: CDH1 Gene Expression and Epigenetic Blockage. *Curr. Cancer Drug Targets* **2014**, *14*, 115–127.
1. Hu, Y.-H.; Zhang, C.-Y.; Tian, Z.; Wang, L.-Z.; Li, J. Aberrant Protein Expression and Promoter Methylation of P16 Gene Are Correlated with Malignant Transformation of Salivary Pleomorphic Adenoma. *Arch. Pathol. Lab. Med.* **2011**, *135*, 882–889. [CrossRef]
2. Li, J.; El-Naggar, A.; Mao, L. Promoter Methylation of P16INK4a, RASSF1A, and DAPK Is Frequent in Salivary Adenoid Cystic Carcinoma. *Cancer* **2005**, *104*, 771–776. [CrossRef]
3. Shargh, S.A.; Sakizli, M.; Khalaj, V.; Movafagh, A.; Yazdi, H.; Hagigatjou, E.; Sayad, A.; Mansouri, N.; Mortazavi-Tabatabaei, S.A.; Khorram Khorshid, H.R. Downregulation of E-Cadherin Expression in Breast Cancer by Promoter Hypermethylation and Its Relation with Progression and Prognosis of Tumor. *Med. Oncol.* **2014**, *31*, 250. [CrossRef]
4. Li, G.; Liu, Y.; Yin, H.; Zhang, X.; Mo, X.; Tang, J.; Chen, W. E-Cadherin Gene Promoter Hypermethylation May Contribute to the Risk of Bladder Cancer among Asian Populations. *Gene* **2014**, *534*, 48–53. [CrossRef]
5. Xia, L.; Hu, Y.; Gu, T.; Wang, L.; Tian, Z. Promoter Hypermethylation May Contribute to E-cadherin Repression in the Human Salivary Carcinoma Ex Pleomorphic Adenoma. *Int. J. Oncol.* **2018**, *52*, 496–504. [CrossRef]
6. Zhang, C.-Y.; Mao, L.; Li, L.; Tian, Z.; Zhou, X.-J.; Zhang, Z.-Y.; Li, J. Promoter Methylation as a Common Mechanism for Inactivating E-Cadherin in Human Salivary Gland Adenoid Cystic Carcinoma. *Cancer* **2007**, *110*, 87–95. [CrossRef]
7. Yan, F.; Shen, N.; Pang, J.; Molina, J.R.; Yang, P.; Liu, S. The DNA Methyltransferase DNMT1 and Tyrosine-Protein Kinase KIT Cooperatively Promote Resistance to 5-Aza-2′-Deoxycytidine (Decitabine) and Midostaurin (PKC412) in Lung Cancer Cells. *J. Biol. Chem.* **2015**, *290*, 18480–18494. [CrossRef]
8. Lombaerts, M.; van Wezel, T.; Philippo, K.; Dierssen, J.W.F.; Zimmerman, R.M.E.; Oosting, J.; van Eijk, R.; Eilers, P.H.; van de Water, B.; Cornelisse, C.J.; et al. E-Cadherin Transcriptional Downregulation by Promoter Methylation but Not Mutation Is Related to Epithelial-to-Mesenchymal Transition in Breast Cancer Cell Lines. *Br. J. Cancer* **2006**, *94*, 661–671. [CrossRef]
9. Nass, S.J.; Herman, J.G.; Gabrielson, E.; Iversen, P.W.; Parl, F.F.; Davidson, N.E.; Graff, J.R. Aberrant Methylation of the Estrogen Receptor and E-Cadherin 5′ CpG Islands Increases with Malignant Progression in Human Breast Cancer. *Cancer Res.* **2000**, *60*, 4346–4348.
0. Liu, J.; Sun, X.; Qin, S.; Wang, H.; Du, N.; Li, Y.; Pang, Y.; Wang, C.; Xu, C.; Ren, H. CDH1 Promoter Methylation Correlates with Decreased Gene Expression and Poor Prognosis in Patients with Breast Cancer. *Oncol. Lett.* **2016**, *11*, 2635–2643. [CrossRef]
1. Li, Y.-X.; Lu, Y.; Li, C.-Y.; Yuan, P.; Lin, S.-S. Role of CDH1 Promoter Methylation in Colorectal Carcinogenesis: A Meta-Analysis. *DNA Cell Biol.* **2014**, *33*, 455–462. [CrossRef]
2. Sato, T.; Tanigami, A.; Yamakawa, K.; Akiyama, F.; Kasumi, F.; Sakamoto, G.; Nakamura, Y. Allelotype of Breast Cancer: Cumulative Allele Losses Promote Tumor Progression in Primary Breast Cancer. *Cancer Res.* **1990**, *50*, 7184–7189. [PubMed]
3. Cui, H.; Wang, L.; Gong, P.; Zhao, C.; Zhang, S.; Zhang, K.; Zhou, R.; Zhao, Z.; Fan, H. Deregulation between MiR-29b/c and DNMT3A Is Associated with Epigenetic Silencing of the CDH1 Gene, Affecting Cell Migration and Invasion in Gastric Cancer. *PLoS ONE* **2015**, *10*, e0123926. [CrossRef] [PubMed]
4. Dong, C.; Wu, Y.; Wang, Y.; Wang, C.; Kang, T.; Rychahou, P.G.; Chi, Y.-I.; Evers, B.M.; Zhou, B.P. Interaction with Suv39H1 Is Critical for Snail-Mediated E-Cadherin Repression in Breast Cancer. *Oncogene* **2013**, *32*, 1351–1362. [CrossRef] [PubMed]

Journal of
Clinical Medicine

MDPI

Review

Sjögren's Syndrome-Related Organs Fibrosis: Hypotheses and Realities

Margherita Sisto *, Domenico Ribatti and Sabrina Lisi

Department of Basic Medical Sciences, Neurosciences and Sensory Organs (SMBNOS), Section of Human Anatomy and Histology, University of Bari "Aldo Moro", I-70124 Bari, Italy; domenico.ribatti@uniba.it (D.R.); sabrina.lisi@uniba.it (S.L.)

* Correspondence: margherita.sisto@uniba.it; Tel.: +39-080-547-8315; Fax: +39-080-547-8327

Abstract: Sjögren's syndrome (SS) is a systemic chronic autoimmune disorder characterized by lymphoplasmacytic infiltration of salivary glands (SGs) and lacrimal glands, causing glandular damage. The disease shows a combination of dryness symptoms found in the oral cavity, pharynx, larynx, and vagina, representing a systemic disease. Recent advances link chronic inflammation with SG fibrosis, based on a molecular mechanism pointing to the epithelial to mesenchymal transition (EMT). The continued activation of inflammatory-dependent fibrosis is highly detrimental and a common final pathway of numerous disease states. The important question of whether and how fibrosis contributes to SS pathogenesis is currently intensely debated. Here, we collect the recent findings on EMT-dependent fibrosis in SS SGs and explore clinical evidence of multi-organ fibrosis in SS to highlight potential avenues for therapeutic investigation.

Keywords: salivary glands; fibrosis; EMT; Sjögren's syndrome; autoimmunity

Citation: Sisto, M.; Ribatti, D.; Lisi, S. Sjögren's Syndrome-Related Organs Fibrosis: Hypotheses and Realities. *J. Clin. Med.* **2022**, *11*, 3551. https://doi.org/10.3390/jcm11123551

Academic Editor: Tracey A. Newman

Received: 1 June 2022
Accepted: 17 June 2022
Published: 20 June 2022

1. Introduction

Fibrosis is the end result of various chronic autoimmune diseases. Much evidence has been collected demonstrating an abnormal expression of various factors responsible for the activation of fibrotic process in the joints of patients affected by rheumatoid arthritis (RA) [1–4], in inflammatory bowel disease (IBD), and in conjunction with ulcerative colitis and Crohn's disease [5,6]. Additionally, renal fibrosis features have often been encountered linked to systemic lupus erythematosus (SLE) nephritis [7,8]. The common denominator in all these fibrotic manifestations in autoimmune diseases appears to be the activation of an epithelial to mesenchymal transition (EMT) process following chronic inflammatory stimulation. The activation of EMT is essential for accurate embryogenesis and tissue repair, and also plays a significant role in the development of fibrosis in mature organs as an outcome of severe chronic disease. This hypothesis was amply demonstrated by experimental animal models, in which the inhibition of EMT is effective in attenuating the progression of tissue fibrosis [9,10]. The concept that chronic injury often triggers EMT cascade, leading to severe organ fibrosis, was recently linked to the atrophy and fibrosis of salivary glands (SGs) [11–13], which occurs in the chronic inflammatory autoimmune disease Sjögren's syndrome (SS) [14].

Based on the scientific evidence that many autoimmune diseases are characterized by secondary fibrotic manifestations in different organs, this review aims to collect scientific evidence of multi-organ fibrotic phenomena in SS due to an excessive production of inflammatory factors. Data reported in the literature seem to support the idea that SS, in addition to being characterized by SG fibrosis, can be associated with fibrosis found in other organs, thus, confirming that SS is a chronic, multisystem autoimmune condition.

2. Sjögren's Syndrome Features

Sjögren's syndrome (SS) is a systemic chronic autoimmune disorder characterized by the lymphocytic infiltration of the SGs and lacrimal glands that causes glandular damage leading to xerostomia (dry mouth) and xerophthalmia (dry eyes). Furthermore, SS is also known as "sicca syndrome" or "sicca complex", because the disease shows a combination of dryness symptoms found in the oral cavity, pharynx, larynx, and vagina. Thus, SS is a systemic disease, involving virtually any organ system. Impaired function is associated with reduced quality of life and symptoms, such as pain, fatigue, and depression, in a comparable way with other diseases, such as SLE or RA [15].

Infectious agents, especially viruses, and genetic and epigenetic factors are supposed to be involved in SS aetiology. The current SS pathogenic model is increasingly known as "autoimmune epithelitis". This model considers salivary gland epithelial cells as crucial players because they, on the one hand, represent the targets of autoimmune attach and on the other hand, release various pro-inflammatory factors, exacerbating the immune response [16,17]. Various experimental evidence has demonstrated that overexpression of certain cytokines, such as IFN-gamma and tumor necrosis factor-alpha may contribute to the SG dysfunction observed in SS by disrupting the tight junction structure of epithelial cells [18]. Alterations in the cellular junction integrity lead to significant changes in salivary gland epithelial cells polarity and organization that may affect secretory functionality [19] This scenario fits well with the inflammatory-related EMT activation program observed in SS, characterized by a loss of epithelial markers, such as E-cadherin and tight junction proteins [20–22]. All these phenomena, potentially implicated in the reduction of the normal quality and quantity of saliva in SS, resulted in accelerated development of SG inflammation [18,19].

3. Fibrosis and EMT Program Activation

Fibrosis is defined by the accumulation of extracellular matrix (ECM) components, particularly type I collagen and fibronectin by myofibroblasts, at the site of injury [23]. There is a great deal of evidence indicating that myofibroblasts involved in fibrosis are derived from resident epithelial cells that have been transformed through the activation of the EMT program to synthesize ECM factors. The accumulation of fibrotic components can cause malfunction and failure of the organs affected [24–26]. Nevertheless, EMT emerges as a decisive factor in activating a pathological fibrotic cascade in chronic inflammatory diseases Therefore, EMT-dependent fibrosis identifies a condition marked by an uncontrolled and unresolved inflammatory reaction [27]. Furthermore, EMT-dependent fibrosis was found in chronic inflammatory diseases of multiple organs, such as the kidney, liver, lung, intestine, and in SGs [5–14]. Typically, EMT events occur as part of a repair-associated process in order to rebuild tissues following trauma and inflammatory damage. These events are reparative if the injury is moderate and acute. However, in chronic inflammation, abnormal formation of myofibroblasts provokes a progressive fibrosis that often leads to organ parenchymal destruction and loss of function. On the other hand, inflammation is a potent inducer of EMT and, therefore, inflammation and EMT support each other [9,27].

4. Clinical Fibrotic Manifestation in SS

The following paragraphs report the data present in the literature relating to organ fibrosis correlated with SS. The phenomenon has been extensively studied in SGs, where the molecular mechanisms that could trigger fibrosis are now known and have been correlated with EMT. In recent years, cases of secondary fibrosis have also been observed, which could be correlated with the state of chronic inflammation that characterizes SS.

4.1. EMT-Dependent Salivary Gland Fibrosis

A clear link between chronic inflammation and fibrosis has been demonstrated in SGs, recently associated with SG atrophy [28,29]. In SS, fibrosis seems to be involved in the decreased secretory function of SGs, which leads to hyposalivation and xerostomia [12].

It is now widely accepted that the development of a fibrotic program in SS is due to the production of fibrogenic mediators by inflammatory and epithelial cells; among these mediators, a prevailing role is played by TGF-β1 [30]. Sisto et al. demonstrated that TGF-β1 promotes salivary gland epithelial cells transition towards mesenchymal cells through the activation of the EMT-dependent fibrosis [31–33]. Experiments performed on human salivary gland epithelial cells in vitro demonstrated that TGF-β1 was able to shift salivary gland epithelial cells from the classic cobblestone morphology to a more fibroblast-like morphology characterized by a weakening of cell–cell adhesion. This was supported by the observation that SS SG biopsies show an elevated expression of TGF-β1 [34].

The aberrant upregulation of TGF-β1 in the SS SGs causes EMT via the activation of canonical and non-canonical pathways. As recently demonstrated, the TGF-β1/SMAD/Snail signaling pathway was involved, as confirmed by the detection of a wide distribution of TGF-β1, pSMAD2/3, and SMAD4 proteins in the SS SG tissues. Furthermore, in SS SGs, a strong positivity for EMT-cascade factors and mesenchymal markers was also evidenced, such as SNAIL, vimentin, and collagen type I. Additionally, SS SGs were characterized by a decreased expression of typical epithelial markers, such as E-cadherin [11,35] (Figure 1).

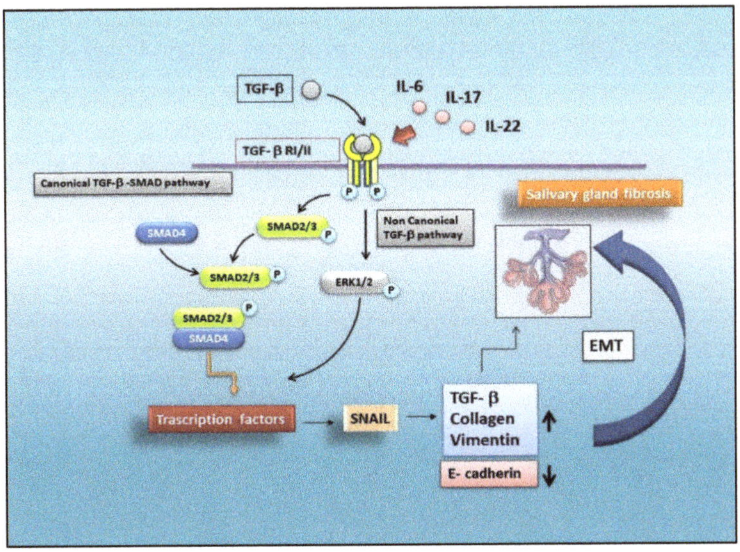

Figure 1. Schematic representation of TGF-β-mediated EMT signalling in SS. In a situation of chronic inflammation, TGF-β activates the canonical SMAD2/3 and the non-canonical ERK-mediated pathways, triggering the EMT process in salivary gland epithelial cells. The activation of transcription factors (such as SNAIL), promotes the prolonged induction of EMT, repressing epithelial marker genes and activating genes linked to the mesenchymal phenotype. Pro-inflammatory cytokines, such as IL-17, IL-22, and IL-6, induce EMT-dependent severe fibrosis in SGs.

A breakthrough in research has recently been made showing that the loss of epithelial markers and the acquisition of mesenchymal markers was strictly correlated with the grade of SG inflammation. Currently, attempts to explain the development of fibrotic phenomena in SS SGs, induced by the initiation of an EMT program, have focused their attention on the role of several pro-inflammatory cytokines. The results are very encouraging; Sisto et al. demonstrated that IL-17 and IL-22 participate in TGF-β1/EMT-dependent SG fibrosis. Both the cytokines are upregulated in SS and linked to low levels of saliva production; in addition, both IL-17 and IL-22 are abundantly secreted in SS SGs and correlated with the inflammatory degree of the glands [36].

Interestingly, in an experimental model represented by healthy salivary gland ep ithelial cells in culture, both IL-17 and IL-22 induce morphological changes compatibl with those observed in EMT. In particular, using IL-17 as stimulus, in healthy salivar gland epithelial cells, the activation of the canonical TGF-β1/Smad2/3 and non-canonica TGF-β1/Erk1/2 pathway was demonstrated [36]. When testing if other pro-inflammator cytokines exert their effect on the activation of EMT-dependent fibrosis pathways in S interesting results were obtained with IL-6, detected at very high levels in SS SGs. The IL- treatment induces a reduced E-cadherin gene transcription and protein synthesis in health salivary gland epithelial cells, accompanied by increased levels of vimentin and collage type I [37] (Figure 1).

4.2. Cardiac Fibrosis

Cardiac fibrosis is the accumulation of scar tissue in the heart, and is defined as th imbalance between production and degradation of ECM protein production. Cardia fibrosis is strongly associated with many cardiac pathophysiologic conditions, and re cently, several interesting studies have detected an increased incidence of cardiovascula disease (CVD) morbidity and mortality in patients affected by rheumatic autoimmun diseases, such as SLE and RA [38,39]. In recent years, substantial evidence has emerge demonstrating a link of SS with an increased risk of cardiovascular manifestations, such as stroke and myocardial infarction [40]. Furthermore, intriguing observations have bee reported that chronic inflammation in SS patients can trigger a coronary event and, thu an increased risk of CVD [40], but this needs further investigation [40,41]. Indeed, it wa also reported that myocardial injury is typically clinically silent in patients with RA, an this could explain the lack of data on cardiac events in patients with SS, since clinical an pathophysiological characteristics are often shared between RA and SS. In recent papers it was a high prevalence of myocardial fibrosis in the patients with SS who underwent t cardiac magnetic resonance imaging (cMRI) was observed, which can be used to obtain quantitative functional evaluation of the myocardium [42,43]. In these studies, emerging data highlight that lymphocytic infiltration into the myocardium is conceivable as a patho logical characteristic of myocardial fibrosis in SS patients. The results clearly highligh that the higher the extent of lymphocytic infiltration into salivary glands, the greater th possibility of development of myocardial fibrosis [42]. In fact, myocardial fibrosis is presen in patients with SS without cardiac symptoms, and alterations in cMRI data were ofte linked with SG focus score (FS) ≥ 3 [42,44]. This study suggests a significant associatio between myocardial fibrosis and the degree of lymphocytic infiltration into the SGs as a important prognosis factor for SS [43]. Yokoe et al., in an interesting study, have obtaine several important results from the observation of a representative number of SS patient by the use of non-contrast cMRI, without cardiovascular clinical symptoms [43]. Thes findings suggest and confirm that cardiac dysfunction and cardiac fibrosis are strongl evident in SS patients. Furthermore, the importance of this study was to demonstrate tha myocardial fibrosis could be considered as an extra-glandular event of SS [43], and tha cMRI could be a useful tool for detecting asymptomatic myocardial fibrosis in patients with SS with a higher SG FS [42].

4.3. Liver Fibrosis

The autoimmune destruction of exocrine glands that occurs in SS often extends t non-exocrine organs. Liver involvement was one of the main extra-glandular event reported in patients with SS [45,46]. In this context, the main causes of liver disease i primary SS are chronic viral hepatitis infections and autoimmune hepatitis [47]. With regards to viral infections, chronic hepatitis C virus infection is often involved in hepati impairment in SS patients deriving from the Mediterranean area, while chronic hepatiti B virus infection seems to be the main cause of liver involvement in Asian SS patients Autoimmune hepatitis is the second leading cause of liver damage in SS patients [47]. Live fibrotic processes depend on the activation of an initial injury of hepatocytes by autoreactiv immunological phenomena; these events lead to the proliferation of myofibroblasts and the activation of stellate cells [48]. These manifestations may, in turn, accelerate the deposition of collagen or glycoproteins in the liver, leading to liver fibrosis that interferes with the liver function and contributes to gradual organ failure [49]. The immunological parallel between SS and autoimmune-related hepatitis increases the progression and the development of liver fibrosis in SS. Thus, the assessment of the presence of liver fibrosis and its severity might have a value as prognostic factor in patients with SS. In a recent study, the transient elastography (TE) technique was used, which represents a new non-invasive method for the assessment of hepatic fibrosis in SS patients with normal liver function and structures, and without manifestations of evident liver diseases [46]. Using this approach, a high percentage of SS patients examined present a substantial liver fibrosis, suggesting that the frequency of potential liver fibrosis may have been underestimated in SS patients without clinical symptoms. Furthermore, this study proposed that TE could be used to evaluate the degree of hepatic fibrosis at an earlier stage of SS disease with a notable precision grade [46].

4.4. Lung Fibrosis

Pulmonary involvement in SS is an understudied condition with important clinical implications. The common pulmonary manifestations of SS are interstitial lung disease (ILD), airway abnormalities, and lymphoproliferative disorders [50]. Among them, ILD represents a frequent extra-glandular manifestation of SS, with the majority of the studies indicating a prevalence of about 20%, and resulting in significant morbidity and mortality [50,51]. This condition is associated with an injured respiratory function that leads to a poor quality of life and, indeed, is considered a significant cause of fatal outcomes in SS [52]. Therefore, the identification of poor prognostic predictive factors is required in order to provide appropriate management in patients with SS-associated ILD. When ILD includes scar tissue and the injury and damage of the walls of the air sacs of the lung, as well as in the tissue and space around these air sacs, this condition is known as pulmonary fibrosis. Pulmonary fibrosis is part of this wide group of more than 200 ILD. Efforts have been made to characterize the relationship between SS and ILD, with an emphasis upon idiopathic pulmonary fibrosis (IPF). Roca et al. highlighted that ILD is observed in a significant percentage of SS patients, and that this condition is associated with severe lung injury that develops versus fibrosis pulmonary [53]. Recently, an interesting study was addressed to systematically evaluate the incidence and characterize ILD fibrosis phenotype in a well-defined SS-ILD cohort [54]. These data have revealed that pulmonary disease is commonly linked with SS, resulting in a wide variety of clinical manifestations [54]. Firstly, symptomatic lung involvement triggers scar tissue and injury, provoking an evolution toward a progressive fibrosing phenotype in the lung identified in 13% of SS patients and so confirming previous investigations [55,56]. The second important implication is the need for effective SS screening in patients presenting apparently idiopathic ILD [54]. Subsequently, recent studies from different countries have, however, all observed that the prognosis of pulmonary involvement is not favorable in patients with SS [57]. Thus, early ILD and IPF detection is very important in SS disease evolution [58]. However, it remains controversial whether all SS patients should undergo a systematic search for lung involvement [59] with the view to redefine disease recognition strategies.

4.5. Kidney Fibrosis

Renal involvement is an extra-glandular condition well recognized in SS patients. The most common histopathological condition is an interstitial lymphocytic infiltrate with tubular atrophy and, consequently, renal fibrosis that leads to a slow progressive deterioration in kidney function [60].

Kidney disease typically manifests 2–3 years after the beginning of the involvement of the exocrine glands, and slowly leads to decreased renal function. Kidney disease occurs in 5% of patients with SS, with a broad range of clinical conditions [60]. The most frequent event of nephropathy in SS is tubule interstitial nephritis (TIN), characterized by lymphoplasmacytic infiltration of the kidney showing similarity to the lymphoid infiltration that occurs in the SGs. Patients with SS associated with TIN have significant renal fibrosis, and as a consequence, show organ impairment and lymphocytic infiltration leading to acute or chronic forms of TIN [61–63]. New emergent observations suggest that infiltration in the renal tubules is mostly caused by CD4+ T lymphocytes, features of the pathophysiological process in SGs [61,64]. Unfortunately, TIN remains a condition often undiagnosed due to its inauspicious clinical course [60,62]. Recently, a wide Taiwanese cohort study indicated that patients with SS are more likely to develop chronic kidney disease as a consequence of TIN and found that a progressive decline in kidney function occurred in 15% of SS patients [62].

A schematic representation of all the identified secondary fibrosis in SS is shown in Figure 2.

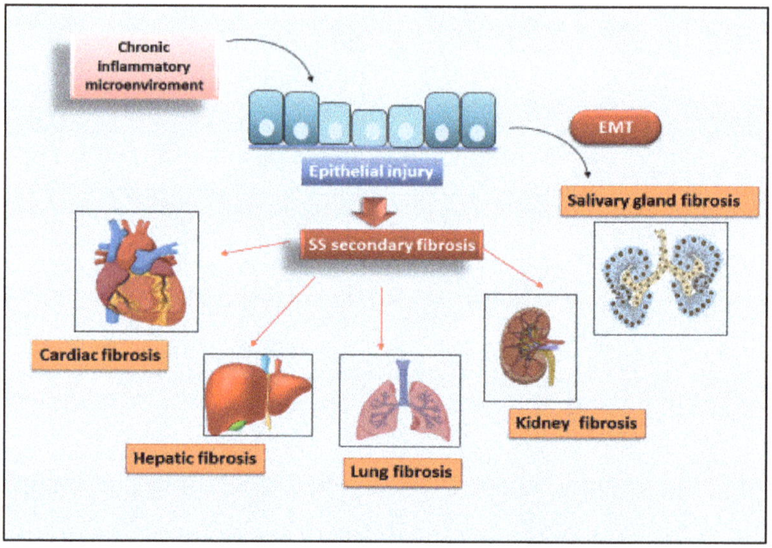

Figure 2. Secondary organ fibrogenesis in SS. Chronic inflammatory microenvironment cooperates for the progression of organ fibrosis in SS patients. Injury events lead to organ damage, inflammation, and fibrosis in the liver, kidney, lung, heart, and SGs.

5. Conclusions

Sjögren's syndrome is a chronic inflammatory autoimmune disease of variable severity and course. Although SS continues to be a challenging disease, there is now a better knowledge of its causes, earlier recognition of its symptoms, and more effective therapeutic treatments. In this review update, we are discussing evolving concepts in SS which is considered, in fact, to be a systemic disease with a fibrotic evolution of SGs. We discuss more recent studies, mostly published within the last 5 years, highlighting the possibility that secondary organ fibrosis could be a feature of SS. The clinical implication of this review article is, therefore, to summarize the current state of knowledge of molecular mechanisms involved in SG fibrosis in SS. The relationship between inflammation, EMT, and fibrosis has been established in several autoimmune diseases. The majority of studies on EMT-dependent fibrosis in SS have been carried out in the SGs, and, actually, the possibility that the same pathways operate during other secondary fibrotic processes in SS, including cardiac, pulmonary, renal, or hepatic fibrosis, has not yet been investigated. The purpose of our review is to draw precise attention to a possible and probable involvement of an EMT program in the fibrotic evolution of secondary diseases associated with SS, and to emphasize that a multidisciplinary approach is needed to identify the secondary fibrotic forms observed in SS disease. These data will help physicians better understand the disease, and to identify novel therapeutic protocols to block fibrosis in SS patients.

Author Contributions: All authors conceived of the presented idea and approved the final version of the manuscript. M.S. and S.L. collected the data reported in the study and take responsibility for their integrity. D.R. performed a critical reading of this review. All authors have read and agreed to the published version of the manuscript.

Funding: This research received no external funding.

Institutional Review Board Statement: Not applicable.

Informed Consent Statement: Not applicable.

Conflicts of Interest: The authors declare no conflict of interest.

References

1. Zvaifler, N.J. Relevance of the stroma and epithelial-mesenchymal transition (EMT) for the rheumatic diseases. *Arthritis Res. Ther.* **2006**, *8*, 210. [CrossRef] [PubMed]
2. Chen, S.Y. Does epithelial-mesenchymal transition happen in rheumatoid joints? *Eur. J. Rheumatol.* **2014**, *1*, 86–87. [CrossRef] [PubMed]
3. Fintha, A.; Gasparics, Á.; Rosivall, L.; Sebe, A. Therapeutic Targeting of Fibrotic Epithelial-Mesenchymal Transition—An Outstanding Challenge. *Front. Pharmacol.* **2019**, *10*, 388. [CrossRef] [PubMed]
4. Lotz, M.; Kekow, J.; Carson, D.A. Transforming growth factor-beta and cellular immune responses in synovial fluids. *J. Immunol.* **1990**, *144*, 4189–4194.
5. Jiang, H.; Shen, J.; Ran, Z. Epithelial–mesenchymal transition in Crohn's disease. *Mucosal Immunol.* **2018**, *11*, 294–303. [CrossRef]
6. Flier, S.N.; Tanjore, H.; Kokkotoum, E.G.; Sugimoto, H.; Zeisberg, M.; Kalluri, R. Identification of epithelial to mesenchymal transition as a novel source of fibroblasts in intestinal fibrosis. *J. Biol. Chem.* **2010**, *285*, 20202–20212. [CrossRef]
7. Liu, Y. New insights into epithelial-mesenchymal transition in kidney fibrosis. *J. Am. Soc. Nephrol.* **2010**, *21*, 212–222. [CrossRef]
8. Rastaldi, M.P. Epithelial-mesenchymal transition and its implications for the development of renal tubulointerstitial fibrosis. *J. Nephrol.* **2006**, *19*, 407–412.
9. López-Novoa, J.M.; Nieto, M.A. Inflammation and EMT: An alliance towards organ fibrosis and cancer progression. *EMBO Mol. Med.* **2009**, *1*, 303–314. [CrossRef]
10. O'Connor, J.W.; Gomez, E.W. Biomechanics of TGFβ-induced epithelial-mesenchymal transition: Implications for fibrosis and cancer. *Clin. Trans. Med.* **2014**, *15*, 3–23. [CrossRef]
11. Sisto, M.; Lisi, S.; Ribatti, D. The role of the epithelial-to-mesenchymal transition (EMT) in diseases of the salivary glands. *Histochem. Cell Biol.* **2018**, *150*, 133–147. [CrossRef] [PubMed]
12. Leehan, K.M.; Pezant, N.P.; Rasmussen, A.; Grundahl, K.; Moore, J.S.; Radfar, L.; Lewis, D.M.; Stone, D.U.; Lessard, C.J.; Rhodus, N.L.; et al. Minor salivary gland fibrosis in Sjögren's syndrome is elevated, associated with focus score and not solely a consequence of aging. *Clin. Exp. Rheumatol.* **2018**, *112*, 80–88.
13. Ficarra, B.J. Submandibular salivary gland fibrosis. *J. Med.* **1996**, *27*, 103–113. [PubMed]
14. Sisto, M.; Lorusso, L.; Ingravallo, G.; Tamma, R.; Ribatti, D.; Lisi, S. The TGF-β1 Signaling Pathway as an Attractive Target in the Fibrosis Pathogenesis of Sjögren's Syndrome. *Mediat. Inflamm.* **2018**, *2018*, 1965935. [CrossRef] [PubMed]
15. Lendrem, D.; Mitchell, S.; McMeekin, P.; Bowman, S.; Price, E.; Pease, C.T.; Emery, P.; Andrews, J.; Lanyon, P.; Hunter, J.; et al. Health-related utility values of patients with primary Sjogren's syndrome and its predictors. *Ann. Rheum. Dis.* **2014**, *73*, 1362–1368. [CrossRef]
16. Selmi, C.; Gershwin, M.E. Chronic autoimmune epithelitis in Sjogren's syndrome and primary biliary cholangitis: A comprehensive review. *Rheumatol. Ther.* **2017**, *4*, 263–279. [CrossRef]
17. Ittah, M.; Miceli-Richard, C.; Eric Gottenberg, J.; Lavie, F.; Lazure, T.; Ba, N.; Sellam, J.; Lepajolec, C.; Mariette, X. B cell activating factor of the tumor necrosis factor family (BAFF) is expressed under stimulation by interferon in salivary gland epithelial cells in primary Sjogren's syndrome. *Arthritis Res. Ther.* **2006**, *8*, R51. [CrossRef]
18. Ewert, P.; Aguilera, S.; Alliende, C.; Kwon, Y.J.; Albornoz, A.; Molina, C.; Urzúa, U.; Quest, A.F.; Olea, N.; Pérez, P.; et al. Disruption of tight junction structure in salivary glands from Sjogren's syndrome patients is linked to proinflammatory cytokine exposure. *Arthritis Rheum.* **2010**, *62*, 1280–1289. [CrossRef]
19. Barrera, M.J.; Bahamondes, V.; Sepulveda, D.; Quest, A.F.; Castro, I.; Cortés, J.; Aguilera, S.; Urzúa, U.; Molina, C.; Pérez, P.; et al. Sjogren's syndrome and the epithelial target: A comprehensive review. *J. Autoimmun.* **2013**, *42*, 7–18. [CrossRef]
20. Sisto, M.; Ribatti, D.; Lisi, S. ADAM 17 and Epithelial-to-Mesenchymal Transition: The Evolving Story and Its Link to Fibrosis and Cancer. *J. Clin. Med.* **2021**, *10*, 3373. [CrossRef]
21. Sisto, M.; Ribatti, D.; Lisi, S. Organ Fibrosis and Autoimmunity: The Role of Inflammation in TGFβ-Dependent EMT. *Biomolecules* **2021**, *11*, 310. [CrossRef] [PubMed]

22. Sisto, M.; Ribatti, D.; Lisi, S. SMADS-Mediate Molecular Mechanisms in Sjögren's Syndrome. *Int. J. Mol. Sci.* **2021**, *22*, 320 [CrossRef] [PubMed]
23. Li, M.; Luan, F.; Zhao, Y.; Hao, H.; Zhou, Y.; Han, W.; Fu, X. Epithelial-mesenchymal transition: An emerging target in tissu fibrosis. *Exp. Biol. Med.* **2016**, *241*, 1–13. [CrossRef] [PubMed]
24. Iwano, M.; Plieth, D.; Danoff, T.M.; Xue, C.; Okada, H.; Neilson, E.G. Neilson Evidence that fibroblasts derive from epitheliu during tissue fibrosis. *J. Clin. Investig.* **2002**, *110*, 341–350. [CrossRef] [PubMed]
25. Radisky, D.C.; Kenny, P.A.; Bissell, M.J. Fibrosis and cancer: Do myofibroblasts come also from epithelial cells via EMT? *J. Ce Biochem.* **2007**, *101*, 830–839. [CrossRef]
26. Wynn, T.A.; Ramalingam, T.R. Mechanisms of fibrosis: Therapeutic translation for fibrotic disease. *Nat. Med.* **2012**, *18*, 1028–104 [CrossRef]
27. Thiery, J.P.; Acloque, H.; Huang, R.Y.; Nieto, M.A. Epithelial-mesenchymal transitions in development and disease. *Cell* **200** *139*, 871–890. [CrossRef]
28. Koski, H.; Janin, A.; Humphreys-Beher, M.G.; Sorsa, T.; Malmström, M.; Konttinen, Y.T. Tumor necrosis factor-alpha and recepto for it in labial salivary glands in Sjögren's syndrome. *Clin. Exp. Rheumatol.* **2001**, *19*, 131–137.
29. Skopouli, F.; Li, L.; Boumba, D.; Stefanaki, S.; Hanel, K.; Moutsopoulos, H.M.; Krilis, S.A. Association of mast cells with fibros and fatty infiltration in the minor salivary glands of patients with Sjögren's syndrome. *Clin. Exp. Rheumatol.* **1998**, *16*, 63–65.
30. Zavadil, J.; Bottinger, E.P. TGF-β and epithelial-to-mesenchymal transitions. *Oncogene* **2005**, *24*, 5764–5774. [CrossRef]
31. Hall, B.E.; Zheng, C.; Swaim, W.D.; Cho, A.; Nagineni, C.N.; Eckhaus, M.A.; Flanders, K.C.; Ambudkar, I.S.; Baum, B. Kulkarni, A.B. Conditional overexpression of TGF-β1 disrupts mouse salivary gland development and function. *Lab. Investi* **2010**, *90*, 543–555. [CrossRef] [PubMed]
32. Woods, L.T.; Camden, J.M.; El-Sayed, F.G.; Khalafalla, M.G.; Petris, M.J.; Erb, L.; Weisman, G.A. Increased expression of TGF- signaling components in a mouse model of fibrosis induced by submandibular gland duct ligation. *PLoS ONE* **2015**, *10*, e012364 [CrossRef] [PubMed]
33. González, C.R.; Amer, M.A.; Vitullo, A.D.; González-Calvar, S.I.; Vacas, M.I. Immunolocalization of the TGFB1 system i submandibular gland fibrosis after experimental periodontitis in rats. *Acta Odont. Latinoam.* **2016**, *29*, 138–143.
34. Mason, G.I.; Hamburger, J.; Bowman, S.; Matthews, J.B. Salivary gland expression of transforming growth factor beta isoforms i Sjogren's syndrome and benign lymphoepithelial lesions. *Mol. Pathol.* **2003**, *56*, 52–59. [CrossRef] [PubMed]
35. Sisto, M.; Lorusso, L.; Ingravallo, G.; Ribatti, D.; Lisi, S. TGFβ1-Smad canonical and -Erk non-canonical pathways participate i interleukin-17-induced epithelial–mesenchymal transition in Sjögren's syndrome. *Lab. Investig.* **2020**, *100*, 824–836. [CrossRe [PubMed]
36. Sisto, M.; Lorusso, L.; Tamma, R.; Ingravallo, G.; Ribatti, D.; Lisi, S. Interleukin-17 and -22 synergy linking inflammation an EMT-dependent fibrosis in Sjögren's syndrome. *Clin. Exp. Immunol.* **2019**, *198*, 261–272. [CrossRef] [PubMed]
37. Sisto, M.; Tamma, R.; Ribatti, D.; Lisi, S. IL-6 Contributes to the TGF-β1-Mediated Epithelial to Mesenchymal Transition in Huma Salivary Gland Epithelial Cells. *Arch. Immunol. Ther. Exp.* **2020**, *68*, 27. [CrossRef] [PubMed]
38. Lee, Y.H.; Choi, S.J.; Ji, J.D.; Song, G.G. Overall and cause-specific mortality in systemic lupus erythematosus: An update meta-analysis. *Lupus* **2016**, *25*, 727–734. [CrossRef]
39. Solomon, D.H.; Karlson, E.W.; Rimm, E.B.; Cannuscio, C.C.; Mandl, L.A.; Manson, J.E.; Stampfer, M.J.; Curhan, G.C. Cardiovasc lar morbidity and mortality in women diagnosed with rheumatoid arthritis. *Circulation* **2003**, *107*, 1303–1307. [CrossRef]
40. Wu, X.F.; Huang, J.Y.; Chiou, J.Y.; Chen, H.H.; Wei, J.C.; Dong, L.L. Increased risk of coronary heart disease among patients wit primary Sjögren's syndrome: A nationwide population-based cohort study. *Sci. Rep.* **2018**, *8*, 2209. [CrossRef]
41. Beltai, A.; Barnetche, T.; Daien, C.; Lukas, C.; Gaujoux-Viala, C.; Combe, B.; Morel, J. Cardiovascular morbidity and mortality i primary Sjögren's syndrome: A systematic review and meta-analysis. *Arthritis Care Res.* **2020**, *72*, 131–139. [CrossRef] [PubMed
42. Nishiwaki, A.; Kobayashi, H.; Ikumi, N.; Kobayashi, Y.; Yokoe, I.; Sugiyama, K.; Matsukawa, Y.; Takei, M.; Kitamura, N. Salivar Gland Focus Score Is Associated with Myocardial Fibrosis in Primary Sjögren's Syndrome Assessed by a Cardiac Magneti Resonance Approach. *J. Rheumatol.* **2021**, *48*, 627. [CrossRef] [PubMed]
43. Yokoe, I.; Kobayashi, H.; Nishiwaki, A.; Nagasawa, Y.; Kitamura, N.; Haraoka, M.; Kobayashi, Y.; Takei, M.; Nakamura, H Asymptomatic myocardial dysfunction was revealed by feature tracking cardiac magnetic resonance imaging in patients wit primary Sjögren's syndrome. *Int. J. Rheum. Dis.* **2021**, *24*, 1482–1490. [CrossRef] [PubMed]
44. Voulgarelis, M.; Tzioufas, A. Pathogenetic mechanisms in the initiation and perpetuation of Sjögren's syndrome. *Nat. Re Rheumatol.* **2010**, *6*, 529–537. [CrossRef] [PubMed]
45. Kaplan, M.J.; Ike, R.W. The liver is a common non-exocrine target in primary Sjögren's syndrome: A retrospective review. *BM Gastroenterol.* **2002**, *2*, 21. [CrossRef]
46. Lee, S.W.; Kim, B.K.; Park, J.Y.; Kim, D.Y.; Ahn, S.H.; Song, J.; Park, Y.B.; Lee, S.K.; Han, K.H.; Kim, S.U. Clinical predictors c silent but substantial liver fibrosis in primary Sjogren's syndrome. *Mod. Rheumatol.* **2016**, *26*, 576–582. [CrossRef]
47. Zeron, P.B.; Retamozo, S.; Bové, A.; Kostov, B.A.; Sisó, A.; Ramos-Casals, M. Diagnosis of Liver Involvement in Primary Sjögre Syndrome. *J. Clin. Transl. Hepatol.* **2013**, *1*, 94–102.
48. Liedtke, C.; Nevzorova, Y.A.; Luedde, T.; Zimmermann, H.; Kroy, D.; Strnad, P.; Berres, M.L.; Bernhagen, J.; Tacke, F Nattermann, J.; et al. Liver Fibrosis-From Mechanisms of Injury to Modulation of Disease. *Front. Med.* **2022**, *8*, 81449 [CrossRef]

49. Jiao, J.; Friedman, S.L.; Aloman, C. Hepatic fibrosis. *Curr. Opin. Gastroenterol.* **2009**, *25*, 223–229. [CrossRef]
50. Fairfax, A.J.; Haslam, P.L.; Pavia, D.; Sheahan, N.F.; Bateman, J.R.; Agnew, J.E.; Clarke, S.W.; Turner-Warwick, M. Pulmonary disorders associated with sjogren's syndrome. *Q. J. Med.* **1981**, *50*, 279–295.
51. Dong, X.; Zhou, J.; Guo, X.; Li, Y.; Xu, Y.; Fu, Q.; Lu, Y.; Zheng, Y. A retrospective analysis of distinguishing features of chest HRCT and clinical manifestation in primary sjogren's syndrome-related interstitial lung disease in a Chinese population. *Clin. Rheumatol.* **2018**, *37*, 2981–2988. [CrossRef] [PubMed]
52. Kamiya, Y.; Fujisawa, T.; Kono, M.; Nakamura, H.; Yokomura, K.; Koshimizu, N.; Toyoshima, M.; Imokawa, S.; Sumikawa, H.; Johkoh, T.; et al. Prognostic factors for primary Sjögren's syndrome-associated interstitial lung diseases. *Respir. Med.* **2019**, *159*, 105811. [CrossRef] [PubMed]
53. Roca, F.; Dominique, S.; Schmidt, J.; Smail, A.; Duhaut, P.; Lévesque, H.; Marie, I. Interstitial lung disease in primary Sjögren's syndrome. *Autoimmun. Rev.* **2017**, *16*, 48–54. [CrossRef] [PubMed]
54. Sogkas, G.; Hirsch, S.; Olsson, K.M.; Hinrichs, J.B.; Thiele, T.; Seeliger, T.; Skripuletz, T.; Schmidt, R.E.; Witte, T.; Jablonka, A.; et al. Lung Involvement in Primary Sjögren's Syndrome-An Under-Diagnosed Entity. *Front. Med.* **2020**, *7*, 332. [CrossRef]
55. Palm, O.; Garen, T.; Berge Enger, T.; Jensen, J.L.; Lund, M.B.; Aalokken, T.M.; Gran, J.T. Clinical pulmonary involvement in primary sjogren's syndrome: Prevalence, quality of life and mortality–a retrospective study based on registry data. *Rheumatology* **2013**, *52*, 173–179. [CrossRef]
56. Belenguer, R.; Ramos-Casals, M.; Brito-Zeron, P.; del Pino, J.; Sentis, J.; Aguilo, S.; Font, J. Influence of clinical and immunological parameters on the health-related quality of life of patients with primary sjogren's syndrome. *Clin. Exp. Rheumatol.* **2005**, *23*, 351–356.
57. Gao, H.; Sun, Y.; Zhang, X.Y.; Xie, L.; Zhang, X.W.; Zhong, Y.C.; Zhang, J.; Hou, Y.K.; Li, Z.G. Characteristics and mortality in primary Sjögren syndrome-related interstitial lung disease. *Medicine* **2021**, *100*, e26777. [CrossRef]
58. Kakugawa, T.; Sakamoto, N.; Ishimoto, H.; Shimizu, T.; Nakamura, H.; Nawata, A.; Ito, C.; Sato, S.; Hanaka, T.; Oda, K.; et al. Lymphocytic focus score is positively related to airway and interstitial lung diseases in primary Sjögren's syndrome. *Respir. Med.* **2018**, *137*, 95–102. [CrossRef]
59. Lin, W.; Xin, Z.; Zhang, J.; Liu, N.; Ren, X.; Liu, M.; Su, Y.; Liu, Y.; Yang, L.; Guo, S.; et al. Interstitial lung disease in Primary Sjögren's syndrome. *BMC Pulm. Med.* **2022**, *22*, 73. [CrossRef]
60. Aiyegbusi, O.; McGregor, L.; McGeoch, L.; Kipgen, D.; Geddes, C.C.; Stevens, K.I. Renal Disease in Primary Sjögren's Syndrome. *Rheum. Ther.* **2021**, *8*, 63–80. [CrossRef]
61. Maripuri, S.; Grande, J.P.; Osborn, T.G.; Fervenza, F.C.; Matteson, E.L.; Donadio, J.V.; Hogan, M.C. Renal involvement in primary Sjögren's syndrome: A clinic pathologic study. *Clin. J. Am. Soc. Nephrol.* **2009**, *4*, 1423–1431. [CrossRef] [PubMed]
62. Kidder, D.; Rutherford, E.; Kipgen, D.; Fleming, S.; Geddes, C.; Stewart, G.A. Kidney biopsy findings in primary Sjögren syndrome. *Nephrol. Dial. Transplant.* **2015**, *30*, 1363–1369. [CrossRef]
63. Goules, A.; Geetha, D.; Arend, L.J.; Baer, A.N. Renal involvement in primary Sjögren's syndrome: Natural history and treatment outcome. *Clin. Exp. Rheumatol.* **2019**, *118*, 123–132.
64. Evans, R.D.R.; Laing, C.M.; Ciurtin, C.; Walsh, S.B. Tubulo interstitial nephritis in primary Sjögren syndrome: Clinical manifestations and response to treatment. *BMC Musculoskelet. Disord.* **2016**, *17*, 2. [CrossRef] [PubMed]

Journal of
Clinical Medicine

MDPI

eview

E-Cadherin Signaling in Salivary Gland Development and Autoimmunity

Margherita Sisto *, Domenico Ribatti and Sabrina Lisi

Department of Basic Medical Sciences, Neurosciences and Sensory Organs (SMBNOS), Section of Human Anatomy and Histology, University of Bari "Aldo Moro", 70124 Bari, Italy; domenico.ribatti@uniba.it (D.R.); sabrina.lisi@uniba.it (S.L.)
* Correspondence: margherita.sisto@uniba.it; Tel.: +39-080-547-8315; Fax: +39-080-547-8327

Abstract: E-cadherin, the major epithelial cadherin, is located in regions of cell–cell contact known as adherens junctions. E-cadherin contributes to the maintenance of the epithelial integrity through homophylic interaction; the cytoplasmic tail of E-cadherin directly binds catenins, forming a dynamic complex that regulates several intracellular signal transduction pathways, including epithelial-to-mesenchymal transition (EMT). Recent progress uncovered a novel and critical role for this adhesion molecule in salivary gland (SG) development and in SG diseases. We summarize the structure and regulation of the E-cadherin gene and transcript in view of the role of this remarkable protein in SG morphogenesis, focusing, in the second part of the review, on altered E-cadherin expression in EMT-mediated SG autoimmunity.

Keywords: E-cadherins; salivary glands; morphogenesis; EMT; Sjögren's syndrome; autoimmunity

Citation: Sisto, M.; Ribatti, D.; Lisi, S. E-Cadherin Signaling in Salivary Gland Development and Autoimmunity. *J. Clin. Med.* **2022**, *11*, 2241. https://doi.org/10.3390/jcm11082241

Academic Editor: Eng Ooi

Received: 11 March 2022
Accepted: 15 April 2022
Published: 17 April 2022

Publisher's Note: MDPI stays neutral with regard to jurisdictional claims in published maps and institutional affiliations.

1. Introduction to Cadherins

Cadherins are transmembrane or membrane-associated glycoproteins that mediate Ca^{2+}-dependent cell–cell adhesion and have mainly been described for their instrumental role during morphogenesis [1]. Cadherins' functions extend to multiple aspects of morphogenesis, ranging from polarization of simple epithelia to the formation of tissues and organs architecture, the conference of resistance to detachment and the control of cellular tissue organization and cohesion [1]. Cadherins expression occurs through a dynamic process and is regulated by a great number of developmental factors and cellular signals. From the analysis of the sequence similarity, cadherins were divided into five subfamilies: classical types I and II (E-, P-, N- and VE-cadherin), atypical (T-cadherin), desmosomal (desmogleins, desmocollins), protocadherins and cadherin-related proteins [2]. The family of classical cadherins includes E (epithelial)-, N (neural)-, P (placental)-, VE (vascular-endothelial)-, R (retinal)- and K (kidney)-cadherins; among these, E-cadherin is essential for the formation of adherens junctions (AJs) in epithelial cells. E-cadherin mediates strong, homotypic adhesion between neighboring epithelial cells, thereby, safeguarding epithelial barrier integrity [2,3]. The lack of a functional, tight junction and desmosome formation in the absence of E-cadherin emphasizes its central role in the regulation of epithelial cell–cell contacts [2].

2. E-Cadherin Discovery

E-cadherin, a type-I cadherin, is generally considered the prototype of all cadherins because of its early identification and its thorough characterization both in normal and in pathological conditions. In 1977, Takeichi [4] proposed the existence of a physiological Ca^{2+}-dependent cell–cell adhesion that could explain the adhesive properties of a lung cell line in addition to the more known modality of Ca^{2+}-independent agglutination. Takeichi discovered a surface protein of about 150 kDa involved in the Ca^{2+}-dependent cell–cell adhesion, reporting, for the first time, the E-cadherin adhesion potential. At the same time, other research groups investigated in this field, reaching results that, only later, were linked together. François Jacob's group, in 1980, described a specific cell-surface glycoprotein named uvomorulin, the 84 kDa fragment of which was responsible for the Ca^{2+}-dependent compaction of mouse embryonal cells [5]. By the use of antibodies against this 84 kDa fragment, cell–cell interactions were perturbated, and the compaction of embryos before implantation was prevented. Using experiments based on subsequent trypsinizations, the same research group deduced that a short-lived precursor was produced by cells from which a stable form of 120 kDa is derived; this 120 kDa protein, in presence of Ca^{2+}, was cleaved, giving rise to the 84 kDa active fragment. Electron microscopy revealed that uvomorulin was localized in the intermediate junctions or AJs of intestinal epithelial cells [6], and, nowadays, it is established that the 84 kDa fragment corresponds to the ectodomain of E-cadherin. Concurrently, Wheelock's group [7] reported the identification and purification of a protein, expressed by epithelial cell lines and tissues, that was named cell-CAM 120/80. This identification was achieved using antibodies directed against an 80 kDa protein that was released into serum-free medium by MCF-7 human breast cancer cells [7,8]. These antibodies caused disruption of cell–cell junctions in mouse epithelial cells and enabled characterization of the cell-surface form of the antigen as a glycoprotein of 120 kDa from which the 84 kDa fragment was released. Complementary studies, performed by Begemann and colleagues [9], demonstrated the presence of a 124 kDa cell adhesion glycoprotein in chicken liver epithelial cells named L-CAM, which was converted into an 81 kDa protein by trypsinization in the presence of Ca^{2+}. Interestingly, these antibodies did not affect aggregation of retinal cells expressing R-cadherin instead of E-cadherin. Once all these pioneering studies were reconciled, in 1984, the name "cadherins" was introduced [10] to identify this class of cell–cell adhesion molecule. The prefix "E" (for epithelial) was adopted for cadherin expressed by epithelial cells, and subsequent experiments performed by Takeichi's group revealed the existence of other cadherins which have distinct cellular expression patterns, such as N- and P-cadherins [11]. Once E-cadherin was definitely individuated as a cell–cell adhesion protein, the subsequent phases led to the cloning of the E-cadherin cDNA [12], the individuation of the tertiary structure of E-cadherin extracellular domain [13], the study of the E-cadherin/catenin complexes [14] and the demonstration of a key role of E-cadherin-mediated regulation of cellular replication [15,16].

3. E-Cadherin Structure

E-cadherin is a single-span transmembrane protein. E-cadherin protein precursor is a polypeptide with a short signal sequence for import into the endoplasmic reticulum, a pro-peptide of about 130 amino acid residues (AA) and a mature polypeptide of about 728 AA (Figure 1). The mature E-cadherin contains a transmembrane domain, a cytoplasmic domain of 150 AA and an ectodomain of 550 AA comprising five tandemly repeated domains. Four of these domains are known as cadherin repeats (EC1 to EC4), whereas EC5 is characterized by four conserved cysteines [17]. E-cadherin forms calcium-dependent, homotypic cell–cell adhesion structures known as AJs that mediate intercellular adhesion [18], cell polarity, cell–cell communication, cell survival, cell differentiation and tissue development [19–22]. The extracellular domain is responsible for homophilic interactions between cadherin molecules expressed at the surface of neighboring cells [17]. Cadherin cytoplasmic tails bind to proteins p120-catenin and β-catenin (alternatively, its homolog γ-catenin in some cell types), while p120-catenin regulates the stability of cadherin–catenin complexes at the plasma membrane [23], and β-catenin interacts with the actin-binding protein α-catenin which contains an actin-binding domain and physically links AJ complexes to the actin cytoskeleton [23,24]. The integrity of the cadherin–catenin complex and the association with the cytoskeletal actin represent prerequisites for cell–cell adhesion [23,24].

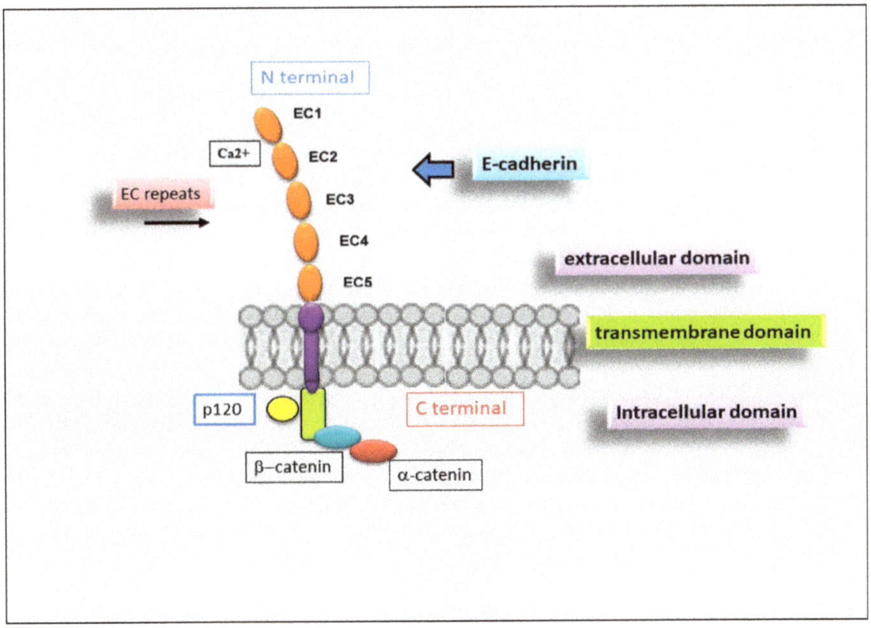

Figure 1. Schematic representation of E-cadherin protein. E-cadherin contains 5 extracellular cadherin (EC) repeats linked by Ca^{2+} binding sites, a transmembrane domain and an intracellular domain that binds p120-α-catenin and β-catenin.

4. Development of Submandibular Gland

The submandibular gland (SMG) development occurs through branching morphogenesis [25–29]. Through the use of comparative studies, it is now known that the development of human and mouse salivary glands (SGs) occurs through the same developmental pattern [30,31]. In the mouse, the first stage of SG morphogenesis shows only the initial thickening of the oral epithelium characterizing the prebud stage, which occurs at embryonic day (E) 11.5 [28,32]. The SMG placode is visible as a localized thickening of the oral epithelium adjacent to the tongue. The epithelial thickening gives rise to the initial bud structure by E12.5. By this time in development, the salivary proof enlarges and invaginates into the underlying mesenchyme, which begins to condense, resulting in the formation of a primary bud linked to the oral surface by a duct that will become the major secretory duct. The cells deriving from the neural crests arrange themselves to surround the epithelial sketches, giving rise to the submandibular parasympathetic ganglia. The signals that initiate this neural–epithelial interaction have not been fully described yet [28,33,34]. By E13, known as the pseudoglandular stage, the final part of the bud grows in size and undergoes rounds of clefting and new bud formation, resulting in approximately 3–5 epithelial buds. The lumen formation already starts at this stage by removing the epithelial cells from the center of the solid stalks through programmed cell death apoptosis [28,32,35]. Branching morphogenesis then progresses, and the majority of the ducts develop a lumen at the canalicular stage from about E15.5. Around E17.5, the branches and terminal buds are delved to form the ductal and acinar system, and, at this point, the terminal bud stage is completed and exhibits differentiated terminal end buds and a presumptive ductal system [32].

5. The Pivotal Role for E-Cadherin in Salivary Gland Morphogenesis

Although the E-cadherin adhesion receptor mediates different, acknowledged functions during epithelial branching morphogenesis, relatively little is known of how E-cadherin, in addition to directly mediating intercellular adhesion, impacts the development of salivary acini and ducts. Recent studies showed that, during embryonic SMG morphogenesis, E-cadherin plays a decisive role in determining the differentiation of epithelial progenitor cells into acinar or ductal cells in a specific stage of embryonic development and in guiding the development of glandular structures until maturation [36]. In vitro SMG organogenesis experiments from isolated SMG cells confirmed that E-cadherin is predominantly involved in the structuring of the branching morphogenesis of SGs [37]. Clarifying the mechanism responsible for E-cadherin-mediated SMG development will have important implications for the general understanding of branching morphogenesis in the context of epithelial tissue development. It is now clear that the E12.5 SMG contains two distinct cellular populations that present a different E-cadherin junctional organization which conditions the subsequent phases of cellular differentiation [38]. The external cellular layer located in contact with the basement membrane consists of closely packed epithelial cells surrounding the polymorphic cells located in the region of the internal glandular bud. The role of E-cadherin in SMG development was investigated by inducing E-cadherin inhibition by the use of both specific antibodies against E-cadherin and siRNAs-mediated E-cadherin gene silencing. These interesting experiments revealed that the disorganized cells in the initial bud express E-cadherin and β-catenin uniformly and diffusely over their surface [26,39]; in addition, another columnar cell population was recognized in the outer layer of the initial bud, in contact with the basement membrane, characterized by distinct E-cadherin junctions, likely to be linked to the columnar morphology. When the glandular bud grows and branches, these highly organized columnar cells remain in the outermost part. Strangely, during the E-cadherin inhibition experiments, the columnar organization of these outer cells was not lost. Probably, the lack of E-cadherin was compensated by N-cadherin, which is highly expressed in these cells. On the contrary, the cells of the inner region of the bud did not present well-structured E-cadherin junctions and also expressed markers typical of ductal cells, suggesting that they were probably destined to give rise to the ducts. The cells that gave rise to the ducts were identifiable as early as E13.5, arranged along the proximal–distal axis and characterized by a large number of F-actin filaments and by the expression of cytokeratin ductal marker K7 [36]. Only later, these ductal precursors acquired defined E-cadherin junctions, first detected at the apical–lateral borders of ductal cells, and appeared coincident with lumen formation [36]. At this stage of glandular development, ZO-1 expression was also detected at sites apical to E-cadherin junctions, suggesting that ductal cells are linked through tight junctions [36,39]. Therefore, a lower expression of E-cadherin in the interior layer of the glandular bud appears to be necessary to ensure cellular rearrangement; when ductal lumens are formed, the presence of E-cadherin appears to be necessary to ensure stabilization of the ducts in the developing gland (Figure 2). Through inhibition studies performed by the use of siRNA and specific antibodies, the fundamental role of E-cadherin junctions in the ductal precursor fate was demonstrated during the lumenization process; they probably act by the modulation of apoptotic cascade [32,40].

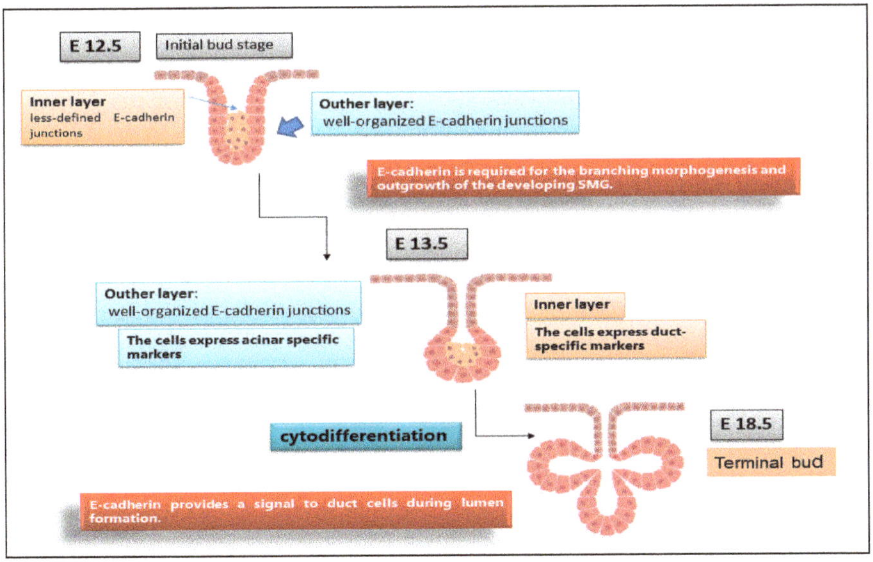

Figure 2. Organization of E-cadherin junctions during SGs morphogenesis. E12.5, E13.5, E18.5 represent stages of SGs embryonic development. At the initial E12.5, E-cadherin was localized to the lateral surfaces of the columnar cells that comprised the outer layer while, in the interior cells, was diffuse, indicating that these cells have less organized E-cadherin junctional structures. By E13.5, outer cell layer expressed a biochemical acinar marker demonstrating that acinar cells begin to differentiate very early in SGs development. The acinar progenitor layer completes the cytodifferentiation at E18.5, expressing E-cadherin in the peripheral cell layer.

6. E-Cadherin Localization in Adult Normal Salivary Glands

In normal SGs, E-cadherin is localized to the cell membrane of acinar and ductal cells, similar to the expression observed for the mammary gland. It is interesting to note that the infoldings of the plasma membrane at the basal site of the duct cell are strongly positive. In excretory ducts, high columnar cells show the strongest reaction for E-cadherin at the basal aspect, and ductal basal cells are weakly positive or negative, supporting those two cell types to obtain different cellular functions. It is possible that the stage of cellular differentiation may be a factor in the expression of E-cadherin, and ductal basal cells are possible progenitor cells of salivary gland tumors [41]. The basement membrane zone lacks staining. Modified myoepithelial cells and plasmacytoid cells seem not to express E-cadherin [42].

7. The Epithelial-to-Mesenchymal Transition (EMT) Process

Epithelial–mesenchymal transition (EMT) is a reversible cellular program that is known to be crucial for embryogenesis, wound healing and malignant progression [43,44]. During EMT, the epithelial cells lose their junctions, present drastic changes in cell polarity, restructure their cytoskeleton and cell–extracellular matrix interactions are remodeled. This process leads to the detachment of epithelial cells from each other and the underlying cellular membrane [45]. Therefore, the cells undergo changes in the transcriptional programs that specify cell shape and reprogram gene expression which lead to enhanced motility of individual cells, promoting the mesenchymal fate [46]. In this context, the epithelial cells progressively lose their cobblestone, epithelial appearance, co-express epithelial and mesenchymal biomarkers, adopt a spindle shape and transiently acquire a quasi-mesenchymal cell state [47,48]. Interestingly, EMT may be induced to varying extents, producing a wide spectrum of intermediate states ("partial EMT"), and may be reversible through mesenchymal-to-epithelial transitions (MET) [47]. Based on these characteristics, recentl these dynamic processes were widely defined as "epithelial–mesenchymal plasticity" [4 EMT is regulated at various levels by inflammatory stimuli, including cytokines such a transforming growth factor-β (TGF-β), fibroblast growth factor family, epidermal growt factor and hepatocyte growth factor [44,48,50,51]. These EMT-inducing signals upregula specific transcription factors (TFs) called EMT-TFs (e.g., Snail, Twist and ZEB) to repres E-cadherin expression and induce mesenchymal gene expression [52]. In line with thi small, non-coding, single-stranded RNAs (microRNAs or miRNAs) act in concert with TF to modulate the induction or repression of the EMT signaling process. The main initiatio signals of EMT are, therefore, represented by downregulation of E-cadherin, the expressio of which is decreased during EMT, and the loss of function of this protein promotes th EMT transition. The transcriptional repression of E-cadherin has long been considered critical step during EMT [53].

8. E-Cadherin and EMT

E-cadherin, as one of the most important molecules in cell–cell adhesion of epithelia cells [54], is considered the main effector of EMT and a unique start signal. Therefore, it i also considered a potent tumor suppressor because aberrant regulation of E-cadherin i often found in a multitude of malignant epithelial cancers [55,56]. E-cadherin is importan in conserving the epithelial phenotype and regulating homeostasis of tissues by modulatin various signaling pathways [56]. Loss of E-cadherin is constantly shown at sites of EM during development and cancer [56,57], and this event enhances cancer cell invasivenes in vitro and contributes to the transformation of adenoma to carcinoma in animal mo els [58]. Therefore, the expression level of E-cadherin often is inversely correlated wit tumor grade and stage. In some cases, E-cadherin-negative cell lines showed the most de astatingly high levels of tumorigenicity in nude mice. Furthermore, the loss of E-cadheri can be the result of different mechanisms, such as the inactivating mutations of the huma E-cadherin gene discovered in about 50% of infiltrating breast carcinomas [58]. Promote methylation, a type of epigenetic alteration, is considered to be the predominant mechanism of inactivation of the E-cadherin gene. This mechanism has been recognized in many soli tumors; in fact, patients who present inactivation of the E-cadherin gene and altered expre sion of its protein are considered at high risk of developing diffuse gastric carcinoma an thus, by these criteria at least, E-cadherin is considered a tumor suppressor gene [58,59]. E cadherin CDH1 gene promoter possesses several regulatory sequences that mediate CDH transcriptional repression in mesenchymal cells, especially during EMT [60]. In additio the methylation of CpG sites located in the CDH1 enhancers correlates with low gen expression [61]. DNA methylation is catalyzed by DNA (cytosine-5)-methyltransferase (DNMTs) [62]. Recent studies revealed the aberrant hypermethylation of CDH1 in he atocellular carcinomas [63,64]. This hypermethylation seems to involve the activation o DNMT1, DNMT3A1 and DNMT3A2, and the hypermethylation of CpG sites is significantl associated with gene and protein E-cadherin suppression [65]. More details were provide by Hermann et al., who demonstrated a central role for Snail in the CpG methylation o the E-cadherin promoter through the recruitment of DNMT1 [66]. In salivary adenoi cystic carcinoma (SACC), one of the most common malignant SG neoplasms, a reduction o E-cadherin reactivity was also recorded in the solid variant, especially in the periphera cells that are more likely to cause metastases. The phenotypical alterations observed i these cells suggest the involvement of the EMT process in the progression of SACCs [65]. In terestingly, the expression levels of circRNAs, member of the non-coding RNA family, wer upregulated in cancer tissues of SACC patients; cell transfection techniques, used to inhib the expression of circRNA members in SACC cell lines, demonstrated that the proliferativ invasive and migratory abilities of SACC cells were significantly decreased, and the EM process was inhibited, affecting E-cadherin expression [67]. Recent findings highlighte another interesting phenomenon called "cadherin switch", in which the normal expressio of E-cadherin is substituted by the abnormal expression of N- or P-cadherin [55,56,68

This downregulation of E-cadherin is linked with the release of β-catenin that induces the WNT signaling pathway. There is evidence that the malfunction of the E-cadherin/catenin complex permits the separation of malignant cells from the primary tumor mass, thus, provoking tumor progression and metastasis [69]. Several studies demonstrated that reduced expression of E-cadherin and catenins is critical in the development and progression of human carcinomas [69–71], while, on the contrary, E-cadherin alone acts as a suppressor molecule in cancer invasion and metastasis [21]. However, the use of E-cadherin/β-catenin as prognostic markers in SG tumors, for instance, may have no predictive value; Furuse and colleagues [70] demonstrated that such molecules may be immunoexpressed, for example, in healthy SGs, as well as in malignant SG neoplasia, invasive or not. Interestingly, the role of E-cadherin in EMT is still debated, and some authors argue that the loss of E-cadherin is not causal nor a necessity for EMT, and restoration of E-cadherin expression in E-cadherin-negative malignant cells does not reverse the EMT [72]. Nilsson et al. also demonstrated that E-cadherin loss is consequential rather than causal for c-erbB2-induced EMT in non-malignant mammary epithelial cell lines [73]. Loss of E-cadherin alone was demonstrated to be insufficient to trigger the EMT program in non-malignant breast cell lines [74]. In addition, loss of E-cadherin expression seems to be an oversimplification because, surprisingly, several metastases still contain high levels of E-cadherin, and epithelial cells expressing E-cadherin can become invasive and metastasize, notably in patients with prostate cancer [75], ovarian cancer [76] and glioblastoma [77]. Interestingly, the dual role of E-cadherin is possibly due to the existence of two forms of E-cadherin, which are membrane-tethered E-cadherin and soluble E-cadherin (sE-cadherin) [78]. sE-cadherin was initially discovered by Wheelock et al. [7], and subsequent studies were carried out to investigate the propriety of sE-cadherin as a cancer biomarker [79]. sE-cadherin interferes with AJs and promotes invasion and metastasis as a paracrine/autocrine signaling molecule in the progression of various types of cancer such as gastric cancer. Therefore, it induces the activity of a dysintegrin and metalloprotease (ADAM) and matrix metalloproteinases (MMPs), as well as modulates several signaling pathways [77–80]. Furthermore, interesting studies demonstrated that sE-cadherin is highly expressed in ovarian cancer patients, where sE-cadherin induces tumor angiogenesis via activation of β-catenin and NF-κB signaling, thus, causing a carcinoma metastatic spread [80].

9. The Role of E-Cadherin in Salivary Gland Pathogenesis: Lesson from Sjögren's Syndrome

The main aspects related to the organization of epithelia in SGs are relevant to understanding the pathophysiological alterations observed in primary Sjögren's syndrome (pSS), where the protective function of epithelia is lost. pSS is, essentially, a chronic inflammatory autoimmune epithelitis characterized by complex pathogenesis, that affects mainly the lachrymal glands and SGs [81,82]. In this scenario, E-cadherin, which is the main actor in maintaining epithelial tissue integrity and giving strength to conserve polarization of the epithelial cell layers [83], seems to play an important role in the molecular mechanisms involved in pSS [84–86]. Preliminary studies reported that tight junction proteins and AJs are downregulated in human minor SGs with pSS, thus, determining a marked disorganization of the apical pole of these cells in pSS patients [87]. Nevertheless, in pSS SGs, lymphocytes invade the epithelial tissue, and this invasion causes a dramatic, decreased exocrine secretion that leads to dry mouth [88]. In fact, the interactions between lymphocytes and the salivary epithelium could potentially determine the loss of glandular tissue and might compromise the epithelial integrity [89]. In this context, recent findings highlighted that the arrangement of apical factors in points proximal and distal to lymphocytic infiltration in SGs remained intact in a mouse model of pSS [89]. It was observed that E-cadherin distribution remained intact in areas without lymphocytic infiltration, while E-cadherin immunoexpression was absent in areas presenting infiltrating lymphocytes, so, contributed to the loss of glandular tissue organization [89]. Altered expression of E-cadherin also seems to have had a fundamental role in the recent line of research that studied the phenomenon of the EMT-dependent fibrosis observed in pSS SGs [84–86]. An increased expression of proinflammatory cytokines, such as IL-6, IL-17 and IL-22, in pSS has a pivotal role in the development of EMT-dependent SG fibrosis characterized by the progressive loss of E-cadherin and by the growing increased expression of the mesenchymal markers by SG cells accompanied by dramatic morphological changes [84–86]. These studies elucidated that, in pSS SGs' inflammatory microenvironment, increased expression of TGF-β determines the activation of EMT involving both the canonical SMAD2/3 pathway and the non-canonical MAPK pathway [84–86] (Figure 3). These discoveries were enriched by a recent study investigating serum levels of sE-cadherin in relation to infiltrating lymphocytes in pSS to characterize the expression of E-cadherin and integrin αEβ7/CD103 in the pSS SG epithelium [90]. Interestingly, serum levels of sE-cadherin were significantly increased in pSS compared to controls. In addition, membrane-bound E-cadherin and clusters of αEβ7/CD103-positive cells were located, in particular, in acinar and ductal cells in epithelium tissue both in pSS and controls. These findings indicate a suggestive role for the αEβ7/CD103 and E-cadherin interaction in pSS SGs, and the sE-cadherin fragment may also play a role in the tissue destruction, resulting, thus, in the accumulation of fibrotic SG tissue and pSS disease progression [90].

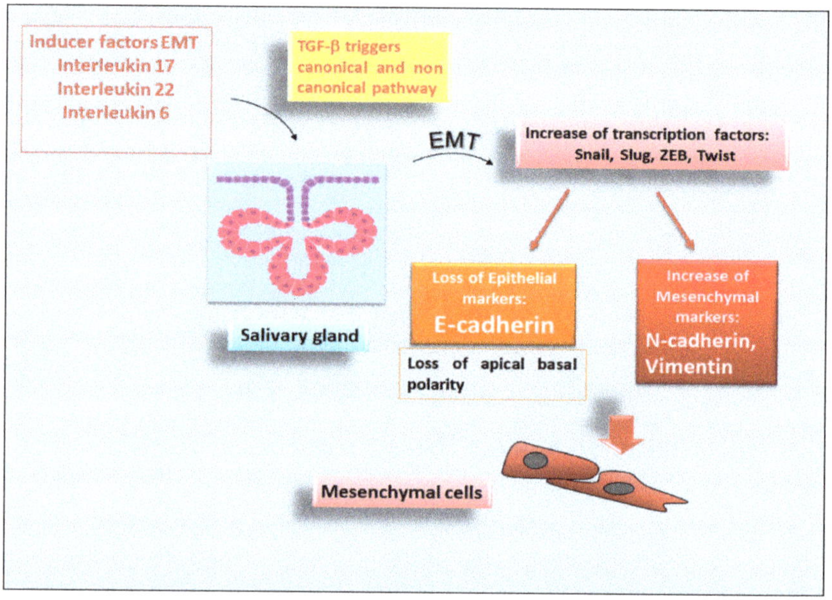

Figure 3. Role of E-cadherin during the epithelial-mesenchymal transition (EMT) process in pSS. In pSS, the transition of epithelial cells versus a mesenchymal phenotype is triggered by several proinflammatory factors and is characterized by the loss of cellular contact and cellular polarity. During EMT, the loss of epithelial marker E-cadherin and an increase of mesenchymal markers occur, through the upregulation of transcriptional factors [i.e., SNAIL, TWIST, Zinc finger E-box-binding homeobox (ZEB), Slug]. The acquisition of mesenchymal markers led to the stabilization of the newly acquired phenotype.

10. Conclusions

Unquestionably, E-cadherin is deeply involved in establishing cell polarity and differentiation and, thereby, in the establishment and maintenance of tissue homeostasis during the SGs' development. In this review, we sought to discuss the impact of mechanisms of E-cadherin on SG morphogenesis. Several parameters can contribute to differences in cell adhesion energies, including, but not limited to, the intrinsic, biophysical properties of

E-cadherin bonds and E-cadherin surface expression levels. A key question, thus, remains as to whether cell segregation during SG development can be explained solely in terms of the intrinsic properties of the E-cadherin ectodomain or whether it is also necessary to incorporate cellular properties, including biomechanics and functional responses to E-cadherin ligation. Providing a picture of these interactions proposes many interesting future research avenues to consider. Since E-cadherin is the major determinant of the epithelial phenotype, it represents the main driver of the EMT program, and the characterization of E-cadherin multifaceted expression corroborates the interpretation of E-cadherin's roles during the EMT activation cascade. Only the codifying of its expression in relation to the cell phenotype and the timing of its loss during the transition of normal ductal epithelium versus the de-differentiated mesenchymal-like state will allow us to better understand the molecular mechanisms in terms of chronic inflammatory diseases such as autoimmune diseases.

Author Contributions: All authors were involved in drafting the article or revising it critically for important, intellectual content, and all authors approved the final version for publication. M.S. and S.L. have full access to the data collected in the study and take responsibility for their integrity. D.R. performed a critical reading of this review. All authors have read and agreed to the published version of the manuscript.

Funding: No external funding was involved in this review.

Institutional Review Board Statement: Not applicable.

Conflicts of Interest: The authors declare no conflict of interest.

References

1. Patel, S.D.; Chen, C.P.; Bahna, F.; Honig, B.; Shapiro, L. Cadherin-mediated cell-cell adhesion: Sticking together as a family. *Curr. Opin. Struct. Biol.* **2003**, *13*, 690–698. [CrossRef] [PubMed]
2. Jaiganesh, A.; Narui, Y.; Araya-Secchi, R.; Sotomayor, M. Beyond Cell-Cell Adhesion: Sensational Cadherins for Hearing and Balance. *Cold Spring Harb. Perspect. Biol.* **2018**, *10*, 029280. [CrossRef] [PubMed]
3. Pal, M.; Bhattacharya, S.; Kalyan, G.; Hazra, S. Cadherin profiling for therapeutic interventions in Epithelial Mesenchymal Transition (EMT) and tumorigenesis. *Exp. Cell Res.* **2018**, *368*, 137–146. [CrossRef] [PubMed]
4. Takeichi, M. Functional correlation between cell adhesive properties and some cell surface proteins. *J. Cell Biol.* **1977**, *75*, 464–474. [CrossRef]
5. Peyriéras, N.; Hyafil, F.; Louvard, D.; Ploegh, H.L.; Jacob, F. Uvomorulin: A nonin-tegral membrane protein of early mouse embryo. *Proc. Natl. Acad. Sci. USA* **1983**, *80*, 6274–6277. [CrossRef]
6. Boller, K.; Vestweber, D.; Kemler, R. Cell-adhesion molecule uvomorulin is localized in the intermediate junctions of adult intestinal epithelial cells. *J. Cell Biol.* **1985**, *100*, 327–332. [CrossRef]
7. Wheelock, M.J.; Buck, C.A.; Bechtol, K.B.; Damsky, C.H. Soluble 80-kd fragment of cell-CAM 120/80 disrupts cell-cell adhesion. *J. Cell Biochem.* **1987**, *34*, 187–202. [CrossRef]
8. Kjeldsen, T.B.; Laursen, I.; Lykkesfeldt, A.; Briand, P.; Zeuthen, J. Monoclonal anti-bodies reactive with components in serum-free conditioned medium from a hu-man breast cancer cell line (MCF-7). *Tumor Biol.* **1989**, *10*, 190–201. [CrossRef]
9. Begemann, M.; Tan, S.S.; A Cunningham, B.; Edelman, G.M. Expression of chicken liver cell adhesion molecule fusion genes in transgenic mice. *Proc. Natl. Acad. Sci. USA* **1990**, *87*, 9042–9046. [CrossRef]
10. Yoshida-Noro, C.; Suzuki, N.; Takeichi, M. Molecular nature of the calcium-dependent cell-cell adhesion system in mouse teratocarcinoma and embryonic cells studied with a monoclonal antibody. *Dev. Biol.* **1984**, *101*, 19–27. [CrossRef]
11. Takeichi, M. The cadherins: Cell-cell adhesion molecules controlling animal morphogenesis. *Development* **1988**, *102*, 639–655. [CrossRef] [PubMed]
12. Mohan, R.; Lee, B.; Panjwani, N. Molecular cloning of the E-cadherin cDNAs from rabbit corneal epithelium. *Curr. Eye Res.* **1995**, *14*, 1136–1145. [CrossRef] [PubMed]
13. Parisini, E.; Higgins, J.; Liu, J.-H.; Brenner, M.B.; Wang, J.-H. The Crystal Structure of Human E-cadherin Domains 1 and 2, and Comparison with other Cadherins in the Context of Adhesion Mechanism. *J. Mol. Biol.* **2007**, *373*, 401–411. [CrossRef] [PubMed]
14. Curtis, M.W.; Johnson, K.R.; Wheelock, M.J. E-Cadherin/Catenin Complexes Are Formed Cotranslationally in the Endoplasmic Reticulum/Golgi Compartments. *Cell Commun. Adhes.* **2008**, *15*, 365–378. [CrossRef]
15. Rahnama, F.; Thompson, B.; Steiner, M.; Shafiei, F.; Lobie, P.E.; Mitchell, M.D. Epigenetic regulation of E-cadherin controls endometrial receptivity. *Endocrinology* **2009**, *150*, 1466–1472. [CrossRef]
16. Georgopoulos, N.T.; Kirkwood, L.A.; Walker, D.C.; Southgate, J. Differential regulation of growth-promoting signalling pathways by E-cadherin. *PLoS ONE* **2010**, *5*, e13621. [CrossRef]

17. Zheng, K.; Laurence, J.S.; Kuczera, K.; Verkhivker, G.; Middaugh, C.R.; Siahaan, T.J. Characterization of Multiple Stabl Conformers of the EC5 Domain of E-cadherin and the Interaction of EC5 with E-cadherin Peptides. *Chem. Biol. Drug Des.* **200** *73*, 584–598. [CrossRef]
18. Hirano, S.; Nose, A.; Hatta, K.; Kawakami, A.; Takeichi, M. Calcium-dependent cell-cell adhesion molecules (cadherins): Subclas specificities and possible in-volvement of actin bundles. *J. Cell Biol.* **1987**, *105*, 2501–2510. [CrossRef]
19. Grunwald, G.B. The structural and functional analysis of cadherin calcium-dependent cell adhesion molecules. *Curr. Opin. Ce Biol.* **1993**, *5*, 797–805. [CrossRef]
20. Marrs, J.A.; Nelson, W.J. Cadherin Cell Adhesion Molecules in Differentiation and Embryogenesis. *Int. Rev. Cytol.* **199** *165*, 159–205. [CrossRef]
21. Wheelock, M.J.; Johnson, K.R. Cadherins as Modulators of Cellular Phenotype. *Annu. Rev. Cell Dev. Biol.* **2003**, *19*, 207–23 [CrossRef] [PubMed]
22. Halbleib, J.M.; Nelson, W.J. Cadherins in development: Cell adhesion, sorting, and tissue morphogenesis. *Genes Dev.* **200** *20*, 3199–3214. [CrossRef] [PubMed]
23. Huber, A.H.; Stewart, D.B.; Laurents, D.V.; Nelson, W.J.; Weis, W.I. The cadherin cytoplasmic domain is unstructured in th absence of β-catenin: A possible mecha-nism for regulating cadherin turnover. *J. Biol. Chem.* **2001**, *276*, 12301–12309. [CrossRe
24. Mège, R.M.; Ishiyama, N. Integration of Cadherin Adhesion and Cytoskeleton at Adherens Junctions. *Cold Spring Harb. Perspec Biol.* **2017**, *9*, a028738. [CrossRef] [PubMed]
25. Bernfield, M.; Danerjee, S.D.; Koda, J.E.; Rapraeger, A.C. Remodelling of the base-ment membrane: Morphogenesis an maturation. *Ciba Found Symp.* **1984**, *108*, 179–196. [PubMed]
26. Hieda, Y.; Iwai, K.; Morita, T.; Nakanishi, Y. Mouse embryonic submandibular gland epithelium loses its tissue integrity durin early branching morphogenesis. *Dev. Dyn.* **1996**, *207*, 395–403. [CrossRef]
27. Fernandes, R.P.; Cotanche, D.A.; Lennon-Hopkins, K.; Erkan, F.; Menko, A.S.; Kukuruzinska, M.A. Differential expression c proliferative, cytoskeletal, and adhesive proteins during postnatal development of the hamster submandibular gland. *Histochen Cell Biol.* **1999**, *111*, 153–162. [CrossRef]
28. Jaskoll, T.; Melnick, M. Submindibular gland morphogenesis: Stage-specific expres-sion of TGF-a/EGF, IGF, TGF-b, TNF, an IL-6 signal transduction in normal em-bryonic mice and the phenotypic effects of TGF-b2, TGF-b-3, and EGF-R null mutation *Anat. Rec.* **1999**, *256*, 252–268. [CrossRef]
29. Patel, V.N.; Rebustini, I.T.; Hoffman, M.P. Salivary gland branching morphogene-sis. *Differentiation* **2006**, *74*, 349–364. [CrossRe
30. Kashimata, M.; Sayeed, S.; Ka, A.; Onetti-Muda, A.; Sakagami, H.; Faraggiana, T.; Gresik, E.W. The ERK-1/2 signaling pathwa is involved in the stimulation of branching morphogenesis of fetal mouse submandibular glands by EGF. *Dev. Biol.* **200** *220*, 183–196. [CrossRef]
31. Sakai, T.; Larsen, M.; Yamada, K.M. Fibronectin requirement in branching mor-phogenesis. *Nature* **2003**, *423*, 876–881. [CrossRe [PubMed]
32. Melnick, M.; Jaskoll, T. Mouse sub-mandibular gland morphogenesis: A paradigm for embryonic signal processing. *Crit. Re Oral Biol. Med.* **2000**, *11*, 199–215. [CrossRef] [PubMed]
33. Patel, N.; Sharpe, P.T.; Miletich, I. Coordination of epithelial branching and salivary gland lumen formation by Wnt and FG signals. *Develop. Biol.* **2011**, *358*, 156–167. [CrossRef] [PubMed]
34. Knox, S.M.; Lombaert, I.M.; Haddox, C.L.; Abrams, S.R.; Cotrim, A.; Wilson, A.J.; Hoffman, M.P. Parasympathetic stimulatio improves epithelial organ regeneration. *Nat. Commun.* **2013**, *4*, 1494. [CrossRef] [PubMed]
35. Teshima, T.H.N.; Wells, K.L.; Lourenço, S.V.; Tucker, A.S. Apoptosis in Early Sali-vary Gland Duct Morphogenesis and Lume Formation. *J. Dental Res.* **2016**, *95*, 277–283. [CrossRef] [PubMed]
36. Walker, J.L.; Menko, A.S.; Khalil, S.; Rebustini, I.; Hoffman, M.P.; Kreidberg, J.A.; Kukuruzinska, M.A. Diverse roles of E-cadheri in the morphogenesis of the sub-mandibular gland: Insights into the formation of acinar and ductal structures. *Dev. Dyn.* **200** *237*, 3128–3141. [CrossRef] [PubMed]
37. Wei, C.; Larsen, M.; Hoffman, M.P.; Yamada, K.M. Self-Organization and Branching Morphogenesis of Primary Salivary Epithelia Cells. *Tissue Eng.* **2007**, *13*, 721–735. [CrossRef]
38. Larsen, M.; Wei, C.; Yamada, K.M. Cell and fibronectin dynamics during branching morphogenesis. *J. Cell Sci.* **200** *119*, 3376–3384. [CrossRef]
39. Heida, Y.; Nakanishi, Y. Epithelial morphogenesis in mouse embryonic sub-mandibular gland: Its relationships to the tissu organization of epithelium and mesenchyme. *Dev. Growth Differ.* **1997**, *39*, 1–8. [CrossRef]
40. Mailleux, A.A.; Overholtzer, M.; Schmelzle, T.; Bouillet, P.; Strasser, A.; Brugge, J.S. BIM Regulates Apoptosis during Mammar Ductal Morphogenesis, and Its Absence Reveals Alternative Cell Death Mechanisms. *Dev. Cell* **2007**, *12*, 221–234. [CrossRef]
41. Yamada, K.; Jordan, R.; Mori, M.; Speight, P.M. The relationship between E-cadherin expression, clinical stage and tumou differentiation in oral squamous cell carcinoma. *Oral Dis.* **1997**, *3*, 82–85. [CrossRef] [PubMed]
42. Andreadis, D.; Epivatianos, A.; Mireas, G.; Nomikos, A.; Poulopoulos, A.; Yiotakis, J.; Barbatis, C. Immunohistochemical detectio of E-cadherin in certain types of salivary gland tumours. *J. Laryngol. Otol.* **2006**, *120*, 298–304. [CrossRef] [PubMed]
43. Kalluri, R.; Weinberg, R.A. The basics of epithelial-mesenchymal transition. *J. Clin. Investig.* **2009**, *119*, 1420–1428. [CrossRef [PubMed]
44. Nieto, M.A.; Huang, R.Y.; Jackson, R.A.; Thiery, J.P. EMT: 2016. *Cell* **2016**, *166*, 21–45. [CrossRef]

45. Thiery, J.P.; Acloque, H.; Huang, R.Y.J.; Nieto, M.A. Epithelial-Mesenchymal Transitions in Development and Disease. *Cell* **2009**, *139*, 871–890. [CrossRef]
46. Dongre, A.; Weinberg, R.A. New insights into the mechanisms of epitheli-al-mesenchymal transition and implications for cancer. *Nat. Rev. Mol. Cell Biol.* **2019**, *20*, 69–84. [CrossRef]
47. Leggett, S.E.; Hruska, A.M.; Guo, M.; Wong, I.Y. The epithelial-mesenchymal tran-sition and the cytoskeleton in bioengineered systems. *Cell Commun. Signal.* **2021**, *19*, 32. [CrossRef]
48. Williams, E.D.; Gao, D.; Redfern, A.; Thompson, E.W. Controversies around epithelial-mesenchymal plasticity in cancer metastasis. *Nat. Rev. Cancer.* **2019**, *19*, 716–732. [CrossRef]
49. Yang, J.; Antin, P.; Berx, G.; Blanpain, C.; Brabletz, T.; Bronner, M.; Campbell, K.; Cano, A.; Casanova, J.; Christofori, G.; et al. Guidelines and definitions for research on epithelial-mesenchymal transition. *Nat. Rev. Mol. Cell Biol.* **2020**, *21*, 341–352, Erratum in *Nat. Rev. Mol. Cell Biol.* **2021**, *22*, 834. [CrossRef]
50. Zavadil, J.; Böttinger, E.P. TGF-beta and epithelial-to-mesenchymal transitions. *Oncogene* **2005**, *24*, 5764–5774. [CrossRef]
51. Thiery, J.P.; Sleeman, J.P. Complex networks orchestrate epithelial-mesenchymal transitions. *Nat. Rev. Mol. Cell Biol.* **2006**, *7*, 131–142. [CrossRef] [PubMed]
52. Lamouille, S.; Xu, J.; Derynck, R. Molecular mechanisms of epithelial–mesenchymal transition. *Nat. Rev. Mol. Cell Biol.* **2014**, *15*, 178–196. [CrossRef] [PubMed]
53. Aban, C.E.; Lombardi, A.; Neiman, G.; Biani, M.C.; La Greca, A.; Waisman, A.; Moro, L.N.; Sevlever, G.; Miriuka, S.; Luzzani, C. Downregulation of E-cadherin in pluripotent stem cells triggers partial EMT. *Sci. Rep.* **2021**, *11*, 2048. [CrossRef] [PubMed]
54. Rodriguez-Boulan, E.; Macara, I.G. Organization and execution of the epithelial polarity programme. *Nat. Rev. Mol. Cell Biol.* **2014**, *15*, 225–242. [CrossRef] [PubMed]
55. Loh, C.Y.; Chai, J.Y.; Tang, T.F.; Wong, W.F.; Sethi, G.; Shanmugam, M.K.; Chong, P.P.; Looi, C.Y. The E-Cadherin and N-Cadherin Switch in Epitheli-al-to-Mesenchymal Transition: Signaling, Therapeutic Implications, and Challenges. *Cells* **2019**, *8*, 1118. [CrossRef]
56. Yu, W.; Yang, L.; Li, T.; Zhang, Y. Cadherin Signaling in Cancer: Its Functions and Role as a Therapeutic Target. *Front. Oncol.* **2019**, *9*, 989. [CrossRef]
57. Kang, Y.; Massagué, J. Epithelial-mesenchymal transitions: Twist in development and metastasis. *Cell* **2004**, *118*, 277–279. [CrossRef]
58. Thiery, J.P. Epithelial-mesenchymal transitions in tumour progression. *Nat. Rev. Cancer* **2002**, *2*, 442–454. [CrossRef]
59. Liu, X.; Chu, K.-M. E-Cadherin and Gastric Cancer: Cause, Consequence, and Applications. *BioMed Res. Int.* **2014**, *2014*, 637308. [CrossRef]
60. Gao, L.M.; Xu, S.F.; Zheng, Y.; Wang, P.; Zhang, L.; Shi, S.S.; Wu, T.; Li, Y.; Zhao, J.; Tian, Q.; et al. Long non-coding RNA H19 is responsible for the progression of lung adenocarcinoma by mediating methylation-dependent repression of CDH1 promoter. *J. Cell Mol. Med.* **2019**, *23*, 6411–6428. [CrossRef]
61. Tedaldi, G.; Molinari, C.; Celina, S.; Barbosa-Matos, R.; André, A.; Danesi, R.; Arcangeli, V.; Ravegnani, M.; Saragoni, L.; Morgagni, P.; et al. Genetic and Epige-netic Alterations of CDH1 Regulatory Regions in Hereditary and Sporadic Gastric Cancer. *Pharmaceuticals* **2021**, *14*, 457. [CrossRef] [PubMed]
62. Traube, F.R.; Carell, T. The chemistries and consequences of DNA and RNA meth-ylation and demethylation. *RNA Biol.* **2017**, *14*, 1099–1107. [CrossRef] [PubMed]
63. Yang, B.; Guo, M.; Herman, J.G.; Clark, D.P. Aberrant promoter methylation pro-files of tumor suppressor genes in hepatocellular carcinoma. *Am. J. Pathol.* **2003**, *163*, 1101–1107. [CrossRef]
64. Lee, S.; Lee, H.J.; Kim, J.H.; Lee, H.S.; Jang, J.J.; Kang, G.H. Aberrant CpG island hypermethylation along multistep hepatocarcinogenesis. *Am. J. Pathol.* **2003**, *163*, 1371–1378. [CrossRef]
65. Belulescu, I.C.; Mărgăritescu, C.; Dumitrescu, C.I.; Munteanu, M.C.; Mărgăritescu, O.C. Immuno phenotypical alterations with impact on the epithelial-mesenchymal transition (EMT) process in salivary gland adenoid cystic carcinomas. *Rom. J. Morphol. Embryol.* **2020**, *61*, 175–187. [CrossRef]
66. Hermann, A.; Goyal, R.; Jeltsch, A. The Dnmt1 DNA-(cytosine-C5)-methyltransferase Methylates DNA Processively with High Preference for Hemimethylated Target Sites. *J. Biol. Chem.* **2004**, *279*, 48350–48359. [CrossRef]
67. Wei, H.; Li, J.; Xie, C.; Dong, H. Circular RNA hsa_circ_0011946 promotes the malignant process of salivary adenoid cystic carcinoma by downregulating miR-1205 expression. *Exp. Ther. Med.* **2022**, *23*, 295. [CrossRef]
68. Mitselou, A.; Galani, V.; Skoufi, U.; Arvanitis, D.L.; Lampri, E.; Ioachim, E. Syndecan-1, Epithelial-Mesenchymal Transition Markers (E-cadherin/β-catenin) and Neoangiogenesis-related Proteins (PCAM-1 and Endoglin) in Colorectal Cancer. *Anticancer Res.* **2016**, *36*, 2271–2280.
69. Mitselou, A.; Batistatou, A.; Nakanishi, Y.; Hirohashi, S.; Vougiouklakis, T.; Char-alabopoulos, K. Comparison of the dysadherin and E-cadherin expression in primary lung cancer and metastatic sites. *Histol. Histopathol.* **2010**, *25*, 1257–1267.
70. Furuse, C.; Cury, P.R.; Altemani, A.; dos Santos Pinto, D., Jr.; de Araújo, N.S.; de Araújo, V.C. Beta-catenin and E-cadherin expression in salivary gland tumors. *Int. J. Surg. Pathol.* **2006**, *14*, 212–217. [CrossRef]
71. Nollet, F.; Berx, G.; van Roy, F. The role of the E-cadherin/catenin adhesion com-plex in the development and progression of cancer. *Mol. Cell Biol. Res. Commun.* **1999**, *2*, 77–85. [CrossRef] [PubMed]

72. Hollestelle, A.; Peeters, J.K.; Smid, M.; Timmermans, M.; Verhoog, L.C.; Westenend, P.; Heine, A.A.J.; Chan, A.; Sieuwerts, A.M. Wiemer, E.; et al. Loss of E-cadherin is not a necessity for epithelial to mesenchymal transition in human breast cancer. *Breast Cancer Res. Treat.* **2013**, *138*, 47–57. [CrossRef] [PubMed]
73. Nilsson, G.; Akhtar, N.; Kannius-Janson, M.; Baeckström, D. Loss of E-cadherin ex-pression is not a prerequisite for c-erbB2 induced epithelial-mesenchymal transition. *Int. J. Oncol.* **2014**, *45*, 82–94. [CrossRef] [PubMed]
74. Chen, A.; Beetham, H.; Black, M.A.; Priya, R.; Telford, B.J.; Guest, J.; Wiggins, G.A.; Godwin, T.D.; Guilford, P.J. E-cadherin loss alters cytoskeletal organization and adhesion in non-malignant breast cells but is insufficient to induce an epitheli-al-mesenchymal transition. *BMC Cancer* **2014**, *14*, 552. [CrossRef] [PubMed]
75. Putzke, A.P.; Ventura, A.P.; Bailey, A.M.; Akture, C.; Opoku-Ansah, J.; Çeliktaş, M.; Hwang, M.S.; Darling, D.S.; Coleman, I.M. Nelson, P.S.; et al. Metastatic Progression of Prostate Cancer and E-Cadherin: Regulation by Zeb1 and Src Family Kinases. *Am. J Pathol.* **2011**, *179*, 400–410. [CrossRef]
76. Reddy, P.; Liu, L.; Ren, C.; Lindgren, P.; Boman, K.; Shen, Y.; Lundin, E.; Ottander, U.; Rytinki, M.; Liu, K. Formation of E-cadherin-mediated cell-cell adhesion activates AKT and mitogen activated protein kinase via phosphatidylinositol 3 kinase and ligand-independent activation of epidermal growth factor receptor in ovarian cancer cells. *Mol. Endocrinol.* **2005**, *19*, 2564–2578 [CrossRef]
77. Lewis-Tuffin, L.J.; Rodriguez, F.; Giannini, C.; Scheithauer, B.; Necela, B.M.; Sarkaria, J.N.; Anastasiadis, P.Z. Misregulated E-Cadherin Expression Associated with an Aggressive Brain Tumor Phenotype. *PLoS ONE* **2010**, *5*, e13665. [CrossRef]
78. Hu, Q.-P.; Kuang, J.-Y.; Yang, Q.-K.; Bian, X.-W.; Yu, S.-C. Beyond a tumor suppressor: Soluble E-cadherin promotes the progression of cancer. *Int. J. Cancer* **2015**, *138*, 2804–2812. [CrossRef]
79. Grabowska, M.M.; Day, M.L. Soluble E-cadherin: More than a symptom of disease. *Front. Biosci.* **2012**, *17*, 1948. [CrossRef]
80. Tang, M.K.S.; Yue, P.Y.K.; Ip, P.P.; Huang, R.-L.; Lai, H.-C.; Cheung, A.N.Y.; Tse, K.Y.; Ngan, H.Y.S.; Wong, A.S.T. Soluble E-cadherin promotes tumor angiogenesis and localizes to exosome surface. *Nat. Commun.* **2018**, *9*, 2270. [CrossRef]
81. Mitsias, D.I.; Kapsogeorgou, E.K.; Moutsopoulos, H.M. Sjögren's syndrome: Why autoimmune epithelitis? *Oral Dis.* **2006** *12*, 523–532. [CrossRef] [PubMed]
82. Parisis, D.; Chivasso, C.; Perret, J.; Soyfoo, M.S.; Delporte, C. Current State of Knowledge on Primary Sjögren's Syndrome, an Autoimmune Exocrinopathy. *J. Clin. Med.* **2020**, *9*, 2299. [CrossRef] [PubMed]
83. Stemmler, M.P. Cadherins in development and cancer. *Mol. Biosyst.* **2008**, *4*, 835–850. [CrossRef] [PubMed]
84. Sisto, M.; Ribatti, D.; Lisi, S. ADAM 17 and Epithelial-to-Mesenchymal Transition: The Evolving Story and Its Link to Fibrosis and Cancer. *J. Clin. Med.* **2021**, *10*, 3373. [CrossRef] [PubMed]
85. Sisto, M.; Ribatti, D.; Lisi, S. Organ Fibrosis and Autoimmunity: The Role of In-flammation in TGFβ-Dependent EMT. *Biomolecules* **2021**, *11*, 310. [CrossRef] [PubMed]
86. Sisto, M.; Ribatti, D.; Lisi, S. SMADS-Mediate Molecular Mechanisms in Sjögren's Syndrome. *Int. J. Mol. Sci.* **2021**, *22*, 3203 [CrossRef]
87. Barrera, M.J.; Bahamondes, V.; Sepúlveda, D.; Quest, A.F.; Castro, I.; Cortés, J.; Aguilera, S.; Urzúa, U.; Molina, C.; Pérez, P.; et al Sjögren's syndrome and the epithelial target: A comprehensive review. *J. Autoimmun.* **2013**, *42*, 7–18. [CrossRef]
88. Mavragani, C.P.; Moutsopoulos, H.M. The geoepidemiology of Sjögren's syndrome. *Autoimmun. Rev.* **2010**, *9*, A305–A310 [CrossRef]
89. Mellas, R.E.; Leigh, N.J.; Nelson, J.W.; McCall, A.D.; Baker, O.J. Zonula occludens-1, occludin and E-cadherin expression and organization in salivary glands with Sjögren's syndrome. *J. Histochem. Cytochem.* **2015**, *63*, 45–56. [CrossRef]
90. Jonsson, M.V.; Salomonsson, S.; Øijordsbakken, G.; Skarstein, K. Elevated Serum Levels of Soluble E-Cadherin in Patients with Primary Sjogren's Syndrome. *Scand. J. Immunol.* **2005**, *62*, 552–559. [CrossRef]

MDPI
St. Alban-Anlage 66
4052 Basel
Switzerland
Tel. +41 61 683 77 34
Fax +41 61 302 89 18
www.mdpi.com

Journal of Clinical Medicine Editorial Office
E-mail: jcm@mdpi.com
www.mdpi.com/journal/jcm

www.ingramcontent.com/pod-product-compliance
Lightning Source LLC
Chambersburg PA
CBHW062042220926
51850CB00010B/2643
* 9 7 8 3 0 3 6 5 5 5 6 7 6 *